HEALING
WITH
FOOD

HEALING
WITH
FOOD

*281 Nutritional Healing Plans
for 50 Common Ailments*

Melvyn Werbach, M.D.

HarperPerennial

A Division of HarperCollinsPublishers

FIRST HARPERPERENNIAL EDITION

Designed by Alma Hochhauser Orenstein

The Library of Congress has catalogued the hardcover edition as follows:

Werbach, Melvyn R.
    Healing through nutrition : a natural approach to treating 50 common illnesses with diet and nutrients / Melvyn R. Werbach.—1st ed.
        p.   cm.
    Includes index.
    ISBN 0-06-270033-2
    1. Diet therapy—Encyclopedias.   2. Nutrition—Encyclopedias.
I. Title.
RM216.W494   1993
615.8′54′03—dc20   92-24522

ISBN 0-06-272047-3 (pbk.)
94 95 96 97 98 CC/RRD 10 9 8 7 6 5 4 3 2 1

To Gail, my wife and soul-mate,
and our sons, Adam and Kevin

Contents

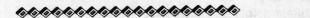

Introduction

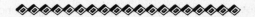

Let thy food be thy medicine, and thy medicine be thy food.
—Hippocrates 460–377 B.C.

Nutritional medicine is both very old and very new. Dietary and herbal treatments are two of the oldest methods of fostering the healing process, with roots extending back to the dawn of civilization. The use of individual nutrients to treat illness, however, is a development of this century, a by-product of our increasing ability to isolate nutritional factors from whole foods.

By definition, nutrients nourish the body. They are natural chemicals used by the body to maintain health and combat illness. Some are essential; others are optional. In the early part of this century, certain nutritional deficiencies were shown to cause specific diseases. Beriberi, for example, was found to be caused by a thiamine deficiency. Scurvy was found to be caused by a vitamin C deficiency.

An *essential* nutrient was defined as a nutrient required by the body to avoid the development of a nutritional deficiency disease. Researchers tried to determine how much of an essential nutrient was needed to protect against the development of the disease. Half a century ago, the consensus of the experts was formalized—for the first time—as nutritional recommendations, which became known as the Recommended Dietary Allowances (RDAs). (See Appendix E for further information on the RDAs.)

Since the formulation of the RDAs, nutritional medicine has developed far beyond this nice, simple model of nutritional deficiency diseases. We now realize that classic nutritional deficiency diseases develop only when deficiencies of essential nutrients are severe. Mild to moderate deficiencies, often called "marginal" deficiencies, do not cause these diseases.

They do, however, promote the development of any of a host of symptoms and numerous other illnesses. They do so because the body is less able to maintain the state of health when it is weakened by marginal nutritional deficiencies, which makes it a more vulnerable target for other illness-producing factors: germs, allergens, stress, genetic weaknesses, aging, environmental chemicals, injuries, etc.

Most nutrients are not essential because they have no known deficiency disease, yet they play a very important role by promoting health and, in the event of illness, healing. We are gradually learning to appreciate and utilize the powerful effects of these non-essential nutrients. We are also gradually learning to appreciate and utilize the powerful effects of nutrients at very high levels of intake. Since, in earlier centuries, nutrients were only available in foods, their dosage was restricted by the limited human capacity of ingesting the food containing them. With our modern ability to isolate and synthesize pure nutrients, this natural ceiling dosage no longer exists.

We initially discovered that a certain quantity of a nutrient can prevent or treat a classic deficiency disease. Then we found that a higher quantity can prevent or treat the features of a marginal nutritional deficiency. Now we are discovering that still higher quantities may prevent or treat many common illnesses.

Whether these megadoses of nutrients are optimal for health remains a topic of intense debate. The argument against ingesting such high quantities is that these unnatural dosages may be unhealthy. Since they are often given at levels which are unobtainable from a reasonable diet, and since they are devoid of their natural relationships with the other substances in foods, they could throw off the body's biochemical balancing mechanisms and thereby cause adverse effects which are not found at lower dosages.

The argument for ingesting nutrients at such high quantities roughly counterbalances the objections: high level nutritional supplementation may provide greater benefits to health and healing than does the minimal level to prevent a deficiency. The question of whether to supplement your diet with an unnaturally high level of a purified nutrient thus becomes: Is the potential benefit worth the potential risk? If you wish to recover from an illness, I believe that the answer is often yes.

While nutrients are at the core of nutritional medicine, the field also has other interests which are closely related. One of these interests is in evaluating patients for exposure to toxic metals such as lead and cadmium. These are natural minerals that promote the development of many illnesses and may interact with nutrients.

In the various chapters of this book I discuss herbal medicines under the heading of "Botanical Factors." While most herbs are not usually considered nutrients, I have included them to make the book more comprehensive. Technically, herbs are non-woody plants that die down to the ground after flowering; however, in herbal medicine, the term is commonly used more broadly, referring to any plant, all or part of which is valued as a healing agent.

If herbs are plants, how do fruits and vegetables differ from medicinal herbs? Generally, plant foods are coveted because eating them gives us pleasure, and because they are sources of nutrients, while medicinal herbs are coveted because of their medicinal qualities. A few medicinal herbs, such as onions, are so safe and flavorful that they are also considered to be foods; others must be used cautiously as they contain potentially harmful ingredients. Just as foods are the original source of essential nutrients, herbs are the original source of many drugs, such as digitalis (made from foxglove) for the treatment of heart failure, and opium for the treatment of diarrhea.

Recent developments in the use of medicinal herbs parallel the breakthroughs regarding foods. Specific chemicals in these herbs are being extracted and individually tested. Those that are found to be therapeutic are becoming available in pure and occasionally standardized forms. As in the case of high dosages of purified nutrients, these herbal medicines are sometimes capable of causing adverse reactions, especially if a prescribed dosage is exceeded.

The diagnosis and treatment of food sensitivities is closely related to nutritional medicine. Certain foods and food additives promote specific illnesses. For example, gluten—found in wheat, rye, oats, and barley—provokes the symptoms of celiac disease. Others promote numerous nonspecific symptoms, but only in susceptible people. While a food reaction is sometimes obvious, often it is a hidden factor responsible for promoting a surprisingly broad range of illnesses, and only special testing procedures will identify the culprit.

Currently, nutritional medicine is embroiled in a good deal of controversy. We have seen how much of the field as practiced today is a product of twentieth century medical science. In the course of this century, the standards of the medical community for what is considered good medical practice have also changed radically. Traditionally, medical treatment was an empirical science; that is, it was the accumulated wisdom born of repeated observations (technically called "open trials") handed down from generation to generation.

This model was severely challenged and is gradually being replaced with a rational one. This rational model recognizes that a change in a patient's clinical course, following an experimental treatment, is not necessarily due to the identified treatment. It may be due to other factors which coexist with the change. Thus a *treatment* is actually a *treatment package* containing hidden ingredients.

These factors include changes—due to supposedly inactive components of the treatment, and to the patient's faith in the treatment—that would have taken place even if the treatment had not been given. The mind has a powerful effect on healing. We have come to realize that a person's belief in the efficacy of the treatment, called the "placebo effect" ("placebo" derived from "to please" in Latin), can be responsible for some or all of the improvement seen following the start of treatment.

In order to rationally separate the true effect of the treatment being studied from these other factors, "controlled" studies are performed. In such studies, changes in patients following delivery of the treatment package are compared to changes in patients when the treatment package is delivered without one or more of its ingredients. This eliminates the effect of the missing factor(s). Patients whose treatment package is missing something form the "control" group.

Because of the important contribution of the placebo effect, a placebo treatment is often given to the control group instead of the experimental treatment. This fake treatment is designed to appear exactly like the experimental treatment. The better controlled studies are "double-blinded"; that is, researchers, as well as patients, do not know who is receiving the experimental treatment and who is receiving the placebo. In this way, researchers cannot inadvertently add or detract from the results of the experimental treatment by somehow communicating their personal beliefs concerning its efficacy to their patients.

Like the empirical model, the rational model is imperfect. By insisting on looking at one factor at a time, the rational model neglects powerful factors that cannot be separated from the healing cauldron without losing efficacy. I could cite many examples, but especially relevant is the case of certain herbal medicines (such as echinacea) whose individual ingredients may be less effective than the whole herb or, as in the example of mistletoe, whose individual ingredients may be more toxic.

In developed countries, the law of the land is now based on the rational model despite its imperfections. Governments commonly prohibit sales of drugs that have not proven to be safe and effective in double-blind, placebo-controlled studies. Even then, to assure proper use, many are only available when prescribed by a physician. Should the same standard be applied to nutritional medicines? The answer is yes and no. Some nutritional medicines are best described as drugs, which certainly do require scientific studies of safety and efficacy as well as professional regulation; others are best described as foods, which only require scientific studies of efficacy. Many nutritional medicines fall somewhere in between.

Moreover, it would seem that, so long as a nutritional treatment is known to be safe, it should not be withheld until it is proven effective. Scientific proof of efficacy is important, but it is not the only consideration in choosing a treatment. Other questions have to be asked, involving cost, side effects, rapidity and duration of action, interactions with concurrent treatments, and patient preference. Only when all relevant issues are addressed can a truly informed decision be made.

We are currently in a transitional phase. The outmoded simplistic practice of arbitrarily dividing nutritional medicines into foods (which are essentially unregulated) or drugs (which are strictly regulated) must give way to recognition of nutritional medicines (which are in-between foods and drugs). A proper system of regulation for nutritional medicines must evolve. Hopefully, the new system will reward supplement companies for investing money in studies to prove the safety and efficacy of nutritional medicines. Until that is done, the field of nutritional medicine cannot fully blossom.

The chapters in this book summarize our existing knowledge of nutritional treatments for fifty common afflictions. I have tried to select treatments which appear to be effective based on current clinical findings. In general, such treatments are far safer than drugs. Nevertheless, this information is provided *for your education only*. If you wish to try these treatments, do so under medical supervision.

Your safety is not the only reason for medical supervision. Nutritionally-trained physicians can properly evaluate your nutritional status and make treatment recommendations based both on those findings and the specifics of your illness. I can only provide general information; it is your doctor who can translate that general information into the specific treatment program which is best for you.

A frequent question about nutritional healing plans is how long they should be tried. The better this question has been addressed in research studies, the better it can be answered. Often, the results of a treatment are assessed after an arbitrary length of time. If the treatment was found to be effective, that length of time would be a reasonable trial period. With further research, however, it may become clear that the treatment works even sooner, or that the results are better if the treatment is continued longer. If my review of the research seems to suggest a reasonable trial period, I have included that information.

When should a nutritional treatment that appears effective be stopped or the dosage reduced? The answer varies with each treatment. In general, if the supplement is being taken to correct a deficiency, once that deficiency is likely to have been corrected (say, after a few months), it would be reasonable to reduce the dosage or stop the supplement and see if symptoms return. If, however, the supplement is being taken because it is only effective at a dosage that is higher than that found in a healthy diet, it may need to be continued indefinitely. A general principle is to emphasize diet over supplements. They are, after all, supplements to—not substitutes for—a nutritious diet.

The organization of each chapter is identical. I first discuss any relationship that has been found between the illness and diet. If a relationship has been found, I suggest a Healing Diet. (Since essentially the same diet has been found to be beneficial in the treatment of many illnesses, I have named it the Basic Healing Diet and discuss both it and its vegetarian sibling in detail in Appendix A.)

In the next section, Nutritional Healing plans, I discuss the various nutritional and botanical factors which appear to be effective for treating the illness. After that, I provide assistance to help you, in consultation with your doctor, to choose from the various dietary and nutritional interventions I have listed. I believe that nutrition is only one of the many natural approaches to healing which should be considered; therefore I have ended many of the chapters by suggesting some of the non-nutritional natural therapies that may also move you toward healing.

Even though you may not be able to purchase it, I have decided to list tryptophan, an essential amino acid, as a Nutritional Healing Plan because of its many established applications as a nutritional supplement. ("Essential" refers to the fact that we must have tryptophan in our diets for proper functioning.) Tryptophan has been available in pure form as a nutritional supplement for many years. In 1990, however, a serious disorder (Eosinophilia-Myalgia Syndrome) became increasingly common, and evidence was found that contaminated tryptophan supplements were responsible, so many countries (including the U.S.) removed tryptophan supplements from the market. It is hoped that tryptophan supplements will be available again as soon as procedures can be instituted to fully protect the public from the contamination of commercial nutritional products.

One other warning: Unless I have specified otherwise, the dosages I have suggested are for average size adults. Children's dosages are much lower, so please consult your pediatrician for proper dosage.

Twentieth century Western medicine, despite its spectacular accomplishments, has dangerously over-emphasized drugs and surgery, and has neglected safer, more natural healing methods. As we draw near to the end of the century, there is a growing consensus among enlightened physicians and their patients that the practice of medicine be brought back into balance. My hope is that this book, as a contribution toward achieving that balance, will help to develop what will soon be the medicine of the twenty-first century.

Commonly Used Abbreviations

FDA	Food and Drug Administration
g	gram (1,000 mg)
gr	grain
IU	International Unit (an internationally accepted amount of a substance; a measurement of vitamin biological activity)
kg	kilogram
l	liter
lb	pound
mcg	microgram
ml	milliliter
mg	milligram (1,000 mcg)
oz	ounce
qt	quart
tsp	teaspoon
tbsp	tablespoon
RDA	Recommended Dietary Allowances set by the National Research Council's Food and Nutrition Board (varies with age and sex; see Appendix E for detailed information)
U.S. RDA	U.S. Recommended Daily Allowances set by the Food and Drug Administration (FDA) (does not vary with age or sex; see Appendix E for detailed information)

The information in this book is presented to enhance your knowledge of nutritional medicine; it is not a substitute for medical evaluation and treatment by a licensed physician. The Healing Diets and Nutritional Healing plans are designed to be part of your general health treatment plan, and should be followed only with the advice and under the supervision of your doctor.

The author has thoroughly researched the most current medical literature in compiling the information contained in this book. Inasmuch as the information and health plans contained in this book should not be implemented without the supervision of a qualified physician, the author and the publisher expressly disclaim responsibility for any consequences resulting directly or indirectly from the use of this book.

Acne

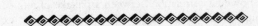

Acne vulgaris, the most common form of acne, is usually a disease of adolescence. It consists of blackheads, whiteheads, pimples, or deep-seated cysts that appear mainly on the face but may also be found on the neck, shoulders, back, and chest. Though almost everyone develops at least a little acne during the teen years, the more serious cases can lead to permanent scarring.

DIETARY FACTORS

As common as acne is, it remains poorly understood. However, there is evidence that it is one of the diseases of civilization, because acne is much less common among members of tribal societies as long as they eat their native diets; when they switch to a modern Western diet, their chances of getting acne increase. Unfortunately, we don't yet fully understand why the Western diet increases the risk of acne. We do know that acne is associated with oily skin due to an excess of *sebum,* the fatty secretion of the sebaceous glands, and that eating fat increases sebum production. Since this increase is moderate in people with normal skin but marked in males with acne, increased sebum may somehow worsen the lesions; thus a diet relatively low in fats may be of some value.[1]

It has also been suggested that natural vegetable oils may be a better source of dietary fat for acne patients than hydrogenated vegetable oils and animal fats, both of which are more saturated. We do know that the more saturated the fat, the more likely it is to solidify at room temperature; if the composition of fat in the diet determines the composition of fat in the sebum, saturated fats would be more likely than unsaturated fats to plug the sebaceous glands and make acne lesions worse.

Eating carbohydrates (which include starches and sugars) also increases sebum production in males with acne. In addition, a survey of 1,000 adults showed a correlation between an intake of refined carbohydrates and sugar, and the risk of skin disorders. However, experiments have failed to prove that limiting sugar intake improves acne.[2,3,4]

The fiber content of the diet of tribal societies is quite high compared to the Western diet in which carbohydrates are refined and most of the fiber is removed. Perhaps, therefore, it is not refined carbohydrates, but the low fiber content of such a diet that contributes to acne. Consistent with this possibility, one clinician found that his acne patients improved when he added an all-bran cereal to their diet. More studies are needed, however, to determine whether a high-fiber diet is a useful acne treatment.[5]

Finally, sensitivities to a number of common foods (especially chocolate, cola drinks, and nuts) have sometimes appeared to explain acne outbreaks. Here is a typical example of how diet appears to affect some acne sufferers, taken from my own practice.

A 13-year-old boy with severe cystic acne consistently had major eruptions the day after eating chocolate, almonds, and possibly other nuts. It would take about one month without eating these foods for his condition to return to the way it was before the outbreak. Additional evidence that he was food-sensitive comes from his history of atopic eczema at age seven, which failed to respond to treatment with topical steroids but responded promptly and permanently to a one-week fruit diet. Avoidance of chocolate and nuts seemed to prevent sudden acne outbreaks but failed to improve his acne any further.

There is, however, no good scientific evidence to prove that such sensitivities exist, and it has been shown that people who believe that their acne is food-sensitive are often mistaken.[6]

THE HEALING DIET

1. Follow the Basic Healing diet as described in Appendix A.
2. Avoid foods found on testing to aggravate acne. *See Appendix B for information about diagnosing food sensitivities.*

NUTRITIONAL HEALING PLANS

Vitamins

Vitamin A

Of all acne remedies, nutritionists are most impressed with the results of vitamin A and its synthetic derivatives. Pilot studies have found that most cases of acne respond within weeks to extremely high dosages (300,000 IU to 500,000 IU) of the vitamin. Such high doses can, however, cause adverse effects because the body stores vitamin A in the liver. You should not, therefore, take vitamin A at high doses (above 10,000 IU) except under a doctor's supervision.[7]

At a lower dosage, vitamin A is safer but less likely to be effective. A partial solution to the problem is to combine vitamin A with vitamin E. Probably because vitamin E slows down the breakdown of vitamin A in the body, 100,000 IU of vitamin A, when taken along with 800 IU of vitamin E, appears to be as effective, and less toxic, than higher doses of vitamin A alone.[8,9]

In recent years, two synthetic forms of vitamin A have been introduced and are now widely prescribed by dermatologists. The first, *isotretinoin* (13-*cis*-retinoic acid), has been proven effective for treating acne, and is especially useful for treating the more severe form of the disease marked by the formation of *cysts,* or abnormal sacs containing semisolid material. Unfortunately, like vitamin A, isotretinoin has considerable potential for serious adverse effects, including birth defects in the children of mothers taking the medication during pregnancy. Other potentially serious effects include elevated blood fats, liver and bowel inflammation, and bone abnormalities. Due to its potential toxicity, the use of isotretinoin has been restricted to people suffering from severe cystic acne that has failed to respond to other forms of treatment.[10]

Tretinoin (vitamin A acid or retinoic acid), the other synthetic vitamin A derivative, is a preparation that is applied directly to the skin. Although tretinoin is fairly effective, its original formulation in an alcoholic solution irritated the skin so badly that it was poorly accepted. Since then, tretinoin has been marketed as a cream and as a gel, and both are much less likely to cause significant irritation.[11]

Because tretinoin is applied to the skin, it is much safer to use than oral forms of vitamin A. Skin irritation is the main side effect. More severe forms of acne, however, may respond only to oral forms of the vitamin.

NUTRITIONAL HEALING PLAN: Vitamin A

Initial Plan

Dosage: 100,000 IU of vitamin A daily

Instructions: Take with 800 IU of vitamin E daily.

Maintenance Plan

To avoid vitamin A toxicity, as soon as improvement is seen reduce the dosage every few weeks until you reach the lowest dose that maintains the improvement.

WARNING

1. Use this plan only while under a physician's care; adverse side effects have frequently been reported at the effective dosage.
2. Do not combine vitamin A with isotretinoin; it increases the risk of adverse side effects.

Other Suggestions

If tretinoin causes skin irritation, use a moisturizing cream or lotion such as Eucerin (R) (Beiersdorf, U.S.) to help reduce the irritation. Otherwise, apply the treatment less frequently.

Trial Period

Results from taking vitamin A may be seen within a few weeks or may take as long as four months.

Vitamin B₆

The results of several studies suggest that supplementation with vitamin B_6 may reduce the symptoms of premenstrual tension syndrome (PMS), including acne flare-ups. For example, acne improved in 72 percent of 106 young women after they took 50 mg of pyridoxine (a form of vitamin B_6) daily for one week prior to and during their menstrual periods.[12]

Although magnesium has not been studied for the treatment of acne, blood magnesium levels, which may be low in those with PMS, can be raised with vitamin B_6. Adding magnesium to a vitamin B_6 supplement is also a good idea.

NUTRITIONAL HEALING PLAN: Vitamin B₆

Preparation

pyridoxine

Dosage: 50 mg daily

Instructions: Take with 400 mg of magnesium daily for 1 week prior to and during menses.

Special Value: premenstrual acne flare-ups

Minerals

Selenium

One common problem in acne is the formation of *pustules,* or little whitish-colored pockets of pus, caused by infected acne lesions. If they are squeezed, the pus drains from them.

In a pilot study, selenium supplementation seemed to be particularly effective for treating acne pustules, possibly because one of the functions of selenium is to help fight infections. The people who did best in this study were those whose blood level of glutathione peroxidase (a selenium-containing enzyme) was low; as the level of this enzyme rose, their acne improved.[13]

Selenium works closely together with vitamin E, and syndromes caused by selenium deficiency overlap those caused by vitamin E deficiency. Because of their close relationship, selenium has often been combined with vitamin E for the treatment of acne (as in the study just discussed) in order to make the treatment more effective.

NUTRITIONAL HEALING PLAN: Selenium

Preparation

organic selenium (such as selenomethionine)

Dosage: 200 mcg daily

Instructions: Take with 400 IU of vitamin E daily.

Special Value: Especially consider this plan if there are pustules.

Zinc

Blood zinc levels are often lower in people who suffer from acne than in people with normal skin—a finding that suggests their body supplies of zinc may be less than optimum to combat the formation of pustules. Even when blood zinc levels are normal, the level of zinc in the skin may be reduced.[14,15]

Some, but not all, double-blind studies have found zinc supplementation to be effective for the treatment of acne. Like selenium, zinc helps the body to fight infections and seems to be particularly effective against acne pustules. It may also reduce the inflammation that is sometimes seen.[16,17,18]

Is zinc as effective as vitamin A for the treatment of acne? More studies are needed; however, in one double-blind study, 135 mg daily of effervescent zinc sulfate was clearly more effective than 300,000 IU daily of vitamin A.[19]

NUTRITIONAL HEALING PLAN: Zinc

Preparation

effervescent (bubbling) zinc sulfate

Dosage: 135 mg of zinc daily

Special Value: Especially consider this plan if the acne is inflamed or if there are pustules.

Trial Period

three months

Other Nutritional Factors

Omega-6 Fatty Acids

The concentration of *linoleic acid,* an essential fatty acid (that is, we require it from food) belonging to the omega-6 family, has been found to be lower in the sebum of acne patients than in the sebum of people with normal skin, which raises the question of whether extra linoleic acid may be beneficial. In an interesting pilot study, people with acne who were placed on a low-fat diet supplemented with corn oil (a good source of linoleic acid) saw their acne improve.[20,21]

NUTRITIONAL HEALING PLAN: Omega-6 Fatty Acids

Preparation

any oil rich in linoleic acid such as corn or safflower oil

Dosage: 1 or 2 tbsp daily

Other Natural Treatments

High-Chromium Yeast

In their skin (but not in their blood), people with acne have difficulty reducing sugar levels through the action of insulin. Some studies of diabetics have found that high-chromium yeast helps normalize blood sugar levels. Moreover, in a pilot study, supplementation with this special yeast appeared to improve acne.[22,23]

High-chromium yeast is a specially grown yeast that is much richer in chromium than ordinary yeast. The efficacy of high-chromium yeast is probably due to *glucose tolerance factor,* a substance that has been shown to improve diabetics' ability to handle sugar and could thus affect sugar metabolism in acne lesions. If further studies confirm these results, perhaps some of the other nutritional treatments that help diabetics handle sugar will be shown to also combat acne.

NUTRITIONAL HEALING PLAN: High-Chromium Yeast

Preparation

high-chromium yeast (200 mcg of chromium per tsp)

Dosage: 1 tsp twice daily

Azelaic Acid

Azelaic acid is not a nutrient; however, since it is found in nature, it is a reasonable alternative to the use of synthetic substances for topical application. A double-blind study found azelaic acid superior to topical benzoyl peroxide (a popular treatment) and tretinoin, as well as to oral tetracycline. Like other topical agents, azelaic acid has a drying effect that can cause skin irritation, although it appears to cause less irritation than most of the alternatives.[24]

NATURAL HEALING PLAN: Azelaic Acid

Preparation

20 percent solution in a cream base

Instructions: Apply lightly to affected areas before going to bed.

Tea Tree Oil

Tea tree oil is the essential oil extracted from a narrow-leafed paper bark tree native to Australia. It consists largely of chemicals with proven antimicrobial effects. Recently, an Australian study compared the effectiveness of a topical application of the oil to the application of benzoyl peroxide lotion. After three months, both treatments produced significant improvement in acne lesions. Although benzoyl peroxide was more effective for noninflamed lesions, people treated with tea tree oil reported fewer side effects.[25]

NATURAL HEALING PLAN: Tea Tree Oil

Preparation

5 percent gel

Instructions: Apply daily to the affected areas.

CHOOSING A PERSONAL PLAN

The Basic Healing diet and any of the Nutritional Healing plans can be tried alone, although those who wish to proceed faster may wish to combine the diet with one or more of the healing plans. If the lesions improve within three months, eliminate one part of the program every two months. If the acne worsens during this period, you can discover whether the worsening was coincidental by returning what you last eliminated to the treatment program; then see if the acne improves again.

Women who suffer from premenstrual acne flare-ups should consider trying the pyridoxine and magnesium combination first. People with pustular acne who wish to try a simple plan should first consider trying the combination of zinc, selenium, and vitamin E.

Prolonged ingestion of either high-dose vitamin A or isotretinoin has potentially serious adverse effects and thus should be avoided except in cases of severe cystic acne that have failed to respond to all other treatment attempts. Even then, treatment should be under medical supervision.

Though you may think that skin lesions such as acne would not respond to purely psychological treatments such as using a placebo instead of an experimental agent, as many as half of all acne patients have been found to respond to placebos. This makes it difficult to know whether nutrititional substances that were not compared to placebos in the acne studies were actually effective against acne. Specifically, the use of selenium, linoleic acid, and high-chromium yeast have not been shown to be more effective than either a placebo or a proven treatment. On the other hand, these substances are so safe that it may be worthwhile to try them. The same can be said for a low-saturated fat, high-fiber diet and specific food eliminations.

Zinc supplementation has been shown to be effective in several placebo-controlled studies. However, other studies have failed to confirm these results and its efficacy is still uncertain.

In addition to or instead of taking supplementation, consider using a natural product that is applied directly to the affected area. Application of either azelaic acid or tea tree oil has been proven effective. Azelaic acid was more effective than benzoyl peroxide, but tea tree oil was less effective; therefore azelaic acid would be my first choice as a topical agent.

ADDITIONAL SUGGESTIONS

1. Wash the affected skin with a washcloth three or more times a day to remove accumulated oil and surface debris.
2. When cleaning the affected skin, use special acne soaps that reduce oiliness.
3. Makeup tends to plug the pores of the oil glands, so it should be used sparingly, if at all. Use a brand that has been specially formulated for people with acne.

Alcoholism

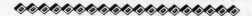

One of the most common diseases in Western societies, alcoholism can be defined as a chronic, compulsive craving for alcohol (ethanol) that causes excessive ingestion. Alcohol in large quantities is a toxic agent, and excessive ingestion eventually results in mental and physical deterioration.

DIETARY FACTORS

A *calorie* is a measure of the energy released by a food when it is broken down in the body. Since alcohol is high in calories, alcoholics can function for many years with alcohol as the major food in their diet. However, the nutritional value of alcohol is very low, so alcoholics commonly develop increasing nutritional deficiencies over time.

Scientists have discovered that despite the toxicity of alcohol (especially to the liver and brain), some diseases associated with alcoholism are caused less by alcohol itself than by alcoholism's effect on eating habits and the absorption and utilization of nutrients. Furthermore, malnutrition increases the adverse effects of alcohol.

It has become an axiom of modern medical practice to place alcoholics on a well-balanced, nutritionally adequate diet, and to try to correct any nutritional deficiencies that have developed. Such a diet improves the alcoholic's health, as the following case illustrates:

> *A 35-year-old longshoreman was a typical "spree" drinker who consumed large quantities of alcohol and ingested very little food during a period of several weeks. He was finally admitted to the hospital with very yellow skin (jaundice) due to liver dysfunction, and his*

10

*liver was enlarged and tender. He immediately began to eat a high-
calorie, high-protein diet. A liver biopsy several days later showed a
moderate amount of fatty change consistent with alcoholic liver
disease.*

*On the diet, he rapidly gained weight, his serum bilirubin concen-
tration (a blood test that measures liver function) returned to normal,
the size of his liver decreased, and its tenderness promptly subsided.
Three weeks after admission, no clinical or laboratory evidence of
liver disease remained. A few days later, a second liver biopsy
showed that the liver was essentially normal.*[1]

In addition, there is preliminary evidence that such a diet may reduce
alcohol craving. For example, when rats were fed a typical "junk food"
diet, they gradually increased their alcohol consumption. However, when
another group of rats were fed a well-balanced, nutritionally adequate
diet, they maintained a low level of alcohol intake. Furthermore, when
caffeine or coffee was added to the diet of either group, the rats increased
their alcohol intake.[2]

The results of a human trial are equally interesting. When people were
placed on a diet in which two-thirds of their calories came from uncooked
natural foods, 80 percent of those who drank or smoked stopped spon-
taneously.[3]

THE HEALING DIET

Follow the Basic Healing Diet as described in Appendix A.

NUTRITIONAL HEALING PLANS

Nutritional healing can benefit alcoholics in three different ways:

1. prevent or reverse the damage done by the overingestion of alcohol
2. reduce the craving for alcohol
3. reduce the symptoms of alcohol withdrawal

NUTRITIONAL HEALING TO COMBAT ALCOHOL TOXICITY

Acetaldehyde Fighters: Niacin, Zinc, and Pantethine

Alcohol is broken down within the body into *acetaldehyde*, a toxic chemical that encourages the development of atherosclerosis, liver disease, and
cardiomyopathy (disease of the heart muscle). As if that isn't bad enough,
acetaldehyde may also encourage alcohol addiction by combining with

other substances present in the body to form certain chemicals that act like narcotic drugs.

One way of reducing the acetaldehyde levels of alcoholics is to give them supplements of niacin or niacinamide (vitamin B_3). Niacin interferes with the production of acetaldehyde from alcohol and thus reduces its level in the body following alcohol ingestion.[4]

The other method of reducing acetaldehyde levels is to boost the activity of *aldehyde dehydrogenase,* the enzyme that breaks acetaldehyde down into harmless acetate. In order to work, this enzyme requires zinc, which is commonly deficient in alcoholics. When rats are given a zinc-deficient diet, they increase their alcohol consumption, possibly because inadequate enzyme activity raises their acetaldehyde levels, which in turn increases their addiction to alcohol. By correcting a zinc deficiency, aldehyde dehydrogenase activity is increased, and acetaldehyde levels should drop.[5]

Another means of increasing aldehyde dehydrogenase activity is by supplementing the diet with *pantethine.* Pantethine, closely related to pantetheine, is derived from pantothenic acid, a member of the vitamin B complex. In contrast to zinc, supplementation with pantethine increases the activity of aldehyde dehydrogenase whether there is an existing deficiency or not.[6]

Pantethine won't help everyone, however. In some individuals, especially people of Mongoloid origin (which includes Asians, Eskimos, and American Indians), aldehyde dehydrogenase is a relatively weak enzyme; thus activating it with pantethine does not make a significant difference in its ability to break down acetaldehyde. (This explains why Asians tend to be more sensitive to the effects of alcoholic beverages than other races.)

There is a simple way to tell whether pantethine is worth a try. Facial flushing and a rapid heart rate after drinking are direct effects of acetaldehyde. If you readily develop these symptoms, your enzyme is weak and pantethine is unlikely to be beneficial.

NUTRITIONAL HEALING PLAN: Acetaldehyde Fighters

Dosages: 250 mg of niacin or niacinamide twice daily

WARNING

Niacin often causes flushing, and other side effects are possible, while niacinamide is better tolerated. Consult your doctor for further information.

---

50 mg of zinc daily

300 mg of pantethine 2 or 3 times daily

Antioxidants: Vitamin C, Vitamin E, Selenium

Another approach to reduce alcohol toxicity is to increase the intake of *antioxidants*. Oxidants, or free radicals, are highly reactive substances that can be very damaging to cells. Vitamin C, vitamin E, and selenium—three antioxidants that are commonly depressed in the blood serum of alcoholics—all appear to reduce the toxic effects of alcohol. They seem especially useful in retarding the development of alcoholic liver disease.

Vitamin C hastens the clearance of alcohol from the bloodstream. Perhaps because of this, supplementation with vitamin C either before or during alcohol ingestion protects the liver against fatty infiltration—the initial change associated with alcoholic liver disease.[7,8]

At least in rats, chronic alcohol ingestion reduces the level of vitamin E in the liver cells. Like vitamin C, when vitamin E is taken either before or during alcohol ingestion, it may prevent fatty infiltration of the liver. In addition, alcohol reduces the level of vitamin E in the heart muscle, and there is evidence from animal studies that supplementation with the vitamin may prevent damage to that muscle.[9,10]

Glutathione peroxidase is an enzyme that protects against alcohol-induced liver damage, and selenium is necessary to activate the enzyme; thus selenium deficiency is associated with active liver disease. Selenium levels may also be depressed in alcoholic myopathy, a disease of the major muscles of the body.[11,12]

NUTRITIONAL HEALING PLAN: Antioxidants

Dosages: 2 g of vitamin C daily and 1 hour prior to alcohol ingestion

400–800 IU of vitamin E daily

200 mcg of selenium daily

Other Nutrients

Thiamine (Vitamin B₁) Deficiency

Neurological and psychiatric complications of alcoholism may result from a thiamine (Vitamin B_1) deficiency, even if the alcoholic is getting what would ordinarily be an adequate amount of thiamine in the diet. Alcoholics are unable to properly absorb and utilize this vitamin. For this reason, although oral supplementation may be beneficial, injections of thiamine are sometimes necessary.[13]

NUTRITIONAL HEALING PLAN: Thiamine Deficiency

Dosage: 100 mg of thiamine daily

Vitamin A Deficiency

Levels of vitamin A are frequently very low in the liver of alcoholics, although blood levels of this vitamin may remain normal for quite some time. Low blood levels are also seen in alcoholic muscle disease.[14,15]

Supplementation with vitamin A has been suggested not only to prevent liver damage but also to correct night blindness and sexual dysfunction. In alcoholics with liver disease, vitamin A supplementation has been shown to improve the senses of taste and smell, possibly by improving the absorption of zinc.[16,17]

NUTRITIONAL HEALING PLAN: Vitamin A Deficiency

Dosage: 10,000 IU of vitamin A daily

WARNING

Vitamin A supplementation should not be combined with heavy drinking; it may **hasten** the development of liver disease.[18]

Magnesium Deficiency

Low blood levels of magnesium are common in chronic alcoholics due to a combination of inadequate diet, poor absorption from the gut, excessive losses in the urine, and a reduced ability of the cells to transfer it in from the outside. A deficiency in magnesium may cause myopathy (muscle disease) in the heart muscle as well as in other muscles; fortunately, it responds rapidly to adequate supplementation.[19,20]

NUTRITIONAL HEALING PLAN: Magnesium Deficiency

Dosage: 500 mg of magnesium daily

NUTRITIONAL HEALING TO REDUCE ALCOHOL CRAVING

We have already discussed how the Basic Healing diet may reduce the alcoholic's craving for alcohol. We also noted that, since the production of acetaldehyde from alcohol can contribute to alcohol craving, any nutritional measure (such as niacin, zinc, or panthethine) that reduces acetaldehyde levels may also reduce such craving.

Thiamine (Vitamin B$_1$)

There have been attempts to discover specific nutrients in the diet that may affect alcohol craving. When rats were given diets deficient in the vitamins of the vitamin B complex, they were more likely to choose alcohol over water. However, after they received supplements of these vitamins, they preferred water over alcohol. More recent animal studies suggest that thiamine may be one member of the vitamin B complex that affects alcohol craving.[21,22]

NUTRITIONAL HEALING PLAN: Thiamine

Dosage: 100 mg of thiamine daily

L-Glutamine

Not only did rats given L-glutamine reduce their intake of alcohol, but nine out of ten alcoholics reported that, after taking glutamine supplements, they had less desire to drink, less anxiety, and slept better. Relatives and friends observing them agreed. When placebos were substituted without their knowledge, only two or three of the ten continued to do well, and none who failed to respond to glutamine responded to the placebo.[23,24]

The following case is an example of the benefits of glutamine supplementation:

A secretary in her early 30s who belonged to Alcoholics Anonymous had been drinking heavily for several years and was extremely despondent. She showed no response to one week of placebos. During the following two weeks she received 1 g of L-glutamine daily. She stopped drinking completely and her outlook improved tremendously.

Without her knowledge, she was shifted back to placebos. By the end of the sixth week, she had started to drink occasionally. By the end of the tenth week, she was drinking as heavily as before taking glutamine and had stopped taking the placebo capsules.

After speaking with the researchers, she agreed to resume the trial and was switched back to glutamine. Her drinking stopped again almost immediately. Over the next three months, she was followed while continuing on glutamine. She reported drinking a little beer occasionally but claimed not to have had hard liquor or to have overindulged at any time. She also commented frequently on her ability to sleep better and on her decreased nervousness.[25]

NUTRITIONAL HEALING PLAN: L-Glutamine

Dosage: 1 g (¼ tsp) of L-glutamine twice daily

NUTRITIONAL HEALING TO REDUCE THE SYMPTOMS OF ALCOHOL WITHDRAWAL

WARNING

Because the symptoms of alcohol withdrawal can be very serious, nutritional healing should be done only under medical supervision.

Omega-6 Fatty Acids

The omega-6 fatty acids are one of the two families of dietary fatty acids which are essential for our bodies. Since the oil from the evening primrose plant is particularly rich in gammalinolenic acid, an important member of that family, it has often been used in studies as a source of these essential nutrients.

The promising results of animal experiments that tested the ability of *evening primrose oil* and related substances to reduce the symptoms of alcohol withdrawal have been confirmed in a human study. For three weeks, patients undergoing alcohol detoxification received Valium as needed along with either evening primrose oil or a placebo. Compared to those who received the placebo, patients who received primrose oil asked for less Valium and showed evidence of a modest but consistent reduction in withdrawal severity, and their liver tests normalized faster.[26]

The following case illustrates the effectiveness of evening primrose oil:

A Norwegian fisherman with severe depression customarily binge-drank for two weeks at a time, consuming a bottle of whiskey a day; then, because he would become sick and run down, he would sober up for one or two weeks. He was given evening primrose oil or a placebo in a double-blind manner (that is, neither he nor the person who gave him the pills knew which he was getting) and told to log each day's alcohol consumption, degree of alcohol craving, and depression on a rating scale. Within a week of starting the primrose oil,

he reported an 80 percent reduction in depression and alcohol crav-
ing, and he consumed no alcohol for 6 weeks for the first time in
years. Shortly after being switched to the placebo, he went on a binge
and dropped out of the study.[27]

NUTRITIONAL HEALING PLAN: Omega-6 Fatty Acids

Preparation

evening primrose oil

Dosage: 1 g 3 times daily

Taurine

There is very early evidence that the amino acid taurine may also reduce the symptoms of alcohol withdrawal in humans. Taurine, by the way, has been shown in test tube and animal studies to be another acetaldehyde inhibitor, although studies in humans still need to be done. This suggests that inhibition of acetaldehyde may be a common mechanism for achieving all of the three types of benefits from nutritional healing: the reduction of alcohol toxicity, craving, and withdrawal symptoms.[28]

NUTRITIONAL HEALING PLAN: Taurine

Dosage: 1 g of taurine 3 times daily

CHOOSING A PERSONAL PLAN

If you are an alcoholic, you should be on the Basic Healing diet, both because of its healing effects and because it may reduce your craving for alcohol. As you probably have difficulty absorbing and utilizing nutrients, additional general nutritional supplementation is advisable. I suggest a high-potency multivitamin/multimineral formula. (These supplements, which are made by a number of smaller companies, are often labeled as "stress" formulas, and their labels suggest that you take at least six tablets or capsules daily.)

Your doctor could order laboratory studies to find out whether, despite a good diet and supplementation, levels of any of the most important nutrients remain low. If so, your doctor can provide you with them by injection until your body has had time to heal.

The B vitamins, especially thiamine, are particularly important to you, as they may reduce your craving for alcohol. If the craving continues despite the above measures, consider a trial of L-glutamine.

Despite these measures, if you remain unable to stop drinking but wish to do whatever you can to protect your body from the toxic effects of alcohol, I suggest you increase your intake of niacin, as recommended above, in order to increase the breakdown of the acetaldehyde that is formed from alcohol. If you don't have a tendency to flush after drinking, you can also try pantethine for the same purpose.

Since you will be on the Basic Healing diet and taking additional daily supplements, you should already have adequate antioxidant protection. However, I would increase vitamin C, one of the major antioxidants, to the level suggested above in order to hasten the clearance of alcohol from your blood.

If you have been drinking heavily and wish some nutritional help while withdrawing from alcohol, evening primrose oil is the best-studied substance for easing withdrawal symptoms. You may wish to combine it with taurine just in case the combination provides you with added benefits, but don't depend upon these nutritional aids to make withdrawal safe and easy. If your alcohol problem is serious, attempt withdrawal only under medical supervision.

ADDITIONAL SUGGESTION

If you can't stop yourself from drinking, consider joining a self-help group such as Alcoholics Anonymous (AA). Active participation in such a group markedly increases your chances of achieving long-term control over your urge to drink.

Allergy and Food Sensitivity

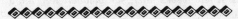

See also: ASTHMA, ECZEMA.

The term *allergy* was coined in the early part of this century to mean altered reactivity to some foreign substance. Today it is often used in the narrower sense of *atopic allergy,* a particular type of over-reaction of the immune system which produces a relatively small number of specific symptoms. Examples are: eye irritation, hives, nasal congestion, postnasal drip, sinus congestion, and wheezing.

When *allergy* is used in this narrow way to refer exclusively to atopic allergy, *sensitivity* is the broad term often used to describe an over-reaction by the body to a specific substance, no matter what the reason. Sensitivities cause an immense variety of reactions that may affect any system of the body—including the brain. In recent years, we have discovered the mechanism underlying atopic allergies; sensitivities, however, appear to have a number of causes, only one of which is atopic allergy and most others of which remain poorly understood. Even people suffering from the typical symptoms of atopic allergy are sometimes found on testing to be sensitive instead of atopic.[1]

DIETARY FACTORS

Sensitivity can develop to essentially any food. If the reaction is immediate, it is easy to recognize. A reaction can be delayed, however, for hours or even for days. It can also be hidden; that is, when a reaction is caused by a commonly eaten food, it may contribute to chronic symptoms without any apparent relationship to when that food is eaten. As the following case illustrates, even the various types of food additives, such as food colorings, can cause reactions:

> *For six weeks a fifty-year-old woman on oral estrogen supplementation suffered from hives which had failed to respond to medication. The rash had begun after she started taking estrogen tablets containing a food coloring, FD&C Yellow No. 5 (tartrazine). It improved when she substituted tartrazine-free estrogen tablets and worsened badly when she resumed use of the original tablets. Strict avoidance of foods and drugs containing tartrazine resulted in rapid resolution of the lesions. A few weeks later, she inadvertently ate a tartrazine-containing relish and developed mild, limited hives and swelling around the eyes.*[2]

THE HEALING DIET

Avoid foods found on testing to provoke symptoms. *See Appendix B for information about diagnosing food sensitivities and allergies.*

NUTRITIONAL HEALING PLANS

Vitamins

Vitamin B₃

Vitamin B_3, both in the form of niacin and niacinamide, has been shown to inhibit the release of histamine, a substance associated with allergic reactions.[3] Antihistamine medications are often quite effective in relieving nasal symptoms; half a century ago, one author noted that injections of niacinamide rapidly relieved symptoms of hay fever.[4] Unfortunately, however, oral niacin has been neglected in modern allergy research, so we know very little about its efficacy.

NUTRITIONAL HEALING PLAN: Vitamin B₃

Preparation

niacin or niacinamide

Dosage: 50 mg twice daily

Pantothenic Acid

While there is little scientific proof, reports suggest that pantothenic acid supplementation may reduce allergic nasal symptoms.[5] It may also benefit other allergic conditions and appears to be as effective as the antihistamines.[6]

> *A physician with allergies took 100 mg of pantothenic acid at bedtime. He found that his nasal stuffiness cleared in less than 15 minutes, and he no longer awakened at 4 or 5 A.M. with a cough and mucous secretions. He subsequently found that many of his patients also noted significant relief from their nasal congestion when they took pantothenic acid supplementation.[7]*

NUTRITIONAL HEALING PLAN: Pantothenic Acid

Dosage: 100–500 mg of pantothenic acid daily as needed

Vitamin B₆

Monosodium glutamate (MSG) is a flavor enhancer. In some people, MSG can cause symptoms such as headache, warmth, stiffness, weakness, tingling, pressure, lightheadedness, heartburn and stomach discomfort. Since Chinese restaurants often use MSG, these symptoms have been labeled the "Chinese restaurant syndrome."

The results of a double-blind study suggest that MSG may cause symptoms by worsening a borderline vitamin B_6 deficiency. Twelve students who became ill after ingesting MSG were given either vitamin B_6 or a placebo (fake pill) daily. After twelve weeks, they were asked to consume MSG again. All except one of the nine students receiving vitamin B_6 showed no response to MSG, while all three students who received placebo still responded.[8]

NUTRITIONAL HEALING PLAN: Vitamin B₆

Special Application

MSG sensitivity

Preparation

pyridoxine

Dosage: 50 mg of pyridoxine daily

WARNING

If this dosage of pyridoxine is taken over many months, there may be a very slight chance of developing symptoms of nerve damage in the hands and feet, such as numbness, "pins and needles," and weakness.

Vitamin B₁₂

Vitamin B$_{12}$

Some people are sensitive to sulfite, a preservative added to foods. If they eat or drink sulfite-containing foods, they may develop symptoms such as nasal or sinus congestion, a runny nose, postnasal drip, an itchy throat, headaches or asthma.

Results of an unpublished double-blind study of 24 sulfite-sensitive people suggest that supplementation with vitamin B$_{12}$ may protect sensitive people from reactions, but only if it is taken 15 minutes before the sulfite exposure. If the vitamin B$_{12}$ is taken sub-lingually (beneath the tongue), it starts to work in as little as 15 minutes; its protection may last a full day.[9]

NUTRITIONAL HEALING PLAN: Vitamin B$_{12}$

Special Application
sulfite sensitivity

Preparation
sublingual vitamin B$_{12}$

Dosage: 2000 mcg daily, dissolved under the tongue

Instructions: Must be taken at least 15 minutes before sulfite exposure.

Vitamin C

Like niacin, vitamin C has been shown to be an antihistamine. Low levels of vitamin C in the plasma (the fluid part of the blood) are found in people with high histamine levels, and vitamin C supplementation reduces blood histamine both in people with low plasma vitamin C levels and in those with high histamine levels.[10]

In a pilot study, vitamin C supplementation often seemed effective in reducing symptoms of hay fever (allergic rhinitis).[11] However, when the vitamin was given in a double-blind study, there was no evidence that it protected people against developing symptoms, or even that it was effective as an antihistamine.[12] Whether vitamin C is effective at a dosage above 4 grams daily is unknown.

There is other evidence that vitamin C supplementation may have some value in the treatment of allergies. Vitamin C has been shown to protect guinea pigs against anaphylaxis, a massive and sometimes fatal allergic reaction, after they were injected with the flavor enhancer MSG.[13] This raises the question of whether it, like vitamin B$_6$, may protect humans against MSG reactions.

NUTRITIONAL HEALING PLAN: Vitamin C

Dosage: unknown but 2 grams of vitamin C three times daily would be reasonable

---

WARNING

May occasionally cause stomach discomfort or loose stools. If these symptoms occur, reduce the dosage.

Minerals

Calcium

In double-blind crossover studies, calcium supplementation has been shown to reduce allergic responses in people suffering from the symptoms of hay fever[14] and bronchial asthma.[15] One study gave calcium intravenously, while the other combined it with vitamin D, so the effective dosage of calcium when given alone remains to be established.

NUTRITIONAL HEALING PLAN: Calcium

Preparation

calcium citrate

Dosage: unknown, but 500 mg daily would be reasonable

Magnesium Deficiency

Chronic magnesium deficiency may make people more vulnerable to classical (atopic) allergic reactions.[16] Inadequate dietary magnesium is common in industrialized societies, and such factors as stress, illness and the use of certain medications can increase the risk of magnesium deficiency.

Laboratory testing will help to diagnose a marginal magnesium deficiency. (Your doctor should be aware that a normal serum magnesium level is not adequate to rule out a deficiency.) Be particularly suspicious if you have other symptoms, such as irritability and muscle spasms, which are associated with a deficiency of magnesium.

NUTRITIONAL HEALING PLAN: Magnesium Deficiency

Dosage: unknown, but 400 mg daily of magnesium would be reasonable

---

Other Nutritional Factors

Essential Fatty Acids

Two classes of fatty acids are considered essential. (Essential means that our bodies need them but cannot make them; thus we require them from foods.) These are the omega-3 and the omega-6 fatty acids. We have evidence that supplementation with fatty acids of either the omega-3[17] or omega-6[18] series may combat the allergic response; however, double-blind studies proving their efficacy remain to be done.

As with magnesium, laboratory testing is the most accurate means of assessing your essential fatty acid nutrition. Since the wrong fatty acid supplement could theoretically be bad for you, treatment with essential fatty acids should be under the guidance of a physician who is knowledgeable about nutrition.

There are a few clues to the presence of a deficiency: People with essential fatty acid deficiencies may be excessively thirsty. Their hair may be dry and lackluster, their skin may be dry with follicular keratoses (thickened skin around hair follicles) and they may be hyperactive and irritable.

A six-year-old boy suffered from chronic nasal congestion with occasional cough and wheezing. He developed hives if licked by a dog and had episodes of irritability and crying after eating sweets. Since infancy he had a history of excessive thirst. He had dry skin, lackluster hair, numerous follicular keratoses, puffiness, a pale, boggy nasal lining, and white spots on his fingernails. Laboratory testing showed elevated eosinophils (an increase in a type of white blood cell suggestive of allergies) and low serum ferritin (suggestive of iron deficiency) in addition to abnormalities in essential fatty acids in the blood.

Based on the essential fatty acid analysis, he was treated with evening primrose oil (EPO) (high in omega-6 fatty acids). After one month, he no longer developed hives when licked by his neighbor's dog, he had less nasal congestion, his skin and hair were less dry, and he appeared calmer. Salmon oil extract (high in omega-3 fatty acids) and an iron supplement were added, and a program of immunotherapy (allergy shots) was started.

Over the next nine months, his hair and skin became lustrous, the eye puffiness disappeared, and he had no congestion or behavioral

problems. Two weeks after EPO was stopped, he became more thirsty; sniffles, a cough, and wheezing developed; his irritability reappeared, and he again developed hives when he had contact with dogs. EPO was restarted and the symptoms disappeared within two weeks.[19]

NUTRITIONAL HEALING PLAN: Essential Fatty Acids

WARNING

Stop immediately if symptoms worsen.

1. Trial of omega-3 fatty acids

Preparation and Dosage

1 g 3 times daily of a cholesterol-free fish oil concentrate
Example: 1 capsule of MaxEPA™ 3 times daily

WARNING

Take under medical supervision.

2. Trial of omega-6 fatty acids

Preparation

evening primrose oil

Dosage: 1 g twice daily

CHOOSING A PERSONAL PLAN

Since a tremendous variety of symptoms have been related to food sensitivities, the only way you can be reasonably certain that your symptoms are affected by hidden reactions to foods is by trying a food elimination diet. (Look in the index under *food sensitivities* for a list of illnesses whose symptoms may be affected by reactions to foods.) Consider a food elimination diet when your symptoms do not appear to be due to tissue damage and cannot be explained other ways. While their observation has yet to be proven, experienced clinicians find that people are more likely to be sensitive to foods that they crave; therefore a strong craving for a particular food should make you more suspicious.

The value of nutritional supplementation for the treatment of atopic allergies is largely unproven. Niacin and vitamin C are antihistamines which, like antihistamine medications, may help to reduce allergic nasal congestion. Pantothenic acid, while not shown to be an antihistamine, may do the same, and calcium has been shown to reduce allergic responses. Any of these supplements can be tried separately, or they could be combined for a single trial.

Although it is reasonably safe to try oral magnesium simply to see if you respond, magnesium supplementation appears to be beneficial only for people who are magnesium-deficient. Your doctor can perform laboratory testing to evaluate your magnesium status. You may also wish to have your diet analyzed by a nutrition professional to see if you are getting at least the RDA of magnesium; if you are not, you should increase the magnesium in your diet.

If you react to MSG (monosodium glutamate), consider a trial of vitamin B_6. If you react to sulfites, consider a trial of sublingual vitamin B_{12}. Finally, don't neglect the essential fatty acids, especially if you have symptoms which suggest that they may be deficient.

OTHER CONSIDERATIONS

The tendency to develop food sensitivities relates to the total load placed on the immune system at any particular time. For example, some people become food-sensitive only during hay fever season, when their atopic allergies act up. In fact, any factors in your life which increase the work your body has to do to keep you healthy, such as stress and air pollution, appear to affect your reactivity to foods.

Anxiety

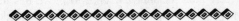

See also: INSOMNIA.

Anxiety is a universal human emotion. It differs from fear, which is a rational response to a real danger, in that it usually lacks a clear or realistic cause. Though some anxiety is normal and healthy, higher levels of anxiety are not only uncomfortable but counterproductive, as they interfere with a person's ability to function.

DIETARY FACTORS

In some people, especially those who are prone to panic attacks, sugar consumption may cause increased anxiety levels. The frequency and cause of this association remain controversial.[1]

Although there are laboratory methods of evaluating the effects of sugar ingestion, they may not tell the full story. Perhaps the best way you can discover whether sugar affects your anxiety is to eliminate all forms of refined sugar from your diet for a two-week trial. Sugar found naturally in foods is generally safe, although if you are motivated it would be best to eliminate those sources of sugar (including lactose, which is found in milk) for the trial period. A number of my patients complaining of high levels of anxiety have found sugar elimination to be remarkably effective, even though it is impossible to tell whether their improvement is simply due to their belief that they have done something useful.

For most of the population, there is no relationship between the amount of caffeine consumed and feelings of anxiety and depression. For people suffering from anxiety with panic attacks, however, the more caffeine they consume, the more anxious and depressed they feel. Double-blind studies have shown that people with anxiety, especially if they are prone to panic attacks, often experience worse symptoms of anxiety after ingesting caffeine. In addition, suddenly stopping regular caffeine ingestion may temporarily worsen anxiety.[2,3]

Some doctors believe that food sensitivities can cause anxiety; however, there is very little scientific evidence to prove this theory. In one study, 30 people complaining of anxiety or other psychological symptoms reported that they felt worse after extracts of certain foods and other substances were placed under their tongues. When fake extracts were placed under their tongues, however, their symptoms were unchanged.[4]

THE HEALING DIET

1. Avoid refined sugars for a trial period of two weeks.
2. Avoid caffeine, which is found in regular coffee, some cola beverages, and some teas, for a trial period of two weeks.
3. Avoid foods found on testing to increase anxiety. *See Appendix B for information about diagnosing food sensitivities.*

NUTRITIONAL HEALING PLANS

Vitamins

All three vitamins that appear to influence anxiety are members of the vitamin B complex.

Niacinamide (Vitamin B₃)

In an animal study, niacinamide, (a form of vitamin B₃) was found to have anti-aggressive, muscle relaxant, and hypnotic effects. The investigators noted that these effects were similar to those of the benzodiazepines, the most commonly prescribed family of tranquilizers for the treatment of anxiety. Though there is scientific indication of niacinamide's efficacy for treating anxiety, double-blind trials have not yet been conducted.[5,6]

NUTRITIONAL HEALING PLAN: Niacinamide

Dosage: not well established, but 500 mg of niacinamide twice daily would be reasonable

---

Thiamine (Vitamin B₁) Deficiency

Anxiety may be caused by a moderate shortage of thiamine (vitamin B_1), a vitamin whose blood level is often inadequate in the elderly. Inadequate thiamine can increase the concentration of lactic acid, and elevated lactate levels are known to be associated with heightened anxiety in predisposed individuals.[7,8,9]

NUTRITIONAL HEALING PLAN: Thiamine Deficiency

Dosage: not well established, but 50 mg of thiamine daily would be reasonable

---

Vitamin B₆ Deficiency

Vitamin B_6 is required for the conversion of *tryptophan,* an amino acid that comes from our diet, into *serotonin,* a neurotransmitter (chemical messenger between nerve cells) that is believed to be involved in the regulation of anxiety. When people with anxiety-related hyperventilation (over-breathing) who also had a marginal deficiency of vitamin B_6 were given supplements of vitamin B_6 and tryptophan in order to increase brain serotonin, their hyperventilation was successfully reduced.[10]

NUTRITIONAL HEALING PLAN: Vitamin B₆ Deficiency

Preparation

pyridoxine

Dosage: not well established, but 40 mg daily would be reasonable

---

WARNING

If this dosage of pyridoxine is taken over many months, there may be a very slight chance of developing symptoms of nerve damage in the hands and feet, such as numbness, "pins and needles," and weakness.

Minerals

Calcium Dysregulation

Medical disorders that reduce the level of calcium in the bloodstream may increase anxiety. This possibility should be suspected if your general anxiety level worsens without reason and stays that way over a period of time. The level of calcium in your bloodstream can be easily evaluated by your doctor. The following case illustrates the reduction of anxiety with calcium supplementation.

> *A 49-year-old postmenopausal vegetarian female with a 30-year history of generalized anxiety complained of an inability to relax and of trembling, sweating, apprehensiveness, insomnia, and occasional depression. She noted that stress would worsen her symptoms.*
>
> *After a year and a half of psychotherapy, her symptoms suddenly increased, seemingly without cause. She was given a tranquilizer, which was of no help. Five weeks later, she developed severe chest pain that was found to be the result of two spontaneous rib fractures. A medical evaluation revealed advanced osteoporosis and a low level of calcium in her blood. After her blood calcium level was normalized and she was placed on estrogen, her anxiety decreased to its former level.[11]*

Magnesium Deficiency

A chronic marginal deficiency of magnesium, common in Western diets, is associated with anxiety along with muscle tension and irritability. Also, about half of all people who experience panic attacks also suffer from a heart condition called mitral valve prolapse; symptoms of this condition may be caused by inadequate dietary magnesium. (For further information, see the chapter on mitral valve prolapse.)

Your physician can test you for a marginal magnesium deficiency by measuring the magnesium levels in your blood cells. (The magnesium level in your blood's serum goes down only if you have a serious medical problem.) The effects of a magnesium deficiency on anxiety is illustrated by the following case from my own practice:

> *An anxious 34-year-old man had a lifetime history of being easily startled—especially when he was relaxed or very tired—that even a slight noise would make him jump or cringe. He also experienced constant calf tension that sometimes became painful. His diet was restricted due to multiple food intolerances; lactose, oils, coarse grains, and most fresh fruits and vegetables would cause him to experience stomach cramps, gas, and diarrhea.*
>
> *Magnesium levels in his white blood cells were abnormally low, and he was placed on a multivitamin/multimineral supplement along with an additional 300 mg of magnesium. Six weeks later, he noted that he was slightly calmer and less tense and that his exaggerated startle response had disappeared. However, he continued to have calf tightness and hypersensitivity to noise.*
>
> *Five months after starting magnesium, there were no further changes, and his white blood cell magnesium levels were unimproved. One measure, but not another, of white blood cell calcium*

*was abnormally low. He was started on 750 mg of calcium daily but
showed no further improvement.*

*He was then given a trial injection of magnesium. Within one hour,
he noted a general feeling of relaxation, and his calf tenseness entirely disappeared for two to three weeks. He subsequently had additional injections whenever his symptoms returned. Each time the
effects lasted longer until the injections were no longer needed.*

NUTRITIONAL HEALING PLAN: Magnesium Deficiency

Dosage: whatever dosage is required to correct the deficiency; 400 mg of magnesium daily would be reasonable

---

Other Nutritional Factors

Omega-3 Fatty Acid Deficiency

It has been argued that *agoraphobia,* or the fear of open spaces, may
sometimes result from a marginal deficiency of the omega-3 family of
essential fatty acids. Though this theory is unproven, it would more likely
apply to people who also have other signs and symptoms of marginal
omega-3 fatty acid deficiency, as shown in the following chart.[12]

OMEGA-3 FATTY ACID DEFICIENCY

dry, cracking skin with areas of patchy dullness on the face
dandruff
stiff, dry hair
"chicken skin" (hyperkeratosis follicularis) on the back of arms and
    thighs
brittle fingernails that grow slowly
tinnitus (ringing in the ears)
fatigue
neuropathies (dysfunction of the nerves)

The following case shows the reduction of agoraphobia with the supplementation of omega-3 fatty acids:

*A 58-year-old man was able to travel in public but suffered from
agoraphobia for 40 years and could not cross an open square or field
by himself without having a severe panic attack. He also had slight
food allergies with alcohol intolerance, slight osteoarthritis, marked
tinnitus, a mild neuropathy, a mild skin rash, and mild fatigue.*

After two to three months of supplementation with linseed oil (an excellent source of omega-3 fatty acids), he reported consistent and definite reduction of agoraphobia and an increased sense of calm.[13]

If you believe you may be low in omega-3 fatty acids, discuss the following Nutritional Healing plan with your doctor. Do not try it on your own, as too high a daily dosage of omega-3 fatty acids, just as too low a dosage, may eventually prove to be unhealthy for you.

NUTRITIONAL HEALING PLAN: Omega-3 Fatty Acid Deficiency

Preparation

linseed oil (pharmaceutical quality)

Dosage: Take a dosage adequate to correct deficiency.

1. Start with 1 tsp with a meal.
2. Increase by 1 tsp every 4 days to a maximum of between 1 and 4 tsp with each meal depending upon your weight. (The higher dosages are only suggested if you are overweight.)
3. Reduce the dosage if you develop any adverse effects, such as diarrhea, muscle aches, skin problems, or mood changes.

WARNING
Take under medical supervision.

Trial Period
initial improvement within two weeks; full benefit within six months

---

Tryptophan

Dietary tryptophan is converted in the body into the neurotransmitter serotonin and may have a mild sedating effect. Its efficacy in anxiety states has not been well tested, although some people find it to be effective.[14]

NUTRITIONAL HEALING PLAN: Tryptophan

Dosage: not well established but ½ to 1 g 3 times daily would be reasonable

Additional Instructions

1. Avoid protein for 90 minutes before and after ingestion.
2. Take with a carbohydrate (such as fruit juice).

Note: Since tryptophan supplements may not be currently available (see Introduction), you may wish to try foods with a high tryptophan to protein ratio (see Appendix A).

CHOOSING A PERSONAL PLAN

Try avoiding refined sugars and caffeine for two weeks, and see if you feel less anxious. If you have other symptoms that suggest food sensitivities, try a food-elimination diet.

Because of their calming effects, niacinamide and tryptophan are worth trying, whereas the other nutrients discussed are beneficial only if you are at least marginally deficient in them. (A nutritionally trained physician can evaluate you for marginal deficiencies.)

ADDITIONAL SUGGESTIONS

Anxiety has many causes, only some of which are nutritional. As in the case of a calcium deficiency, anxiety may result from a medical illness that should be evaluated by your doctor. It may also be caused by psychological conflicts, or it may stem from a primal reaction, a legacy from our primitive past when threats were physical and necessitated a similar response. No matter what the cause, relaxation training can be very effective for teaching you how to reduce your anxiety levels. If you suffer from a type of phobic anxiety, consider behavior therapy. When you need a physical outlet for your feelings, a program of aerobic exercise can be very helpful. If you sense that your anxiety is due to a psychological problem, consider psychotherapy and/or trials of appropriate psychotherapeutic medications.

When considering treatments for anxiety reduction, remember that your anxiety may have more than one cause, and more than one treatment may be beneficial.

Asthma

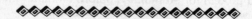

See also: ALLERGIES.

Bronchial asthma is a reversible obstructive disease of the airways that causes episodes of coughing, shortness of breath, and wheezing. Though we know that these episodes can be triggered by a variety of stimuli, the underlying cause of asthma is poorly understood.

DIETARY FACTORS

In the early thirteenth century, the eminent physician Maimonides prescribed a special diet for asthmatics. He suggested a variety of fruits and vegetables (and highly recommended chicken soup). We have learned a great deal about how foods can affect asthma since then. Today we can often achieve dramatic results through a simple program of nutritional treatment.

If you suffer from recurrent attacks of bronchial asthma, it is quite possible that you could experience a dramatic improvement simply by changing your diet. One group of 25 asthmatics, for example, avoided meat, fish, eggs, dairy products, apples, citrus, soybeans, peas, coffee, ordinary tea, chocolate, sugar, salt, and tap water. In addition, they restricted potatoes and either severely restricted or eliminated all grains from their diets. Within 4 months, 71 percent of them had improved; by the end of one year on the diet, almost all of them (92 percent) had improved.[1]

34

Similarly spectacular results were reported by Dutch researchers. One hundred and eighteen asthmatics, most of whom had no known history of food sensitivity, were given various foods to eat. Most experienced worsening of their symptoms sometime between 20 minutes and 56 hours after ingesting a particular food. All but 8 of the 118 experienced a distinct decrease in asthmatic symptoms after avoiding test-positive foods for 6 to 12 months.[2]

In another study, 21 hospitalized, severe asthmatics with symptoms that occurred all year long were put on a liquid diet that was almost entirely free of food antigens (the components of food that can cause symptoms), while 17 similar patients drank a liquid consisting of the regular hospital diet blended to have a similar taste and texture as the experimental diet. Both groups also received their doctors' usual medical treatment during the study.

After only two weeks, there were major differences between the two groups. Nine of the 21 asthmatics on the antigen-free diet improved—3 of them dramatically—and none of them got worse. In the other group, only 1 of the 17 improved, while 5 got worse. The researchers were so impressed by their findings that they suggested that similar patients try an antigen-free diet, even if they have little or no evidence of allergies. You can't help but wonder how much better the experimental group might have done if the diet had been continued longer.[3]

It would be a mistake to conclude from such studies that food reactions are responsible for most asthma attacks. Other studies have found food sensitivity in asthmatics to be less common, and there is evidence that both parents and physicians sometimes overdiagnose food reactions in asthmatics.[4]

Whether or not your asthma is brought on by allergies, you should minimize the amount of salt in your diet. Asthma is set off by the release of *histamine,* a substance produced by the body which, when released by cells, can cause allergic reactions. It has been found that the greater the intake of dietary salt, the more reactive bronchial tubes are to histamine. In one study, for example, ten asthmatics were asked to double their salt intake. After one month, nine of the ten showed increased bronchial reactivity to histamine.[5,6]

THE HEALING DIET

1. Avoid foods found on testing to provoke attacks of asthma. *See Appendix B for information about diagnosing food sensitivities.*
2. Minimize salt consumption.

NUTRITIONAL HEALING PLANS

Vitamins

Vitamin B₆

Levels of vitamin B_6 have been found to be lower in the blood of asthmatics than in nonasthmatics. When 76 asthmatic children took 200 mg of vitamin B_6 daily, their symptoms improved, and their doctors were able to reduce the dosages of bronchodilators and steroids. Similarly, when 7 adult asthmatics were given 50 mg of vitamin B_6 twice daily, they all experienced a dramatic decrease in the frequency, duration, and severity of their asthmatic attacks, and their wheezing stopped after 1 week.[7,8,9]

NUTRITIONAL HEALING PLAN: Vitamin B₆

Preparation

pyridoxine

Dosage: 50 mg twice daily

Instructions: Take with vitamin B complex "50." (Vitamin B complex "50" is a mixture of members of the vitamin B complex containing either 50 mg or 50 mcg of each of the B vitamins.)

WARNING

If this dosage of pyridoxine is taken over many months, there may be a very slight chance of developing symptoms of nerve damage in the hands and feet, such as numbness, "pins and needles," and weakness.

Vitamin B₁₂

When given as intramuscular injections in large doses, vitamin B_{12} also seems to reduce asthmatic symptoms. Of a group of roughly 50 asthmatic children under age 10, about 60 percent stopped wheezing entirely following an intensive course of B_{12} injections, 20 to 30 percent had substantial relief, and only 10 percent had fair to poor results.[10]

A recent study suggests that vitamin B_{12} may be especially helpful to the many people (perhaps as many as 1 in 500) who develop asthma after eating food treated with sulfites. When the vitamin was given to sulfite-sensitive asthmatics before they were exposed to sulfites, it proved to be even more effective than drugs in blocking asthmatic reactions, and its effects lasted longer.[11]

The following case illustrates the benefits of vitamin B_{12} for asthma.

When Dr. Jonathan Wright first saw Rory at age three, he was receiving maximum doses of bronchodilators and inhalers, yet his asthma was getting worse. Prednisone controlled his wheezing but made him swell up. Dr. Wright initially started him on daily injections of vitamin B$_{12}$. After two injections, Rory was breathing more easily. Within two weeks, his wheezing was so much less that his parents stopped his inhaler. After three weeks, they stopped his bronchodilator. When Dr. Wright saw Rory after one month, he was doing "just fine," and the doctor lessened the frequency of the injections. He also began treating Rory for food sensitivities and a low level of stomach acid.

During the next nine years, Rory wheezed only one other time—at age five, when his vitamin B$_{12}$ injections probably had been reduced too much and his foods were not being adequately restricted. He was prescribed bronchodilators again for a short time, and he recovered quickly with the resumption of daily B$_{12}$ shots and strict dietary control. His stomach acid levels were normal when he was tested at age nine, and the infrequent B$_{12}$ injections were stopped. On follow-up at age 12, Rory was fine. [12]

NUTRITIONAL HEALING PLAN: Vitamin B$_{12}$

Consult your doctor about giving you a trial of vitamin B$_{12}$ injections.

Vitamin C

Asthmatics may have reduced levels of vitamin C in their blood.[13] Moreover, the lower the amount of vitamin C in the diet and the lower the amount of the vitamin in the blood serum, the more likely it is that you suffer from wheezing.[14]

Supplementation with vitamin C has been found to reduce asthmatic attacks. In one study, for example, asthmatics receiving 1 gram of vitamin C daily had fewer than one-fourth as many asthmatic attacks as those receiving placebo.[15] Vitamin C has also been shown under scientific (double-blind) conditions to protect people from asthma attacks who tend to have attacks when exercising.[16]

Though we don't yet know why vitamin C is effective, it may work by lowering the level of histamine in the blood. Histamine is a substance the body produces which, when released from mast cells, can cause allergic reactions, including asthma. Many or perhaps most asthmatics have lower blood levels of vitamin C than normal. Among people with low levels of vitamin C, the lower the vitamin C level, the higher the histamine level; when they take vitamin C, their histamine levels fall. In fact, even when vitamin C is not low, but histamine levels are high, vitamin C supplementation will cause histamine levels to fall.[17]

NUTRITIONAL HEALING PLAN: Vitamin C

Dosage: 1 g twice daily

Magnesium

Magnesium is the magic mineral for asthmatics. Its blood level may be reduced in one out of four asthmatics and in one out of two asthmatics during an attack.[18] When given by inhalation[19] or injection,[20] it has proven beneficial in stopping asthmatic attacks and improving lung function. Unfortunately, the efficacy of oral magnesium supplements remains unexplored although, since reduced blood levels are so common, it could well be of some value.

NUTRITIONAL HEALING PLAN: Magnesium

Dosage: 500 mg daily

Hydrochloric Acid Deficiency

One reason why so many asthmatics are food sensitive was discovered over half a century ago. In 1931, Dr. George Bray studied the secretion of hydrochloric acid by the stomach in 200 asthmatic children and compared it to that of children without asthma. Four out of five asthmatic children had reduced levels of stomach acid compared to only one out of ten of the non-asthmatic children. When the asthmatic children with low stomach acid levels were given special hydrochloric acid supplements before or during meals—while they continued to avoid foods to which they were sensitive—they had immediate improvements in appetite, weight, sleep, and asthmatic attacks—which became less severe and shorter in duration.[21]

> **NUTRITIONAL HEALING PLAN: Hydrochloric Acid (HCl)
> Deficiency**
>
> *Preparation:* betaine or glutamic HCl 10 grain capsules
> *Directions:* 1 to 5 capsules as tolerated immediately after
>   eating
> (Before starting, see Appendix C for instructions.)

TRYPTOPHAN: A WARNING

Tryptophan, an essential amino acid, should *not* be used as a nutritional supplement by asthmatics as it is the precursor of serotonin, a neurotransmitter known to cause bronchoconstriction in asthmatics. In one study,[22] when tryptophan was removed from a standard diet, asthmatics actually improved. (It is possible that vitamin B_6 supplementation is effective because it corrects the metabolic defect in tryptophan metabolism commonly found in asthmatics, who often have high levels of serotonin in both blood and saliva.)

COMBINATION TREATMENT

Nutritional healing plans can, of course, be used in combination. Dr. Alan Gaby reports that acute asthma attacks may resolve within a few minutes following an injection of niacinamide, pantothenic acid, vitamin B_6, vitamin B_{12}, vitamin C, calcium, magnesium, and niacinamide.[23] He also reports excellent long-term results from combining nutritional supplementation with the avoidance of inciting foods:

> *In a single year, a young asthmatic boy, who was five when treatment was started, had visited an emergency room twenty times and had been hospitalized several times for asthma and twice for bronchial pneumonia. Dr. Gaby placed him on a food elimination diet and gave him daily supplements of pantothenic acid, vitamin B_6, vitamin C, calcium and magnesium.*
>
> *He quickly became symptom-free but would develop symptoms within hours after ingesting milk or wheat. After one year, he caught a cold which caused moderately severe wheezing and coughing. Dr. Gaby gave him an injection of vitamins, and his wheezing and coughing subsided within three minutes.[24]*

CHOOSING A PERSONAL PLAN

All asthmatics should minimize their salt intake. Since several studies have shown that food sensitivities are a cause of bronchial asthma, find out whether foods provoke their symptoms. If you do find that you are food-sensitive, investigate supplementation with betaine or glutamic HCl.

As to nutritional supplements, I would suggest trying vitamin B_6, vitamin C, and magnesium together along with a vitamin B complex tablet. For children, a series of vitamin B_{12} injections may well be worth a trial.

Breast Disease

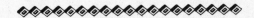

See also: CANCER, PREMENSTRUAL TENSION SYNDROME (PMS).

At least 20 percent of premenopausal women have noncancerous lumpy, tender breasts, most often as the result of fibrocystic breast disease. The condition may be stable, or it may worsen before the menstrual period. Though the disorder is usually not dangerous, some types of breast changes that cause these symptoms are precancerous and increase the risk of developing breast cancer.

DIETARY FACTORS

The more fat in your diet, the greater the risk of benign breast disease. When women with severe breast symptoms related to their menstrual cycles reduced dietary fat to only 15 percent of their caloric intake, breast tenderness, swelling, and lumpiness were reduced.[1]

In addition to a low-fat diet, avoidance of methylxanthines, which are found in coffee, chocolate, cola beverages, and some teas and drugs, may be beneficial. Though some women may notice a difference by simply reducing methylxanthines, others improve only if they completely avoid any food or beverage containing them.[2,3]

THE HEALING DIET

1. Follow the Low-Fat diet as described in Appendix A.
2. Avoid methylxanthines (caffeine and theobromine), which can be found in:

- ▸ regular coffee
- ▸ teas
- ▸ cola beverages
- ▸ chocolate
- ▸ pain relievers
- ▸ muscle relaxants
- ▸ "alertness" tablets
- ▸ diuretics
- ▸ cold/allergy remedies

NUTRITIONAL HEALING PLANS

Vitamins

Vitamin A

Only one pilot study of vitamin A supplementation has been reported, but the results appear promising. Twelve women with moderate to severe breast pain that had failed to respond to mild painkillers or caffeine withdrawal were supplemented with large doses of vitamin A. Ten reported reduced breast pain; in 5, breast masses decreased at least 50 percent. Eight months later, the responding women showed continued benefit.[4]

Because of the potential toxicity of large doses of vitamin A, it should be given only under close medical supervision and after other treatments have proven ineffective. In the one trial, two of the ten women who responded had to stop supplementation because of severe headaches, and three had mild side effects. If supplementation proves effective, an attempt should be made to reduce or eliminate it as soon as possible, since liver storage of the vitamin increases over time and increases the risk of toxic side effects.

NUTRITIONAL HEALING PLAN: Vitamin A

Dosage: 150,000 IU of vitamin A daily

WARNING

High doses of vitamin A may cause serious side effects and therefore should be taken only under the supervision of a knowledgeable physician.

Vitamin E

Studies investigating supplementation with vitamin E have had mixed results, with some showing impressive benefits and others reporting a lack of efficacy. The reason for such differing outcomes is unknown.[5,6,7,8,9]

The following case provides an example of the possible benefits of vitamin E supplementation:

> *A woman who had suffered from breast tenderness for 25 years found complete relief by taking 400 IU of vitamin E daily. Eliminating the supplement, or even reducing the dosage, resulted in return of the tenderness.*[10]

NUTRITIONAL HEALING PLAN: Vitamin E

Dosage: 600 IU of vitamin E daily

Trial Period

three months

Minerals: Iodine

When rats, especially older rats, are deficient in iodine, they develop breast lesions that, under the microscope, resemble human fibrocystic breast disease. The conditions under which iodine deficiency causes the disease in humans is unknown, although supplementation with **special forms** of iodine has been found effective for the treatment of the symptoms of fibrocystic breast disease in roughly 90 percent of women.[11]

WARNING

The iodine in your medicine cabinet is poisonous if swallowed.

If inorganic iodides (such as potassium iodide) are taken, the tissue changes within the breast, known as *fibrosis,* and the potential for cancerous changes remain. Aqueous iodine appears to be superior since it not only relieves pain within two to eight weeks, but also gradually resolves the fibrosis.[12] However, it may not be available.

Once inorganic iodide supplementation is effective, it should not be stopped. If it is discontinued, there is a 90 percent chance of symptoms returning within 9 months.[13] However, your doctor would need to monitor you to be sure that you do not develop iodine toxicity.

NUTRITIONAL HEALING PLAN: Iodine

Note: Only available by prescription. Dosages of two of the preparations your doctor may choose are given as examples.

Preparation

potassium iodide

Dosage: 1 drop daily

Preparation

aqueous (diatomic) iodine

Dosage: 3 to 6 milligrams daily

Other Nutritional Factors

Omega-6 Fatty Acids

Supplementation with evening primrose oil, a good source of omega-6 fatty acids, has been reported to be effective for the relief of breast pain, whether or not the women have breast lumps. Results are better in women whose pain and tenderness are related to their menstrual cycle.[14,15]

NUTRITIONAL HEALING PLAN: Omega-6 Fatty Acids

Preparation

evening primrose oil

Dosage: 1 g 3 times daily

Trial Period

three months

CHOOSING A PERSONAL PLAN

Every woman with benign breast disease should be on a low-fat diet, and avoidance of methylxanthines is certainly worth a trial. As for the Nutritional Healing plans, none of them is well proven. I suggest combining the Healing diet with supplements of evening primose oil (omega-6 fatty acids) and vitamin E. If, after three months your problem persists, see a physician trained in nutritional medicine who can help you with trials of vitamin A and/or iodine.

The following case provides an example of the benefits of nutritional supplementation for breast disease:

A 26-year-old woman began to note a slight premenstrual lumpiness in her breasts while in college. A mammogram showed benign cysts. Two years prior to her evaluation, her symptoms gradually worsened until the cysts remained throughout her cycle; although the cysts were somewhat reduced after her periods, her breasts were sore and tender for one week before her period. Her diet included several cups of coffee daily.

Premenstrual examination revealed numerous small, tender breast cysts throughout both breasts, in addition to dry skin, dandruff, excess earwax, and white spots on her fingernails. She was told to avoid methylxanthines and to improve her diet, and was given supplements of evening primrose oil, vitamin E, zinc gluconate, iodine, a vitamin B complex, and vitamin C. Six months later, she reported that the large majority of the cysts had disappeared in the first 90 days after starting treatment, and that she was no longer having problems with breast cysts.[16]

One final thought: Ginseng may aggravate the symptoms and should not be taken. This popular Chinese herb has been found to cause breast pain and soreness in some women, probably because it contains small quantities of estrogenic female hormones.[17,18]

Cancer

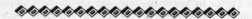

See also: Breast Disease, Cervical Dysplasia.

Cancer refers to tumors whose growth and dissemination within the body is uncontrolled. It is the second most common killer disease; one out of three people will be diagnosed with it in their lifetimes. Roughly half of all cancers are believed to be associated with nutritional factors, especially breast and uterine cancer in women, prostate cancer in men, and gastrointestinal cancer.

DIETARY FACTORS

Fat intake, more often than any other dietary factor, has been repeatedly found to be related to the risk of cancer, and some of the studies suggest that the amount of saturated fat in your diet may be particularly important. Similarly, the higher the intake of cholesterol in your diet, the higher your risk of cancer.[1,2]

Conversely, the higher your intake of dietary fiber, the lower your risk of breast cancer, perhaps because fiber increases the removal of estrogen (a female hormone) through the feces. Fiber intake also lowers the risk of colon cancer, perhaps because it reduces the concentration of cancer-causing agents in the gut, or because it encourages the production of beneficial substances. When added to the diet of people who are genetically prone to develop rectal polyps (which may be precancerous), it inhibits the polyps from developing.[3,4,5]

The consumption of dark green and yellow-orange vegetables (those high in beta-carotene) has been found to reduce cancer risk, as has the consumption of tomatoes and strawberries.[6]

It is not surprising that a vegetarian diet—which is low in fat and high in both fiber and carotenoids—is associated with a reduced risk of breast, colon, and stomach cancer. Vegetables also provide *phytosterols,* which are plant substances that have a structure much like cholesterol and protect against experimental colon cancers in animals. Also, at least in regard to the risk of colon cancer, the amount of cholesterol you eat may not be as important as the ratio of dietary cholesterol to dietary phytosterols.[7,8,9]

Sugar intake has been shown to increase the death rate from breast cancer in animals. In humans, a high sugar intake increases the risk of breast cancer as well as the risk of colorectal cancer. When healthy people were given additional sugar in their diets, intestinal transit time decreased while the amount of fecal bile acids increased—changes that are associated with an increased risk of colorectal cancer.[10,11,12,13]

Alcohol intake, even when modest, is associated with an increased risk of breast cancer, and there is limited evidence of an association with other cancers as well. Smoked, pickled, and salt-cured foods contain nitrosamines and polycyclic aromatic hydrocarbons, which are not only *carcinogenic* (cancer-producing) in animals but are also linked statistically with human esophageal and stomach cancers.[14,15]

Because of conflicting results, numerous studies have failed to clarify the relationship between coffee consumption and cancer risk. In animal studies, caffeine can either increase or decrease cancer cell development depending upon the carcinogen it is used with, the type of host cell, and the stage of the cell cycle in which it is introduced.[16]

Even the hardness of your drinking water affects your risk of getting cancer. Because soft water is so acidic, cadmium and other toxic elements may be leached from pipes in soft water areas, causing them to appear in higher levels in the drinking water. Water hardness is usually due to dissolved calcium and magnesium. In hard water areas, not only are there lower levels of toxic elements in the drinking water but, due to competition from calcium and magnesium ions, the absorption of toxic elements in the intestines is reduced. The harder your drinking water, the lower your risk of getting cancers of the digestive tract.[17,18]

Drinking water is commonly chlorinated to kill any germs it may contain, but chlorination may not be entirely without risk. A study found that the longer people drank chlorinated water, the greater their risk of getting bladder cancer. This finding is consistent with the results of other studies, which found that chlorine disinfection produces toxic by-products. It suggests that safe sources of nonchlorinated drinking water are preferable to water that has been disinfected with chlorine.[19]

THE HEALING DIET

There is no evidence that dietary factors influence the course of human cancer once it is established. There is considerable evidence, however, that dietary factors affect cancer risk. Since treating an established cancer is quite a different matter than preventing cancer from developing in normal tissue, it is questionable whether there is truly a Healing diet for cancer. Nevertheless, I suggest the following diet because it is safe, beneficial to your overall health, and someday may be found to have healing properties.

1. Follow the Basic Healing diet as described in Appendix A.
2. Emphasize fruits and vegetables.
3. Drink hard water that does not require chlorinization for disinfection.

NUTRITIONAL HEALING PLANS

Most research on the relationship between nutritional factors and cancer has concerned cancer prevention. Several nutritional factors have been shown to affect the risk of developing cancer, and we are starting to identify nutrients that can reverse precancerous changes. Compared to our knowledge about the value of nutrition in preventing cancer, we know very little about healing established cancer through nutrition.

Cancer and cancer chemotherapy cause nutritional deficiencies, which should be monitored by your physician and, if possible, corrected. Moreover, certain nutritional factors can reduce the often serious adverse side effects of chemotherapy and radiation.

In recent years, pilot studies suggested that certain nutritional factors, sometimes alone and sometimes combined with conventional treatments, have the potential of favorably influencing the course of certain cancers. However, as the potential of these nutritional cancer treatments needs to be studied further, and because the decision to use them should be made with your physician, Nutritional Healing plans for these specific treatments are not presented.

Vitamins

Folic Acid (Folate)

Women with untreated cervical cancer have reduced levels of folate (another name for folic acid) in their blood. However, this association does not tell us whether low folate levels promote the cancer or low folate levels are a result of the cancer. In any case, localized deficiency of folic acid in the lining of the uterine cervix is associated with the development of *cervical dysplasia* (abnormal tissue changes in the cervix), which can progress to cervical cancer. Women on oral contraceptives are especially vulnerable. (For more detailed information, see *Cervical Dysplasia*.)[20]

Oral folate supplementation is sometimes effective for reversing cervical dysplastic changes associated with localized cervical folate deficiency and may thus prevent the progression to cervical cancer. It may also reverse the abnormal cell changes in another precancerous condition, bronchial squamous metaplasia, which is mainly seen in cigarette smokers.[21,22]

NUTRITIONAL HEALING PLAN: Folic Acid

Suggested Use

reverse precancerous conditions (cervical dysplasia; bronchial squamous metaplasia)

Dosage: 10 mg of folic acid daily

WARNING

This high a dose of folic acid should be taken under a doctor's supervision.

Niacin (Vitamin B₃)

Niacin (Vitamin B_3)

Though there is no evidence that niacin supplementation is beneficial in the prevention or treatment of cancer, it may reduce the adverse effects of chemotherapy. Adriamycin is a popular chemotherapeutic agent that has toxic effects on the heart. When mice were given adriamycin, niacin supplementation reduced the drug's toxicity to the heart without interfering with its antitumor effect. Additional studies will show whether niacin is also effective in humans, and whether it is effective for other toxic effects of chemotherapy.[23]

Niacin and aspirin have both been shown to reduce the tendency toward clotting within blood vessels. In the hope that their combined administration would increase survival in cancer patients treated with radiation therapy (perhaps by improving the circulation), half of a group of people who were receiving a combination of surgery and gamma-ray radiation for advanced bladder cancer also received niacin and aspirin. After five years, people receiving the niacin and aspirin combination had a much lower relapse rate and a much higher survival rate. More studies are needed to discover whether this combination is equally effective for other cancers treated with radiation.[24]

NUTRITIONAL HEALING PLAN: Niacin

To Minimize the Toxicity of Chemotherapy
Dosage: not well established, but 500 mg of niacin 3 times daily would be reasonable

To Minimize Injury from Gamma-Ray Radiation
Dosage: 500–1000 mg of niacin 3 times daily
Instructions: Take with 500 mg of aspirin daily.

WARNING
Because of possible adverse side effects, high-dose niacin supplementation should be taken only under medical supervision.

Vitamin A and the Retinoids

Vitamin A, which the body can derive from the plant version of vitamin A known as *beta-carotene,* has repeatedly been shown in laboratory studies to have potent anticancer effects. However, at doses that humans can tolerate, the vitamin has shown only limited anticancer activity; therefore synthetic derivatives (*retinoids*) that can be better tolerated are being developed. The retinoids have been shown to stimulate definite anticancer activity in a number of precancerous tumors as well as in certain cancers that were unresponsive to chemotherapy.[25]

One double-blind study investigated the effects of weekly doses of vitamin A and beta-carotene on members of the Philippine Ifugao tribe, who chew *betel quid,* a tobacco-like plant mixture that promotes cellular damage. After 9 weeks, the percentage of cells from inside the cheek that had genetic damage decreased from 4 to 2 percent in the vitamin A group, and from 3.5 to 1 percent in the beta-carotene group.[26]

Since the retinoids are prescription drugs and beta-carotene is much safer as a source of supplemental A than vitamin A itself, supplementation with vitamin A is indicated only when doctors need to provide very high supplementary levels for specific treatment purposes.

Vitamin B$_6$

Since the body requires vitamin B$_6$ to make thymidine, a deficiency of which can increase the natural tendency of occasional cells to become abnormal, a deficiency of B$_6$ could theoretically make us more prone to developing cancer. Indeed, mice that are B$_6$-deficient and are exposed to a carcinogenic virus are more susceptible to developing tumors, and the tumors they develop are larger in size. Cancer patients often have low blood levels of vitamin B_6, but it is not known whether this finding is a cause or an effect of the cancer.[27,28,29]

A vitamin B_6 deficiency is not uncommon in Western diets, so it may be protective to take 25 mg daily of vitamin B_6, which is available as pyridoxine, as a supplement, even though it would be best to ensure that you are getting adequate vitamin B_6 from the foods in your diet. *(See Appendix D for food sources of vitamin B_6.)*

Vitamin C

The more vitamin C in your diet, and the higher your blood level of the vitamin, the lower your risk of getting a wide variety of cancers. This vitamin can protect against the development of stomach cancer by blocking the formation of cancer-causing nitrosamines, and supplementation with vitamin C may enhance the beneficial effects of both chemotherapy and radiation treatment.[30,31,32,33]

Though pilot studies suggest that high-dose vitamin C supplementation (in the range of perhaps 3 g 4 times daily) may increase the survival time of terminal cancer patients, better evidence is needed before vitamin C therapy for established cancers will gain wide scientific acceptance. Marginal vitamin C deficiencies are so common in people eating Western diets that, if you can't be sure that you are getting the RDA of vitamin C *(see Appendix E)*, supplementation with 50 mg daily of vitamin C may be protective.[34,35] *(See Appendix D for food sources of vitamin C.)*

Vitamin D

The higher the blood levels of partially activated (25-hydroxy) vitamin D, the lower the risk of colon cancer, and early evidence suggests that supplementation with fully activated (1,25-dihydroxy) vitamin D may inhibit cancer cells from multiplying. Still uncertain is whether the vitamin is too toxic at effective doses to be useful and exactly which cancers it is capable of inhibiting.[36,37,38]

Vitamin E

The higher your blood level of vitamin E, the lower your cancer risk. Like vitamin C, supplementation blocks the formation of carcinogenic nitrosamines in the stomach. *Mutagens* are substances capable of changing the genetic structure of cells and therefore may contribute to the development of cancer; supplementation with vitamin E dramatically reduces their level in the stool. When animals were exposed to agents capable of causing cancer, vitamin E prevented liver and breast cancers, and caused skin cancers to shrink.[39,40,41,42,43,44]

Vitamin E also appears to reduce the toxicity of at least some anticancer drugs. In one study, 69 percent of people receiving vitamin E who were treated with the popular chemotherapeutic drug adriamycin had no hair loss; those who experienced hair loss received the vitamin too late for it to be effective. To be effective, vitamin E must be started one week before chemotherapy is begun.[45]

NUTRITIONAL HEALING PLAN: Vitamin E

Suggested Use

minimize the toxicity of chemotherapy

Preparation

dl-alpha-tocopherol acetate

Dosage: 1600 IU daily

WARNING

High-dose vitamin E should be taken under a doctor's supervision.

Minerals

Calcium

Calcium helps to regulate the proliferation of cells in the lining, or *mucosa,* of the colon. The higher your calcium intake, the lower your risk of colon cancer. In one study, ten people whose rectal mucosal cells were rapidly proliferating—just like the cells of people with familial colon cancer— were given calcium supplements. After two to three months, the abnormal pattern was largely replaced by patterns found in people at low risk for colon cancer.[46,47]

Although it is questionable whether calcium alone will inhibit tumor growth once cancer has developed, a Russian study reported that a calcium salt enhanced the efficacy of radiation therapy for treating tumors of the bones and vulva, while other calcium salts combined with vitamin D enhanced the efficacy of chemotherapy for treating Hodgkin's disease and lung cancer.[48]

NUTRITIONAL HEALING PLAN: Calcium

Suggested Use

reduce an elevated risk of colon cancer

Preparation

calcium citrate

Dosage: 1.5 g daily

Note: As a test of its availability for absorption from the gut, a calcium tablet should dissolve within 30 minutes after being placed in a dish of vinegar.

Magnesium

The higher the magnesium levels in your food, the lower your risk of cancer. In studies with experimental cancer in animals, magnesium-deficient diets increased cancer development, while excess dietary magnesium reduced it.[49]

There is no evidence that magnesium supplementation is effective for treating cancer. However, you should be sure to get enough magnesium in your diet to minimize your cancer risk. (Whole grains and green vegetables are good sources of magnesium.) The alternative for the sizable percentage of people eating Western diets, which are well below the RDA for magnesium, is to take a daily supplement containing 400 mg of magnesium. *(See Appendix E for information about RDAs.)*

Selenium

Most evidence suggests that the higher your selenium intake, the lower your cancer risk. Both test tube studies and studies of experimental cancer in animals demonstrated that selenium supplementation may prevent the development of cancer.[50,51]

No human trials of selenium supplementation have been completed, so selenium supplementation is not an established cancer treatment. However, since marginal selenium deficiency is not uncommon, if you cannot be certain of getting adequate selenium in your diet (particularly if you live in an area where the level of selenium in the soil is very low), consider supplementation with 70 mcg of selenium daily to reduce your cancer risk.

Zinc

Of all the trace elements, the amount of zinc in the diet is most strongly linked to the risk of developing esophageal cancer. Also, people with esophageal cancer have reduced blood zinc levels, although we don't know if this is a cause or a result of the illness.[52,53]

In men with cancer of the prostate, zinc is reduced both in the prostate and in the prostatic secretions. Though this may be simply due to the cancer, it is equally possible that zinc protects against prostate cancer.[54]

We know that zinc protects us from the toxic effects of the metal cadmium, which has been shown to stimulate the growth of the prostate at low concentration. Compared to other groups, men with the most malignant form of prostate cancer have the highest cadmium levels and the lowest zinc levels.[55,56]

Since zinc is often inadequate in Western diets, you can decrease your cancer risk by ensuring that you consume the RDA of zinc (12 mg daily for women; 15 mg daily for men). If this is not possible, take a daily zinc supplement containing 15 mg of zinc.

Other Nutritional Factors

Alkylglycerols

Shark liver oil is richer in alkylglycerols than any substance in our bodies outside of bone marrow and breast milk. When alkylglycerols are given prior to, during, and after radiation therapy for the treatment of uterine cancer, radiation injuries have been reduced by as much as two-thirds. Furthermore, when they are given prior to radiation therapy for uterine cancer, alkylglycerols have been shown to enhance the success of the treatment.[57,58]

NUTRITIONAL HEALING PLAN: Alkylglycerols

Suggested Use

minimize injury from radiation therapy

Preparation

shark liver oil concentrate (85 percent free alkylglycerols)

Dosage: 200 mg 3 times daily

Instructions: Start seven days prior to radiation therapy. Continue during radiation therapy and for one to three months afterward.

Beta-Carotene

Beta-carotene is a precursor to vitamin A. The higher your dietary intake of beta-carotene, the lower your risk of lung and certain other cancers. Though serum beta-carotene levels are often lower in cancer patients (even prior to diagnosis) than in healthy people in control groups, this finding could result from malnourishment rather than from the cancer.[59,60]

Experimental studies have found that beta-carotene protects animals from developing some types of experimental tumors. As for human cancer, the Inuits of northwestern Canada were selected for a pilot study because they use smokeless tobacco (which makes them more susceptible to mouth cancer) and also have low beta-carotene levels. To discover whether beta-carotene could reverse the cell damage that may precede the development of mouth cancer, researchers measured how often cells from inside the mouth contained micronuclei. After the Inuits had taken beta-carotene supplements for ten weeks, cells containing micronuclei were significantly less common, providing evidence that beta-carotene may have a protective effect against the development of cancer.[61,62]

To reduce the risk of cancer, make sure there is adequate beta-carotene in your diet by eating plenty of dark green and orange-yellow vegetables. *(See Appendix D for a list of foods rich in beta-carotene.)*

Butyric Acid

Butyric acid is a fatty acid produced by the normal bacteria of the human colon. It serves as a major energy source for the lining of the colon and rectum. When dietary fiber reaches the colon and is exposed to colonic bacteria, butyric acid is the major substance produced.

Test tube studies have shown that exposure to butyric acid may cause cancer cells to transform into more normal-appearing cells; thus it may be an important protector against cancer. Earlier we discussed the importance of dietary fiber in preventing colon cancer. Perhaps one way in which dietary fiber inhibits the development of colon cancer is by encouraging butyric acid production. Whether supplementation with butyric acid is effective for treating colon cancer remains to be investigated.[63,64]

Cartilage Anti-Angiogenesis Factor

For a cancer to develop, new blood vessels must form that lead to the cancer and travel within it, providing the necessary nourishment for its cells to live and multiply. A substance that inhibits the development of these new blood vessels (an *anti-angiogenesis* substance) might be able to combat the cancer. Such a factor has been discovered in animal cartilage and has been derived from the cartilage of cows and, more recently, sharks.[65,66]

Catrix, a substance derived from the tracheal cartilage of cows, was found effective in the test tube against various cancers at concentrations safe for humans. When tested on people with cancer, the dosage of eight 375 mg capsules of Catrix every 8 hours appeared to treat a variety of cancers both safely and effectively. Several years after starting treatment with Catrix, 90 percent of a group of 31 people improved, and 61 percent of their cancers went into complete remission. Diseases that apparently responded to treatment included glioblastoma multiforme (a rapidly growing, inoperable brain tumor); cancers of the cervix, lungs, ovary, pancreas, prostate, rectum, and thyroid; and inoperable squamous cancer of the nose.[67,68]

The following case illustrates the benefits of Catrix supplementation:

A 69-year-old jaundiced woman was found to have a carcinoma of the head of the pancreas, with lymph node involvement. Surgery was performed, but the surgeon could not remove the entire cancer. The patient refused chemotherapy and was started instead on treatment with Catrix.

Between four and eight months after starting treatment, the level of alkaline phosphatase in her blood increased sharply to ten times normal, suggesting that growth of the cancer had begun to block the flow of bile from the liver. Then the level began to decline. After 26 months, the level had returned to normal. The patient's weight increased steadily from 106 pounds at the onset of treatment, to 136 pounds 2 years later, and subsequently remained steady. Eight years after starting treatment, her physical exam and blood chemistries were normal and she felt well.[69]

Since the angiogenesis-inhibiting factor is one thousand times more concentrated in shark cartilage than in calf cartilage, shark cartilage may prove to be a better source. The results of clinical trials with shark cartilage, however, have not yet been published.[70]

Coenzyme Q_{10}

Coenzyme Q_{10} is a naturally occurring molecule that plays an important role in the production of energy from food. Its administration may reduce the toxic effects of adriamycin, a popular chemotherapeutic drug. Specifically, it may protect the cardiovascular system and reduce hair loss.[71]

NUTRITIONAL HEALING PLAN: Coenzyme Q_{10}

Suggested Use

minimize the toxicity of chemotherapy

Dosage: 30 mg of coenzyme Q_{10} daily

Omega-3 Fatty Acids: Fish Oils

Studies in which animals were exposed to cancer-causing agents as well as test tube studies suggest that fish oils that are high in *eicosapentaenoic acid* (EPA), an omega-3 fatty acid, may reduce the risk of cancer. It is too early, however, to reach a verdict about this nutrient, as it has yet to be studied in humans for this purpose.[72,73]

Omega-6 Fatty Acids: Gamma-Linolenic Acid (GLA)

The omega-6 family of essential fatty acids are derived from linoleic acid. So far, studies of linoleic acid and cancer have had mixed results; some have found it to have an inhibitory effect, while others have found it to promote cancer.[74,75]

By contrast, the evidence is growing that administration of gamma-linolenic acid (GLA), which can be derived from linoleic acid, may inhibit cancer development. In one study of 21 patients with untreatable cancers, administration of six to twelve 500 mg capsules of evening primrose oil, a rich source of GLA, 3 times daily produced marked improvement in the way patients felt, and some of the patients demonstrated objective improvement. Also, administration of evening primrose oil combined with vitamin C doubled the mean survival time for 11 patients with primary hepatic carcinoma (liver cancer).[76,77]

Not all trials have been successful, however, In one study, 54 patients with colorectal cancer failed to benefit. More studies are needed before the therapeutic value of GLA supplementation in cancer can be established. In the meantime, it may be worthwhile to add GLA to conventional treatments because of its lack of toxicity.[78]

Botanical Extracts

Bromelain

Results of a number of studies suggest that the administration of *bromelain,* which is derived from the stem of the pineapple plant, may inhibit the development of cancer. It has caused human leukemic cells to transform to more normal-appearing cells. When cancer was induced in mice, the administration of bromelain decreased the development of lung metastases (the spread of cancer to the lung). Whether it will prove effective in treating human cancer is unknown.[79,80]

Garlic and Onions

Garlic (*Allium sativum*) and onions, (*Allium cepa*) closely related herbs, may have a beneficial effect against cancer. One study found that the residents of a certain county in China who regularly eat up to 20 g of garlic daily have the lowest *gastric* or stomach cancer death rate in the country, whereas the residents of another county who rarely eat garlic have the highest death rate. In another study, when healthy volunteers ate the equivalent of two bulbs of garlic daily for three weeks, their natural killer cells, which are important to the body's defense against cancer, killed many more cancer cells. Also, studies in which cancer was induced in animals have found beneficial effects from both garlic and onions. Human trials with cancer patients are needed to prove whether garlic or onions can influence the course of human cancer.[81,82,83]

Lentinan

The substance *lentinan* comes from the shiitake mushroom, the most popular edible mushroom in Japan. Several studies have demonstrated its efficacy as an adjunct to chemotherapy for patients with advanced or recurrent gastric and colorectal cancers. It has also been proven to be beneficial, when combined with surgical removal of the ovaries and the adrenal glands, for patients with advanced or recurrent breast cancers.[84,85]

Beneficial Bacteria: Lactobacillus Acidophilus

The high-fat, low-fiber Western diet causes alterations in the enzyme activity of stool bacteria, which encourages the development of colon cancer. *Lactobacillus acidophilus,* a bacterium that is a normal inhabitant of the human colon, has been shown to normalize bacterial enzyme activity. Moreover, it breaks down cancer-causing nitrites and nitrosamines into harmless substances. Because of these actions, it should be effective in reducing the risk of colon cancer.[86]

NUTRITIONAL HEALING PLAN: Lactobacillus Acidophilus

Suggested Use

reduce the risk of colon cancer

Dosage: depends on the specific preparation

Examples: one glass of acidophilus milk, or one cup of acidophilus yogurt, once or twice daily

Note: To be effective, yogurt must contain viable (living) acidophilus cultures. (Many commercial yogurts do not contain acidophilus.)

CHOOSING A PERSONAL PLAN

Though nutritional measures that inhibit the development of an illness are often effective in affecting the course of an established illness, cancer is a

CHOOSING A NUTRITIONAL HEALING PLAN FOR CANCER

To Aid in the Treatment of Cancer
        vitamin A
        vitamin C
        vitamin D
        vitamin E
        calcium
        bromelain
        butyric acid
        cartilage anti-angiogenesis factor
        evening primrose oil (gamma linolenic acid)
        lentinan
        shark liver oil (alkylglycerols)

To Reverse a Precancerous Condition
        beta-carotene
        folic acid

To Minimize the Toxicity of Chemotherapy
        niacin
        vitamin E
        coenzyme Q_{10}

To Minimize Internal Injury from Radiation Therapy
        niacin
        shark liver oil (alkylglycerols)

To Minimize Cancer Risk
        beta-carotene
        calcium
        garlic and onions
        Lactobacillus acidophilus

        AVOID DEFICIENCIES OF:
        folic acid
        vitamin A
        vitamin B_6
        vitamin C
        vitamin E
        calcium
        magnesium
        selenium
        zinc

more complicated situation. Nutrition clearly exerts a powerful influence on the events that cause normal tissue to become cancerous. However, once a cancer has developed, the body has lost control of major regulatory mechanisms, which cannot be easily re-established. In other words, nutritional interventions that may be quite powerful in preventing cancer may prove to be entirely ineffective for fighting cancer.

Even so, as long as they have not been proven ineffective, safe nutritional practices may be worth adding to standard treatments for whatever benefit they may provide. This is certainly true of the Basic Healing diet. I have suggested a diet that, based on our current knowledge, appears to be the most effective dietary program to prevent cancer. Though we do not know how effective it is in changing the course of an established cancer, it will strengthen the body's ability to counterattack and therefore is worth following.

Generally, the efficacy of the Nutritional Healing plans for cancer is also poorly documented and should be supervised by your physician. Your consideration of any of them depends upon your goal, as shown in the chart on the previous page.

Canker Sores

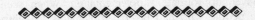

The most common ulcerative disease of the soft tissues of the mouth, canker sores (aphthous stomatitis) are localized, painful, relapsing ulcerations. They most frequently occur on the mucosal lining inside the cheek but can involve any area of the *oral mucosa* (the wet, pink tissue inside the mouth), including the tongue.

DIETARY FACTORS

Though many observers report an apparent relationship between eating certain foods and the development of canker sores, there is very little scientific documentation of this association. One intriguing double-blind study tested the white blood cells of 60 people with recurrent canker sores to discover which foods caused them to release histamine. When those foods were eliminated, 30 percent of the group had fewer canker sores. When foods that had been eliminated were returned to their diets, 30 percent of those foods caused canker sores to increase.[1]

THE HEALING DIET

Avoid foods found on testing to provoke canker sores. *See Appendix B for information about diagnosing food sensitivities.*

NUTRITIONAL HEALING PLANS

Deficiencies of Nutrients

A minority of people suffering from recurrent canker sores are deficient in folic acid, vitamin B_{12}, or iron. For example, 18 percent of a group of 130 people were found to be deficient in 2 or more of these nutrients and were given appropriate supplementation. When seen after one year, all the people who had taken supplements had improved, and two-thirds had had a complete remission, while only one-third of the people who had normal levels of folic acid, vitamin B_{12}, and iron had improved.[2]

Consult a nutritionally trained physician for guidance in diagnosing and treating these deficiencies. Because all three deficiencies are common causes of anemia, a complete blood count should also be performed, in addition to specific tests for folic acid, vitamin B_{12}, and iron. In addition, there are physical signs—soreness of the tongue (glossitis) or painful cracks at the corners of the month (cheilitis)—that make it more likely a nutritional deficiency exists. The following case illustrates the improvement of canker sores with the correction of a deficiency:

> *A woman had repeated episodes of canker sores along with glossitis. She was found to be absorbing less than 1 percent of her dietary intake of vitamin B_{12}, her serum level of the vitamin was well below the normal range, and she was anemic. Injections of vitamin B_{12} produced immediate improvements, with complete and lasting remission of the canker sores, glossitis, and anemia.[3]*

Minerals: Zinc

In pilot studies, zinc supplementation appears to be an effective treatment for canker sores. Laboratory testing of zinc levels may be helpful, but it is unclear whether zinc is effective only when its level in the body is low. For example, when a group of 17 patients were given zinc supplements, all 9 patients with lower serum zinc levels improved, compared to only 3 of the 8 patients with higher zinc levels.[4,5]

NUTRITIONAL HEALING PLAN: Zinc

Dosage: 100 mg of zinc daily

Other Nutritional Factors

Licorice Root

Several studies have shown that licorice root speeds the healing of ulcerations in the lining of the gut. For the treatment of recurrent canker sores, a form of licorice root, used as a mouthwash, appeared to completely heal the canker sores of 15 out of a group of 20 people. They noted a 50 to 75 percent improvement within one day and complete healing of their ulcers by the third day.[6]

NUTRITIONAL HEALING PLAN: Licorice Root

Preparation

fluid extract
> *Instructions:* Use as a mouthwash three or more times daily.

Lactobacillus Acidophilus

Lactobacillus acidophilus is a healthy bacterium that commonly resides in the moist mucus membranes of the gut and vagina. Preliminary reports suggest that with or without *Lactobacillus bulgaricus* (a similar organism), it may be effective in treating canker sores. Acidophilus is applied locally to the ulcerations, then sometimes swallowed. Although a double-blind study failed to find evidence that acidophilus reduces the duration of healing, the subjects in that study were severely mentally retarded, so its effect on pain could not be evaluated.[7,8]

The following case illustrates the benefits of Lactobacillus for canker sores:

> *A 39-year-old woman continually developed canker sores following treatment with an antibiotic 2 years earlier. The sores failed to respond to any medication that her husband, a physician, was able to obtain. He finally decided to give her tablets containing Lactobacillus acidophilus and Lactobacillus bulgaricus, which she dissolved in her mouth along with milk four times a day. Her symptoms promptly disappeared.[9]*

NUTRITIONAL HEALING PLAN: Lactobacillus Acidophilus

Preparations

concentrated L. acidophilus liquid or tablets containing live cultures

Instructions: Four times daily, use the liquid as a mouthwash, or dissolve the tablets in the mouth along with milk.

CHOOSING A TREATMENT PLAN

Consider trying a food-elimination diet, especially if you have other symptoms that could be related to food sensitivities. If you are suspicious that you develop one or more canker sores within a day of eating a specific food, try avoiding that food.

The Nutritional Healing plans presented in this chapter are not scientifically proven. If, however, you are anemic and deficient in vitamin B_{12}, folic acid, or iron, the evidence suggests that your canker sores may respond to appropriate supplementation to correct your anemia.

Despite a lack of scientific proof of its efficacy, mouthwashes containing acidophilus are perfectly safe and therefore worth trying if the approaches suggested above are not helpful. Finally, if no other healing plan is effective, zinc supplementation is reasonably safe and can be tried for a few months.

Carpal Tunnel Syndrome

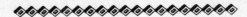

See also: MUSCLE CRAMPS.

A painful disorder of the wrist, *carpal tunnel syndrome* involves compression of the median nerve as it passes through the "tunnel" formed by the wrist bones. In addition to pain, weakness, and a feeling of "pins and needles" in the hand, the fingers may be stiff and difficult to bend. Sometimes there are associated symptoms in other parts of the body, such as fluctuating swelling of the feet or ankles, muscle spasms in the arms and legs at night, or pains in the elbows, shoulders, or knees.

NUTRITIONAL HEALING PLANS

Vitamins

Vitamin B₆ Deficiency

As a country doctor in Texas, John Ellis saw many people afflicted with carpal tunnel syndrome. In 1962, based on his clinical suspicions, he began giving injections of pyridoxine, a form of vitamin B_6, to patients with the disorder. The results were so dramatic that Dr. Ellis devoted himself to proving the efficacy of this vitamin ever since, publishing study after study to substantiate his belief and stimulating other researchers to follow his lead.

Since Dr. Ellis began his investigations, evidence confirming his suspicions has mounted. Blood tests have found that people with carpal tunnel syndrome may have a marginal deficiency of vitamin B_6, suggesting that supplementation is correcting a deficiency rather than working as a drug.

In addition to people reporting relief of their symptoms after vitamin B_6 supplementation, objective tests of median nerve function have documented that the compression of the median nerve is relieved.[1,2,3]

Perhaps the best group study to date involved 28 patients treated with pyridoxine hydrochloride. Based not only on physicians' judgments but also upon objective tests of median nerve function, all but 1 person were substantially improved after 5 to 18 weeks. By comparison, only 1 of 4 people treated with a placebo showed improvement 15 to 36 weeks later.[4]

The following case illustrates the improvement of carpal tunnel syndrome with the correction of a B_6 deficiency:

> *Blood studies done on a man with severe carpal tunnel syndrome showed evidence of a vitamin B_6 deficiency. He was started on 2 mg of pyridoxine daily. After 11 weeks, all but his marginal symptoms were relieved, but blood studies showed only a slight improvement. Pyridoxine was then increased to 100 mg daily. After 12 weeks, the patient's blood studies had become entirely normal.*
>
> *Without his knowledge, he was then switched to a placebo. Nine weeks later his symptoms had worsened, and the results of his blood tests once more suggested that he was vitamin B_6-deficient. He was switched back to 100 mg of pyridoxine daily. After 12 weeks, all his symptoms had disappeared and his blood studies had returned to normal.[5]*

NUTRITIONAL HEALING PLAN: Vitamin B_6 Deficiency

Preparation

pyridoxine

Dosage: 40 mg daily

Instructions: Combine with 400 mg of magnesium daily.

Trial Period

three months

Note: If the Nutritional Healing plan is ineffective, a higher dosage of pyridoxine may be needed; however, because such a dosage can occasionally cause a *neuropathy* (disease of the nerves), it should be taken under the guidance of a physician.

Riboflavin (Vitamin B_2) Deficiency

There is preliminary evidence that a deficiency of riboflavin (vitamin B_2) may promote the development of carpal tunnel syndrome, at least in association with a vitamin B_6 deficiency. This is shown in the following case:

> *A person with a three-year history of carpal tunnel syndrome was found to be deficient in both vitamin B_6 and riboflavin. After five months of supplementation with riboflavin, there was a nearly complete disappearance of symptoms, with a significant increase in the strength of hand squeezing, but no improvement in the blood test for vitamin B_6 deficiency. After pyridoxine supplementation, all remaining symptoms disappeared, hand-squeezing strength further improved, and the blood test for vitamin B_6 became normal.[6]*

NUTRITIONAL HEALING PLAN: Riboflavin Deficiency

Dosage: 50 mg of riboflavin daily

Other Factors

Lithium

Carpal tunnel syndrome is a known side effect of lithium therapy. However, since you may need to stay on lithium, don't stop it on your own, but consult your doctor as to what to do.[7]

CHOOSING A PERSONAL PLAN

When carpal tunnel syndrome fails to heal with conservative treatment, an operation can be performed to relieve the nerve compression. However, in addition to its cost, discomfort, and inconvenience, surgery is not always successful; one in five people who undergo it either experience no relief from symptoms or suffer a recurrence afterward. Nutritional therapy is far cheaper, more comfortable, safer, and simpler. It therefore makes good sense to first give the Nutritional Healing plans an adequate trial.[8]

Cataracts

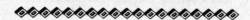

See also: DIABETES, HEART DISEASE, OBESITY.

The lens of the eye is the only transparent organ in the body; a *cataract* is a loss of this transparency that eventually interferes with vision. Worldwide, 50 million people are afflicted with cataracts, including about half the population over age 75.

DIETARY FACTORS

Diabetes, high blood fats (hypertriglyceridemia), and obesity are all associated with a greater risk of developing cataracts. Fortunately, these risk factors are all influenced by diet and can therefore be reduced by dietary means. Nutritional supplements are also beneficial for controlling blood sugar and normalizing blood fats. (See the chapters on diabetes, heart disease, and obesity for specific suggestions.)

Galactose, which is a component of milk sugar (*lactose*), may foster cataract formation in people who have difficulty utilizing it in their bodies due to genetic factors. If these people (who can be identified only with sophisticated blood testing) have a high-lactose intake, they have a significantly increased risk of developing cataracts. Conversely, among people with cataracts, these genetic factors appear to be relatively common.[1,2]

THE HEALING DIET

1. Follow the Basic Healing Diet as described in Appendix A.
2. Restrict the following dairy products that are high in lactose:

   ▸ milk and cream
   ▸ buttermilk
   ▸ cottage cheese
   ▸ ice cream
   ▸ yogurt

Note: Because this diet reduces your calcium intake, you should consider 500 to 1000 mg of supplemental calcium daily.

NUTRITIONAL HEALING PLANS

Vitamins

Antioxidant Vitamins

When they are exposed to light, oxygen molecules may break apart to become oxygen free radicals—unstable substances that can destroy cells. Since the lens is exposed to both light and oxygen, it is vulnerable to damage by this mechanism. The antioxidant vitamins C and E, as well as beta-carotene (which is closely related to vitamin A) are a major defense against such damage.

The lower the blood level of each of the three antioxidant vitamins, the higher the risk of cataracts. When rat lenses were maintained in a solution designed to cause free-radical damage, the addition of either vitamin C or vitamin E protected them. (Beta-carotene was not tested.)[3,4,5]

The concentration of vitamin C in the aqueous humor (the fluid held between the lens and the tissue at the front of the eye) is among the highest of all the body fluids; the lower the intake of this vitamin, the higher the cataract risk. There is even early evidence that vitamin C supplementation may cause early cataracts to regress or disappear. After supplementation with vitamin C, the vision of between 60 and 90 percent of patients with early cataracts improved, sometimes dramatically.[6,7]

The following case illustrates the improvement of cataracts with antioxidant supplementation:

> Four hundred and fifty patients with early (incipient) cataracts received vitamin C along with vitamin A. Though similar patients had previously required surgery after about four years, only a small group of supplemented patients required surgery at that time. The cataracts of some did not progress over 11 years of follow-up.[8]

NUTRITIONAL HEALING PLAN: Vitamin C

Dosage: 350 mg of vitamin C daily

Trial Period

initial improvement in two to eight weeks

The results of giving cataract patients vitamin E or beta-carotene supplements alone have not been reported. However, older people without cataracts were found to ingest significantly more vitamin E than people of the same age who had developed cataracts.[9]

Riboflavin (Vitamin B_2)

A riboflavin (vitamin B_2) deficiency is known to be associated with an increased risk of developing cataracts. One investigator reported that riboflavin supplementation dramatically improved vision in people with early cataracts within 48 hours; 9 months later, he found that the cataracts had disappeared in all 27 people he was treating. (Unfortunately, it appears that this study was never published, and its dramatic results have not yet been confirmed.)[10]

Galactose, which may promote the development of cataracts in certain people, is known to be a riboflavin antagonist; thus a high-lactose intake may be detrimental, not only because some people have difficulty utilizing it properly, but also because it may foster a marginal riboflavin deficiency.[11]

The following case provides an example of the improvement of cataracts with riboflavin supplementation:

A female patient developed cloudy vision in both eyes at age 70 while supplementing her diet with 1.5 g of ascorbic acid, 100 mg of thiamine, 250 mg of pyridoxine, 1.5 g of niacinamide, and 800 IU of vitamin E daily. She was advised to add 25 mg of riboflavin and 3 cod liver oil capsules (for vitamins A and D) daily. One year later, her lenses were clear; three years later no evidence of cataract was seen on optometric examination.[12]

NUTRITIONAL HEALING PLAN: Riboflavin

Dosage: 15 mg of riboflavin daily

Trial Period

initial improvement within 48 hours; improvement may continue for nine months or longer

---

Minerals: Zinc

Cataract patients have lower levels of zinc in the blood than do people of the same age who are free of cataracts. An animal study suggests that zinc may benefit people with early cataracts by stimulating cells in the outer layer of the lens to multiply. Ophthalmologist Gary Price Todd has reported excellent results in his practice with zinc when it is included in a multivitamin supplement. Sixty-seven percent of his patients had improved vision, more than 50 percent of those who initially needed surgery improved to the point where surgery was no longer indicated. The patients who responded usually had a 50 percent improvement in vision.[13,14,15,16]

NUTRITIONAL HEALING PLAN: Zinc

Preparation

zinc sulfate

Dosage: 30 mg of elemental zinc daily

Trial Period

initial improvement within six weeks; improvement may continue for one year or longer

---

COMBINATION TREATMENT

Excellent results in reversing cataracts have been reported with a combined nutritional plan. For example, ophthalmologist Robert Azar, whose clinic treats 25,000 patients annually, places cataract patients on a low-fat, complex-carbohydrate diet that stresses fish, fowl, and fresh produce and is supplemented with vitamin C, water-soluble vitamin E, and zinc for 2 months. If improvement is noted, surgery is delayed. He reports that many people on the program improve enough to make surgery unnecessary.[17]

CHOOSING A PERSONAL PLAN

Everyone who is concerned about preventing or reversing cataracts should follow the Basic Healing diet in order to reduce the factors known to be associated with an increased risk. Since it is difficult to know without blood testing if you are predisposed to problems with milk sugar, the importance of restricting dairy products is uncertain, but you may wish to consider avoiding a high-lactose intake if you or close family members have developed cataracts. (If you wish to be tested by your physician, ask him or her to rule out heterozygous deficiencies of galactokinase and galactose uridyl transferase.)

Although the research is very preliminary, a limited trial of riboflavin, zinc, and the antioxidant vitamins seems quite worthwhile.

ADDITIONAL SUGGESTION

Exposure to the combination of light and oxygen renders the eye lens susceptible to damage. Since sunlight is particularly damaging, consider buying sunglasses that are especially manufactured to protect you from the UVA and UVB rays in sunlight.

Cervical Dysplasia

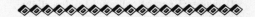

See Also: CANCER.

The *cervix* is the tip of the uterus that extends into the vagina. When a gynecologist takes a Pap smear during a routine examination, cells from the surface of the cervix are examined. *Dysplasia,* the medical term for abnormal cell development, is of concern because the cellular changes are sometimes precancerous. Once the diagnosis of cervical dysplasia is made, effective treatment will prevent the development of cervical cancer.

NUTRITIONAL HEALING PLANS

Vitamins

Folic Acid (Folate) Deficiency

A deficiency of folic acid (otherwise known as folate) in the lining of the cervix appears to be closely related to the development of cervical dysplasia, and women who are taking birth control pills or who are pregnant are especially susceptible to developing a folic acid deficiency. A cervical folate deficiency may be hard to detect because, when the level of cervical folic acid is low, the blood may show no evidence of a generalized folic acid deficiency, or only the level of folate in the red blood cells may be low.

Supplementation with folic acid has been proven to be an effective treatment for cervical dysplasia associated with oral contraceptive use. In a double-blind study, folate supplements successfully reversed mild to moderate degrees of cervical dysplasia in women who were taking birth control pills, even though they remained on the pills.[1,2,3]

NUTRITIONAL HEALING PLAN: Folic Acid Deficiency

Dosage: 5 mg of folic acid twice daily

Trial Period

three months

WARNING

This high a dosage of folic acid should be taken under medical supervision.

Vitamin A and Beta-Carotene Deficiencies

Compared to women with normal Pap smears, women with severe cervical dysplasia are likely to have a lower intake of vitamin A or of *beta-carotene,* which is a precursor form of vitamin A consisting of two molecules of A linked together. Moreover, in both their blood and cervical tissue, these women may have reduced levels of the retinol-binding protein. Since vitamin A (otherwise known as *retinol*) fits into a cleft in this protein to become part of a larger molecule that transfers the vitamin into the cell, a reduced level of retinol-binding protein implies that vitamin A may be less available to the cervical cells.[4]

Oral vitamin A supplementation has not been tested as a treatment for cervical dysplasia, although a form of vitamin A (retinyl acetate) applied directly to the cervix has been shown to increase the levels of both vitamin A and retinol-binding protein in the blood. Also, pilot trials of the cervical application of synthetic vitamin A derivatives have had some success.[5,6,7]

Women with cervical dysplasia have reduced levels of beta-carotene in their blood plasma. Even though oral beta-carotene supplementation, like vitamin A supplementation, has not been tested, it may be preferable to vitamin A because it lacks the potential toxicity of the vitamin. Moreover, a high consumption of carrots and green vegetables (which are rich in beta-carotene) is associated with a low risk of cervical cancer, while a high consumption of milk, liver, and meats (which are high in vitamin A) does not affect cervical cancer risk; this suggests that increasing beta-carotene intake could be more effective than increasing vitamin A.[8,9]

I particularly recommend foods high in beta-carotene as a preventive measure (*see Appendix D for a list of foods rich in beta-carotene*).

Vitamin C Deficiency

Like vitamin A and beta-carotene, the lower the intake of vitamin C, the higher the risk of cervical dysplasia. Women with cervical dysplasia often fail to obtain even half of the U.S. RDA for vitamin C in their diets *(see Appendix E for a discussion of the RDA)*. When these women were compared to women with normal Pap smears, their blood levels of vitamin C were lower.[10,11]

Because it is untested as a treatment for cervical dysplasia, the efficacy of vitamin C is unknown. Given its wide margin of safety, however, a therapeutic trial of the vitamin should be considered.

NUTRITIONAL HEALING PLAN: Vitamin C Deficiency

Dosage: not well established, but 500 mg of vitamin C daily would be reasonable

Trial Period

three months

Minerals: Selenium Deficiency

A selenium deficiency is known to increase the risk of cervical cancer. Moreover, women with cervical dysplasia have significantly lower blood selenium levels than normal women. Despite these intriguing findings, no studies have been completed on the efficacy of selenium supplementation for treating cervical dysplasia.[12,13]

NUTRITIONAL HEALING PLAN: Selenium Deficiency

Dosage: not well established, but 200 mcg of selenium daily would be reasonable

Trial Period

three months

CHOOSING A PERSONAL PLAN

Folic acid stands out as the only nutritional supplement for which there is scientific evidence of efficacy, so it would be the logical choice if you wish to try a single Nutritional Healing plan. However, since all the plans are reasonably safe and are limited to trial periods of three months, you may wish to combine them in an effort to achieve a more powerful effect:

> *The Pap smear of a 26-year-old woman revealed moderate cervical dysplasia. A smear done six months earlier had shown only mild dysplasia, while a smear done three months earlier had also shown a moderate degree of dysplasia. Visual examination of vaginal and cervical tissue was normal. She had been using birth control pills for six years but stopped after the second Pap smear. Since then she noted much heavier menstrual flow, with the last menses lasting eight days.*
>
> *She was given dietary counseling and the following supplements. 5 mg of folic acid 3 times daily; 60,000 IU of vitamin A daily for 2 months, followed by 25,000 IU daily; vitamin B complex "50" twice daily (Vitamin B complex "50" is a mixture of members of the vitamin B complex containing either 50 mg or 50 mcg of each of the B vitamins.); 1 g of vitamin C daily; and 400 IU of vitamin E daily. Two months later the Pap smear was entirely normal and remained so at the four-year follow-up.[14]*

Colds

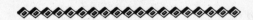

See also: INFECTIONS.

The common cold is an infection of the upper respiratory tract. It is most frequently caused by viruses but is sometimes caused by bacteria. Colds are so common that only 4 to 6 percent of all people are able to avoid catching them. Besides the discomfort of a cold, there is the danger of developing such complications as ear infections, bronchitis, and pneumonia.

DIETARY FACTORS

Yes, chicken soup, at least so long as it is hot and spicy, is good for colds! Modern scientific studies have shown that there is a little bit of truth to this folk remedy. It seems that inhaling the vapor from spicy soups while you consume them stimulates the nasal tissues to produce thin mucus. This can help relieve nasal congestion and thus provide some relief to cold sufferers—while making their mothers feel that they are doing something helpful.

More important, there is no reason to dispute another time-worn principle: Drink plenty of liquids. Fluids relieve congestion and prevent dehydration.

THE HEALING DIET

1. Drink at least eight glasses of water daily.
2. Eat hot, spicy soups.

NUTRITIONAL HEALING PLANS

Vitamin C

Due largely to the prestige of twice Nobel laureate Dr. Linus Pauling, numerous investigators have studied his contention that vitamin C supplementation is an effective method for preventing and treating colds. Using dosages of up to 2 g a day, they found no evidence that vitamin C prevents colds. However, they repeatedly found evidence that vitamin C supplementation can reduce both the severity of colds and their duration. Dr. Pauling recommends much higher doses, but the efficacy of vitamin C at those doses has not been proven.[1]

NUTRITIONAL HEALING PLAN: Vitamin C

Dosage: 500 mg of vitamin C four times daily

Zinc

When George Eby's teen-aged leukemic daughter refused to swallow a zinc gluconate tablet but dissolved it in her mouth, her freshly caught cold disappeared within hours. Mr. Eby, excited about the possible value of zinc gluconate in treating colds, funded a double-blind study to investigate. Sure enough, the study, conducted by experienced researchers, confirmed his observations. While cold sufferers given a useless placebo took 11 days to become symptom-free, cold sufferers who sucked on the zinc lozenges became symptom-free in only four days! In fact, some became asymptomatic within hours, and one in five fully recuperated within one day.[2]

Since then, further studies have been reported, but with conflicting results. Some have confirmed the original findings, whereas others could find no evidence that the treatment was effective. The reasons for the different results are unclear; however, since short-term zinc supplementation appears reasonably safe, it seems worth trying for a week, starting with the first indication of a cold.[3,4]

```
┌─────────────────────────────────────────────────────────┐
│              NUTRITIONAL HEALING PLAN: Zinc               │
│                                                           │
│                       Preparation                        │
│   180-mg zinc gluconate lozenges (containing 23 mg elemen-│
│   tal zinc)                                               │
│     Instructions: Suck on one lozenge for at least ten    │
│     minutes every two hours while awake during the illness.│
│     Maximum Adult Dosage: 12 lozenges daily               │
└─────────────────────────────────────────────────────────┘
```

COMBINATION TREATMENT

Zinc and vitamin C can be used in combination. In addition, a change to a healthier diet and supplementation with other nutrients that bolster the body's immune response (see the chapter on infections), though not yet proven effective for the common cold, may be beneficial, especially when there is evidence of a nutritional deficiency.

ADDITIONAL SUGGESTIONS

About half of all colds are due to *rhinoviruses;* they can spread only when transmitted to the nose or eye of the susceptible person. Children usually infect themselves by rubbing their noses or eyes with contaminated fingers.

Surprisingly, people often catch a rhinovirus cold from a handshake, as 40 percent of people with rhinovirus colds have the virus on their hands, where it can survive for up to 3 hours. However, the main route of rhinovirus transmission is the air—from coughing, sneezing, and nose blowing.[5,6]

Another common cold virus, respiratory syncytial virus (RSV), survives on the skin for only 15 minutes but can survive for hours on other surfaces. In more than 2 out of 3 cases, infection is transmitted by direct contact, though in 40 percent of cases infection results from handling contaminated objects. Sitting in an infected person's room appears to be safe.[7]

The influenza or flu virus survives only ten minutes on the skin but up to three days on nonporous surfaces. This virus is easily spread through the air.[8]

Based on these facts, avoiding people with colds is not the only way you can prevent exposure to cold viruses. You can also prevent a cold by not touching your eyes or nose until you have washed your hands after shaking hands with a person with a cold or after touching objects that were touched that day by a person with a cold.

Constipation

❖◆❖◆❖◆❖◆❖◆❖◆❖◆❖◆❖◆❖◆❖◆❖

See also: IRRITABLE BOWEL SYNDROME.

The term *constipation* is often used to refer to the need to strain in order to pass hard feces, but some definitions also include the inability to pass feces more often than twice a week. It has been estimated that about 10 percent of the population in Western countries suffers from this condition. It becomes more common with advancing age: 3 percent of young adults and at least 20 percent of the elderly complain of it. In Third World countries, however, constipation is almost unknown.

DIETARY FACTORS

In the absence of disease, inadequate fiber in the modern Western diet is believed to be the primary cause for constipation. Undigested fiber absorbs water, which increases the weight and bulk of the stool and makes it softer. These factors activate the bowel muscles, pushing the stool forward more rapidly. Fiber also encourages the growth of gas-producing bacteria in the colon. The gases add to the pressure in the colon to propel the feces forward.[1,2]

Not all dietary fiber is equally effective. In a comparative study, for example, corn bran was found to be more effective for relieving constipation than wheat bran. Though increasing fiber-rich foods in your diet would be preferable, an alternative method would be to add corn bran in increasing amounts.[3]

Note: If you have any disease of the intestinal tract, adding corn bran to your diet should be done only under your doctor's supervision.

Since food sensitivities can interfere with normal intestinal function, constipation may occasionally be a symptom of an adverse reaction to certain foods. (Usually the person who is food-sensitive suffers from other symptoms besides constipation, especially other symptoms of dysfunction of the gastrointestinal tract.[4])

THE HEALING DIET

1. Increase dietary fiber

WARNING

Increased fiber may produce gas and abdominal discomfort, especially until the body has had time to readjust.

- ▶ Preferred Method. A high-fiber diet, as described in Appendix A.
- ▶ Alternative Method. Start with ½ cup of bran (9 g of fiber) daily mixed in with foods, and slowly increase the amount by ½ cup increments, as tolerated, over a few weeks to a maximum of 2 cups of bran daily.
2. Avoid foods found to be constipating. *See Appendix B for information about diagnosing food sensitivities.*

NUTRITIONAL HEALING PLANS

Vitamins

Folic Acid (Folate)

Folic acid (folate) deficiency, though a relatively rare cause of so common a condition as constipation, is the most common of the vitamin deficiencies. As with food sensitivities, if constipation is due to a folic acid deficiency, there usually are other symptoms, which are likely to be neurologic. Tiredness and depression are common, along with restless legs. A neurologic examination by your physician may reveal positive findings, and laboratory tests can be done to discover whether your folic acid levels are low.[5]

NUTRITIONAL HEALING PLAN: Folic Acid

I would recommend that you take folic acid supplementation only under your physician's direction following a medical evaluation. However, you may wish to increase the foods in your diet that are high in folic acid to help prevent a deficiency.

Good sources of folic acid include many fruits (such as cantaloupes and oranges) and vegetables (such as spinach, romaine lettuce, cabbage, Brussels sprouts, broccoli, pinto beans, and chick peas), as well as whole wheat, brewer's yeast, salmon, and organ meats.

Pantothenic Acid

Deficiency of pantothenic acid, another member of the vitamin B complex, is very rare. I mention it because such a deficiency is associated with constipation. Moreover, even in the absence of a pantothenic acid deficiency, there is some evidence that supplementation with this vitamin may stimulate intestinal activity and thus relieve constipation.[6]

NUTRITIONAL HEALING PLAN: Pantothenic Acid

Dosage: 250–500 mg of pantothenic acid daily

Mineral Salts

Certain salts of magnesium, potassium, and sodium are very effective stimulant laxatives; that is, they stimulate the large intestines to push the feces forward. They produce a soft or semiliquid stool in six to eight hours. Milk of magnesia (magnesium hydroxide) is a particularly popular example.[7]

NUTRITIONAL HEALING PLAN: Mineral Salts
Preparation

milk of magnesia

Dosage: 15 to 30 ml

Instructions: Take with one glass of water on an empty stomach.

Botanical Extracts

Cascara Sagrada

Cascara, an extract made from the bark of a deciduous tree, is another stimulant laxative. One of the mildest of its class, it usually produces a soft or formed stool in six to eight hours.[8]

Cascara may impart a yellowish-brown or reddish color to the urine. With prolonged use, the surface lining of the colon may develop a harmless pigmentation that disappears when it is discontinued.[9]

NUTRITIONAL HEALING PLAN: Cascara Sagrada

Dosages:

Extract: 200–400 mg of cascara sagrada daily

Fluid extract: 0.5–1.5 mg daily

Aromatic fluid extract: 5 ml daily

Psyllium

The effectiveness of preparations made from psyllium seeds is due to their high content of *mucilage,* a form of fiber. Like other forms of dietary fiber, psyllium works by increasing the bulk of the feces, rather than by stimulating the colon as the stimulant laxatives do. It may take two or three days to produce results.[10]

NUTRITIONAL HEALING PLAN: Psyllium

Dosages:

Seeds: 2.5–30 g daily

Psyllium hydrophilic colloid: 7 g (1 tsp) 1 to 3 times daily

Additional Instructions: Take one glass of water with each dose.

Senna

A more potent stimulant laxative than cascara, senna was first used by the Arabs in the ninth century. Once it reaches the colon, colonic bacteria break it up into its active components, which stimulate the colon to evacuate. It produces a soft to semifluid stool 6 to 12 hours after ingestion.[11]

NUTRITIONAL HEALING PLAN: Senna

Dosages:

Whole leaf

powdered leaf: 0.5–2 g

fluid extract: 2 ml

syrup: 8 ml

Senna pod

granules: 1 or 2 tsp 1 or 2 times daily

syrup: 2 or 3 tsp 1 or 2 times daily

tablets: 2 to 4 tablets 1 or 2 times daily

Sennosides A and B: 1 or 2 tablets daily

Other Instructions

Take one glass of water with each dose.

Beneficial Bacteria

Lactobacillus Acidophilus

Acidophilus is an important member of the normal bacteria of the colon. When it is successfully implanted, it may relieve constipation from a variety of causes. Its efficacy varies widely from brand to brand due to differences in the strains of the bacteria that are used as well as great variations in strength due to the concentration of organisms.[12]

In contrast to the action of stimulant laxatives, it may take weeks or even months before the benefits of acidophilus are fully realized. If it succeeds in relieving constipation, however, it has probably been successfully implanted and thus may continue to grow on its own. It may then be possible to discontinue its use without experiencing the return of symptoms.

CHOOSING A PERSONAL PLAN

If your constipation is chronic and your doctor has ruled out any disease process complicating it, first try increasing the fiber in your diet. If you find it too difficult to eat enough high-fiber foods, consider adding bran or psyllium to your diet in order to increase its fiber content. You might consider taking an acidophilus preparation at the same time, especially if the constipation began after a course of antibiotics, which may have killed off some of your healthy colon bacteria.

The use of stimulant laxatives tends eventually to make the colon more sluggish as it becomes used to depending on the laxative to become activated. For this reason, it is best not to use them routinely for more than a few weeks. Their intermittent use, however, should not be a problem. (If senna alone is ineffective, the addition of psyllium to senna sometimes produces results.)

As for the use of vitamins, a trial of pantothenic acid is reasonably safe. Since a very high dosage of folic acid may be needed in the unlikely event that the constipation is the result of a folate deficiency, and since such a high dosage may have adverse side effects, the decision to try folic acid supplementation is best left to your doctor.

Finally, consider evaluating yourself for food sensitivities if the above suggestions fail or if there are enough other symptoms of food sensitivities to suggest that they are a possible cause of your constipation.

ADDITIONAL SUGGESTIONS

If nutritional interventions fail, it is quite possible that the constipation is due to mechanical factors preventing the stool from being released during defecation. Some people have unconsciously learned the bad habit of contracting rather than relaxing their muscles surrounding the rectal opening while attempting to defecate, even if they are straining to pass their feces. If you remain constipated after trying nutritional therapy but your stool is soft, this may be your problem. Try to imagine relaxing those muscles and visualize the stool sliding through a wide-open exit.

The poor design of toilet seats also contributes to difficulty in passing feces. Sitting on the seat constricts the anal opening and thus makes defecation more difficult. Try raising yourself off the seat by squatting just above it; if that is too difficult just raise one buttock off the seat. People who have failed to find relief with other methods have sometimes found that this simple measure provides the solution.

Dementia (Senile)

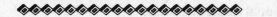

Senile dementia is a progressive degenerative brain disease marked by such symptoms as the loss of recent memories, slowness in thought and movement, and confusion and disorientation. Alzheimer's disease, the most common form, accounts for about half of all cases of senile dementia; its cause is poorly understood. Also common is dementia due to damage caused by a reduced blood supply to the brain, known as multi-infarct dementia.

DIETARY FACTORS

Experts estimate that 10 to 20 percent of all dementias in the elderly are reversible. Malnutrition is one cause of reversible dementia, and it is also possible that malnutrition contributes to the progression of nonreversible dementias. Compared to healthy people of the same age, people with dementia are more likely to be nutritionally deficient.

One reason that nutritional deficiencies occur is that people fail to eat adequate amounts of wholesome foods due to forgetfulness or apathy. Another reason is that nutrients that are ingested may not be well utilized; they may not be absorbed normally from the gut and may not be easily transported from the bloodstream into the brain tissue.[1]

THE HEALING DIET

Follow the Basic Healing Diet as described in Appendix A.

NUTRITIONAL HEALING PLANS

Nutritional Replenishment

Deficiencies of the following nutrients are believed to be possible causes of dementia. A nutritionally trained physician can make a proper evaluation about deficiencies of these nutrients and should supervise nutritional replenishment. Even if a person is not deficient, it is possible, but unproven, that a low dosage of supplementation with these nutrients may prevent or reverse the symptoms of the illness in some people.

Folic Acid (Folate) Deficiency

A folic acid (folate) deficiency is known to be associated with apathy, disorientation, poor concentration, and memory deficits, along with damage to the neurologic system. Although even the healthy elderly may fail to ingest adequate folate, blood levels of folic acid are more likely to be low in people with dementia than in normal people of the same age.[2]

Everyone with dementia should be checked by their doctor for folate deficiency. When it is found, folic acid supplementation may cause at least a partial reversal of both the dementia and any neurologic symptoms, as shown by the following case:

A 75-year-old epileptic woman with severe dementia and neurologic degeneration affecting all her limbs received folate supplementation. Her mental functioning gradually improved, as reflected by improvements in her brain waves. Her neurologic disorder regressed, and her reflexes became normal.[3]

NUTRITIONAL HEALING PLAN: Folic Acid Deficiency

Dosage: 10–20 mg of folic acid daily for 1 week; then 2.5–10 mg daily

---

WARNING

Take under medical supervision.

Niacin (Vitamin B₃) Deficiency

Niacin deficiency is not uncommon in the elderly, despite an adequate dietary intake and oral supplementation. Dementia is one of the three cardinal signs of *pellagra,* the niacin deficiency disease; diarrhea and dermatitis are the other two. Since people with pellagra often have dementia without the other signs, the diagnosis could readily be missed unless blood studies are done.[4,5]

Not only will restoring adequate niacin levels stop a niacin-deficiency dementia from progressing, but sometimes the dementia will prove to be reversible, with full recovery in several weeks.

NUTRITIONAL HEALING PLAN: Niacin Deficiency

Preparation

niacinamide

Dosage: 300 mg daily for the first week; then 100 mg daily

Thiamine (Vitamin B₁) Deficiency

Marginal thiamine (vitamin B₁) deficiency is not uncommon in the elderly. In people with Alzheimer's dementia, the activity of several thiamine-dependent enzymes may be reduced in the brain. In addition to inadequate intake, thiamine deficiency may result from impaired absorption from the gut as well as such conditions as excessive vomiting, gastric (stomach) surgery, and chronic diarrhea.[6,7]

Though the memory deficit associated with thiamine rarely disappears after thiamine supplementation, adequate supplementation prevents further deterioration.

NUTRITIONAL HEALING PLAN: Thiamine Deficiency

Dosage: 1 g of thiamine 3 times daily for the first week; then 100 mg daily

WARNING

Such large dosages should be taken under medical supervision.

Vitamin B_{12} Deficiency

The most common cause of a vitamin B_{12} deficiency in the elderly is not a poor diet but degenerative changes in the gut lining that prevent dietary B_{12} from being absorbed. It is standard practice for physicians to order blood testing for vitamin B_{12} levels when evaluating patients with dementia, as a deficiency is known to be associated with confusion, memory loss, depression, and mental slowness in addition to neurologic problems.[8]

If a vitamin B_{12} deficiency is found, the dementia may or may not be reversible. Supplementation should be provided by injection because absorption through the gut may be poor. Neurologic improvement is usually evident within a few days and is often complete after one month.

Occasionally, vitamin B_{12} supplementation is effective despite normal B_{12} blood levels and the lack of suspicious physical findings—perhaps because of deficient levels of the vitamin in the fluid surrounding the brain or because of the inaccuracy of the standard laboratory test for vitamin B_{12}.[9,10]

The following case is an example of the benefits of B_{12} supplementation despite normal B_{12} blood levels:

A 73-year-old woman experienced several months of increasing forgetfulness, intermittent confusion, joint pains, and occasional tingling in her hands. Her medical work-up, including blood and urine studies, X-rays, and scans, was entirely normal. Despite a normal serum vitamin B_{12} level, she was started on intramuscular vitamin B_{12} injections. Within a few days, she seemed better; by three months all symptoms had cleared.[11]

NUTRITIONAL HEALING PLAN: Vitamin B_{12} Deficiency

Preparation

hydroxycobalamin

Dosage: Take 100 mcg daily by intramuscular injection for 1 week; then reduce dosage to a maintenance level (perhaps 1000 mcg per month).

Zinc Deficiency

In patients with Alzheimer's dementia, zinc concentrations may be reduced in both the blood and the brain. Reduced zinc levels in the brain may lead to the development of dementia by directly causing a loss of *neurons* (nerve cells) in the brain or by causing brain aluminum levels to rise. (See the section about aluminum on p. 93.) In theory, zinc supplementation should be beneficial, although it is just starting to be studied.[12,13,14,15,16]

NUTRITIONAL HEALING PLAN: Zinc Deficiency

Dosage: 50 mg of zinc daily

Neurotransmitter Precursor Therapy

Phosphatidyl Choline

The *cholinergic system* in the brain refers to the system of neurons that uses acetylcholine as a neurotransmitter; that is, as a means of transmitting impulses from one neuron to the next. The cholinergic system is involved in normal memory; a decline in its functioning is found in both normal age-related memory loss and Alzheimer's dementia.

Though acetylcholine is made in the body from nutritional precursors in our diet, supplementation with cholinergic nutrients such as phosphatidyl choline has had, at best, only a modest success in affecting Alzheimer's. The reason is unknown, but it may be because most studies have lasted only six months or less; a longer period of time may be needed before improvement or a slowing of the progression of the disease is seen.[17]

NUTRITIONAL HEALING PLAN: Phosphatidyl Choline

Preparation

95 percent pure phosphatidyl choline

Dosage: 10–20 g daily

Trial Period

six months

Tryptophan

Serotonin, like acetylcholine, is a neurotransmitter, and tryptophan is the amino acid in our diet from which the body makes serotonin. Compared to other people their age, people with senile dementia have lower fasting tryptophan levels in their blood, and studies have found that absorption of tryptophan from the gut into the blood may be reduced.[18,19]

No improvement was found when a group of 28 people with dementia were given tryptophan supplementation for 1 month. However, after the same short time period, two out of four people with both dementia and tryptophan malabsorption who were given tryptophan along with 5-hydroxytryptophan (the substance tryptophan is converted into before becoming serotonin) did improve. As is the case with efforts to enhance brain acetylcholine, longer trials are needed to clarify the possible efficacy of tryptophan supplementation. Also, a patient is more likely to respond if the doctor finds evidence that tryptophan absorption is impaired.[20,21]

NUTRITIONAL HEALING PLAN: Tryptophan

Dosage: L-tryptophan 3 g daily

Instructions: Take with 50 mg of DL-5-hydroxytryptophan daily.

Trial Period

six months

Additional Instructions

1. Avoid protein for 90 minutes before and after ingestion.
2. Take with a carbohydrate (such as fruit juice).

Note: Since tryptophan supplements may not be currently available (see Introduction), you may wish to try foods with a high tryptophan to protein ratio (see Appendix A).

Botanical Extracts: Ginkgo Biloba

In a number of clinical trials, some of which were double-blind, an extract made from the leaves of the *Ginkgo biloba* tree has been proven to be a successful treatment for people suffering from dementia due to reduced blood flow to the brain. Administration of *Ginkgo biloba* extract increases blood flow in the brain and improves brain-wave tracings. With ginkgo biloba supplementation, people with dementia become more alert and sociable, think more clearly, feel better, and remember more.[22,23]

NUTRITIONAL HEALING PLAN: Ginkgo Biloba

Preparation

Ginkgo biloba extract (24 percent potency)

Dosage: 40 mg 3 times daily

Trial Period

six months; initial improvement may be noted in eight to twelve weeks

---

Aluminum Toxicity

The role of aluminum in causing dementia remains controversial. Let us review some of the growing evidence:

1. Aluminum is found within *senile plaques,* which are abnormal formations in the brain found in Alzheimer's dementia. It is not clear whether aluminum contributes to the development of these lesions.[24]
2. Several surveys have found an association between aluminum in drinking water and the number of people with Alzheimer's dementia in the local population.[25]
3. Aluminum causes neurofibrillary tangles (tangles of the small fibers of the nerve cell) in the brains of animals that resemble those seen in Alzheimer's dementia, as well as progressive changes in the animal's behavior that also resemble the changes seen in dementia.[26]

With such evidence, it would seem prudent to reduce aluminum exposure, which can come from a number of sources. Though it is not feasible to avoid all aluminum exposure, it can be reduced considerably by avoiding the things shown in the following chart.

PRODUCTS THAT CAN CONTAIN ALUMINUM

Ingestion

aluminum foil absorbed into foods
aluminum pots and pans
antacids
antidiarrheal agents
aspirin (buffered)
cake and pancake mixes
cheese, processed
cheese, ready-to-sprinkle grated
drinking water
flour, self-rising
frozen doughs
pickles

Inhalation

sprays (Example: certain antiperspirants)

Skin contact

roll-on antiperspirants
douches
hemorrhoidal preparations

Also, as I discussed earlier, adequate zinc intake may help protect against aluminum toxicity.

CHOOSING A PERSONAL PLAN

Every attempt should be made to follow the principles of the Basic Healing diet. Meals should not be skipped. To guard against nutritional deficiencies, I suggest a high-potency multivitamin/multimineral formula. To play it safe, minimize exposure to aluminum.

A medical evaluation, including laboratory testing, should be arranged to rule out deficiencies of folic acid, niacin, thiamine, vitamin B_{12}, and zinc, and any deficiency found should be corrected by supplementation. Since vitamin B_{12} may be beneficial despite normal test results, consider a trial of vitamin B_{12} by injection.

Assuming that there are no nutritional deficiencies, ginkgo biloba, with its excellent record of safety and effectiveness, would be my first choice for a therapeutic trial. Much less is known about the value of tryptophan and phosphatidyl choline, the neurotransmitter precursors, but they may be worth a trial. It may, however, be several months before results are seen.

The following case history illustrates the successful reversal of dementia:

A diabetic with a family history of depression, schizophrenia, and senility suffered a serious head injury at age 6 and was hospitalized in his late 20s for a severe mental breakdown. At age 42, he began to feel weak and irritable. He eventually became unable to work and was diagnosed with depression. A few years later, his mental faculties gradually declined until he would spend weeks sitting in a chair looking at his shoes. A CAT scan, taken when he was around age 50, showed brain atrophy. Three physicians diagnosed him as suffering from Alzheimer's dementia and predicted that he would be dead in seven years.

The patient began a water fast on his own and after five days was able to think more clearly. Medical evaluation revealed widespread food and chemical sensitivities and achlorhydria (lack of stomach acid). He had his silver-mercury fillings replaced with an alternative material but reacted so severely to the replacement material that he had all his teeth extracted. Finally, he began an extensive vitamin and mineral supplementation program along with supplements to increase stomach acidity.

A few months after starting the nutritional program, he began to feel better; after two years, he was clearly in remission. Almost four years after the first CAT scan, a second scan showed definite improvement that was confirmed by several specialists. He subsequently recovered so fully that he was able to return to work as an insurance salesman. While he has returned to his former lifestyle, he must rigidly adhere to his dietary and lifestyle program to minimize symptoms.[27]

Since this man tried to treat his dementia in a number of different ways, we do not know which of them, or which combination, was effective. His deficiency of hydrochloric acid may have made him more prone to developing nutritional deficiencies and food sensitivities, though food sensitivities appear to have only a temporary effect upon mental functioning. Some investigators suspect that toxicity from or sensitivity to the mercury in dental amalgams—the substance used to fill teeth—can adversely affect brain function; however, mercury from dental amalgams has not been shown to cause dementia.

In evaluating the results from any of the Nutritional Healing plans, remember that, though reversing dementia is most desirable, slowing down or stopping its progression is more likely to be accomplished.

Depression

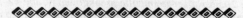

See also: ANXIETY, FATIGUE, INSOMNIA.

Though occasional feelings of sadness are part of the human condition, depression ranges from normal sadness and mourning to an abnormal state of complete disability with overwhelming feelings of hopelessness and suicidal acts. When health professionals speak of depression, they refer to a syndrome that, in addition to a depressed mood, may include disturbed eating, sleeping, and bowel habits, low self-esteem, the inability to derive pleasure from normally pleasurable activities, poor concentration, and feelings of hopelessness.

DIETARY FACTORS

Depression is often associated with an inadequate diet. Depression can cause malnutrition because of a lack of appetite (anorexia), and poor eating habits can cause depression by failing to provide the adequate nutrition necessary for proper functioning.

Depression is also associated with levels of caffeine intake above about 700 mg (about 4 to 5 cups of coffee) daily as well as with higher amounts of refined sugars in the diet. Eliminating caffeine and sugar for as little as one week has been shown to lift depression; resuming sugar and caffeine intake brings the depression back.[1]

Other foods as well as chemicals and molds have been proven to provoke depression in susceptible individuals.[2] The following case provides an example of this:

A 67-year-old woman had suffered from occasional bouts of depression for many years. One episode more than ten years earlier had been severe enough to require hospitalization. She also had a long history of diarrhea with abdominal pain and bloating that was diagnosed as irritable bowel syndrome. When she was placed on an elimination diet, her bowel symptoms disappeared within two weeks. She also reported feeling much more cheerful, alert, and confident; her doctor assumed that this emotional improvement was due to the relief of her bowel symptoms.

When challenged with milk at breakfast, however, her skin became itchy by lunchtime, and she developed severe bloating and diarrhea in the afternoon along with profound depression—even though she now knew that her bowel symptoms could be prevented if she simply avoided drinking milk. The depression lasted two days and then she felt as well as before. She continued on a milk-free diet and, when seen two years later, reported that her depressive episodes had ceased along with her bowel symptoms.[3]

Sometimes, however, people believe that a food causes depression but find on objective testing using placebos that they were wrong.

THE HEALING DIET

1. Follow the Basic Healing diet as described in Appendix A.
2. Avoid caffeine.
3. Avoid foods found on testing to provoke depression. *See Appendix B for information about diagnosing food sensitivities.*

NUTRITIONAL HEALING PLANS

Precursor Therapy (Neurotransmitter Augmentation)

Neurotransmitters are natural substances that transmit messages between nerve cells in the brain. Some neurotransmitters, especially *serotonin* and *norepinephrine,* play an important role in mood regulation. Fortunately, since the body makes these substances from foods in our diet, we can raise levels of neurotransmitters that are too low for optimal functioning by increasing our intake of the foods from which the neurotransmitters are made.

Serotonin

The important neurotransmitter serotonin is derived from L-tryptophan. *Tryptophan* is an essential amino acid, which means that we are unable to make it within our bodies and therefore have to depend on food to supply it to us.

There are many kinds of evidence that suggest that adequate trypto-phan is important for feeling good. When the dietary intakes of tryptophan from several countries were compared, a low-tryptophan intake was found to be associated with a high rate of suicide. People who are hospi-talized due to severe depressions may have low levels of tryptophan in their blood; when they recover, these levels also improve. If people who are recovering from a depression are placed on a low-tryptophan diet, some relapse.[4,5,6]

A component of protein, tryptophan can be increased through diet. However, since it has to compete with many other amino acids to enter the brain, and since it is the least abundant amino acid in foods, tryptophan is best increased through nutritional supplementation. Tryptophan sup-plementation has been extensively studied and, although more proof is needed, appears to be as effective as antidepressant medications.[7]

NUTRITIONAL HEALING PLAN: Tryptophan

Dosage: 2 g of L-tryptophan 3 times daily

Note: Since tryptophan supplements may not be cur-rently available (see Introduction), you may wish to try foods with a high tryptophan to protein ratio (see Appendix A).

Trial Period

two weeks

Additional Instructions

1. Avoid protein for 90 minutes before and after ingestion.
2. Take with a carbohydrate (such as fruit juice).

In order to be converted into serotonin (5-hydroxytryptamine), trypto-phan must first be converted into *5-hydroxytryptophan* (5-HTP), seroto-nin's immediate precursor. Like tryptophan, 5-HTP has been shown to have antidepressant properties that are roughly equal to those of antide-pressant medications. Since 5-HTP is one step closer to serotonin, it is no surprise that there is some evidence that it is even more effective than tryptophan. Its major adverse side effects are gastrointestinal (causing nausea and diarrhea), so it should be taken with meals to minimize irrita-tion to the gut lining.[8,9]

NUTRITIONAL HEALING PLAN: 5-Hydroxytryptophan

Preparation

enteric-coated 5-hydroxytryptophan

Dosage

1. Start with 25 mg daily at mealtime.
2. Increase as tolerated over 10 to 14 days to 75 mg, 3 times daily with meals.

Trial Period

two weeks

Norepinephrine

The important neurotransmitter *norepinephrine* is derived from L-phenylalanine which, like L-tryptophan, is an essential amino acid found in dietary protein. By a different route, L-phenylalanine can also be converted into *phenylethylamine (PEA)* in a reaction that requires vitamin B_6. PEA, a neurotransmitter that has amphetaminelike effects, is abundant in chocolate. (Did you ever wonder why some people are "chocoholics"?)

Though the major role of norepinephrine in depression is well recognized, the role of PEA has been much less explored. In one pilot study, 23 people with major depression who were not receiving medications were found to have low levels of a breakdown product of PEA in the urine. Their moods improved almost as soon as they began supplementation with L-phenylalanine along with vitamin B_6.[10]

In the same study, 31 out of 40 people with major depression seemed to respond to the combination of L-phenylalanine and vitamin B_6. Controlled studies are needed before we can be sure of the benefits of L-phenylalanine. Its major side effects seem related to its stimulant properties: mild headaches, increased anxiety and insomnia, along with mild nausea and constipation.[11]

NUTRITIONAL HEALING PLAN: L-Phenylalanine

Dosage

1. Start with 500 mg of L-phenylalanine upon arising and at noon.
2. Increase by 500 mg daily to about 1500–2000 mg twice daily, as tolerated.
3. Combine each dose with 50 mg of pyridoxine.

WARNING

Should be avoided by phenylketonurics.

Research has also been done on D-phenylalanine and DL-phenylalanine. Each has been shown to be as effective as the antidepressant drug imipramine, and may be effective in many patients with depression. However, none of the three forms of phenylalanine has been tested thoroughly enough to draw final conclusions.[12,13,14]

In order to be converted into norepinephrine, L-phenylalanine must first be converted into tyrosine. Like phenylalanine, tyrosine is an amino acid. Since tyrosine is one step closer to norepinephrine, supplementing it should be beneficial, although it can't be converted into PEA. Indeed, the results of small double-blind studies suggest that tyrosine supplementation may be effective for some depressions.[15]

Vitamin Deficiencies

If a member of the vitamin B complex becomes deficient, a deficiency syndrome develops, and depression is usually part of that syndrome. There may be a downward spiral: Depression may cause a lack of appetite as well as a lack of concern with the nutritional quality of the diet, leading to an inadequate intake of B vitamins and a marginal vitamin B deficiency, which, in turn, may deepen the depression.

Folic Acid (Folate) Deficiency

Folic acid (folate) deficiency is the most common of all the vitamin deficiencies; the average American adult, for example, consumes only 60 percent of the U.S. RDA for folate daily *(see Appendix E for an explanation of the U.S. RDA)*. Folate depletion is commonly associated with depression. Even more important, examination of the serum folate levels of people who are seriously depressed frequently reveals that these levels are reduced and occasionally deficient. Among people who are depressed, the worse the depression, the lower the level of folic acid in the blood. Most often the folate deficiency has developed after the depression, due to such factors as poor diet and the use of alcohol and drugs.[16,17,18,19]

If your doctor finds that your level of folic acid is low, folate supplementation is indicated. (Folate-deficient people who are most likely to respond are those who became depressed because they were tiring too easily.[20])

NUTRITIONAL HEALING PLAN: Folic Acid Deficiency

Dosage: 800 mcg of folic acid daily

Riboflavin (Vitamin B_2) Deficiency

As with the other B vitamins, even though we know that riboflavin (vitamin B_2) deficiency causes depression, we don't know how frequently depressed people are riboflavin-deficient. When 172 people were evaluated for riboflavin deficiency in the order that they were admitted to a psychiatric hospital, more than one-fourth were found to be deficient. Furthermore, it turned out that those patients who had a riboflavin deficiency also had been given a diagnosis of a mood disorder.[21]

NUTRITIONAL HEALING PLAN: Riboflavin Deficiency

Dosage: 40 mg of riboflavin daily

Thiamine (Vitamin B_1) Deficiency

In the earliest stage of thiamine (vitamin B_1) deficiency, otherwise normal people become depressed, irritable, and fearful. Thiamine deficiency is common when mental illness is severe enough to require hospitalization; in one group of 10 patients in a psychiatric hospital, 3 of them (30 percent) were found to be thiamine-deficient.[22,23]

NUTRITIONAL HEALING PLAN: Thiamine Deficiency

Dosage: 40 mg of thiamine daily

Vitamin B_6 Deficiency

I mentioned earlier that vitamin B_6 is required to convert phenylalanine to phenylethylamine (PEA). It is also required to convert dietary tryptophan to serotonin. Laboratory evidence of vitamin B_6 deficiency is common in depression. Of all the possible psychiatric diagnoses, patients in a psychiatric hospital who are B_6-deficient are most likely to have a diagnosis of *endogenous depression,* that is, depression due to factors within the person rather than to outside events. The presence of mild neurologic symptoms such as numbness and "pins and needles" or "electric shock" sensations increases the likelihood of a vitamin B_6 deficiency.[24,25,26]

While researchers have yet to find out how often depressed people improve by boosting their B_6 intake, they have proven that pyridoxine is effective for treating depression caused by taking birth control pills. This is because the hormones in the pills interfere with vitamin B_6 while they speed up the destruction of tryptophan; the result is that the conversion of tryptophan into serotonin is impaired.[27]

NUTRITIONAL HEALING PLAN: Vitamin B_6 Deficiency

Preparation

pyridoxine

Dosage: 40 mg daily

Vitamin B_{12} Deficiency

About 5 percent of people admitted to a psychiatric hospital are deficient in vitamin B_{12}, while perhaps another 10 percent have subnormal levels of the vitamin. Those with lower B_{12} levels are more likely to have a mood disorder than those with adequate levels. Though we don't yet know how effective vitamin B_{12} supplementation is for relieving depression, one group of people complaining of tiredness felt better following a course of vitamin B_{12} injections but not after a course of placebo injections. Since tiredness is often a feature of depression, many of these people were likely to have been depressed.[28,29,30]

NUTRITIONAL HEALING PLAN: Vitamin B_{12} Deficiency

Dosage: 1000 mcg of vitamin B_{12} intramuscularly, weekly to monthly as needed

---

Vitamin C Deficiency

People coming down with *scurvy,* the vitamin C deficiency disease, may first become depressed. Though scurvy is rare in industrialized countries, a mild form may develop that is marked by chronic depression, tiredness, irritability, and vague ill health.[31]

There is some evidence that mild scurvy may not be as uncommon in modern industrialized societies as we may think. When the diets of 12 depressed women who subsequently attempted suicide were compared to those of another 12 women who were not depressed and had no history of suicide attempts, the only significant difference found was a lower intake of vitamin C. Among patients in a mental hospital, plasma vitamin C levels tend to be low; moreover, if they are given vitamin C, it takes longer for their bodies to become saturated with the vitamin than it does for normal people.[32,33,34]

In one study, 40 chronic psychiatric patients randomly received either vitamin C or a placebo. Three weeks later, only the patients given vitamin C were less depressed.[35]

NUTRITIONAL HEALING PLAN: Vitamin C Deficiency

Dosage: 1 g of vitamin C twice daily

Mineral Deficiencies

Iron Deficiency

People with iron-deficiency anemia often feel tired and depressed. Not many people realize that, even after iron supplementation cures the anemia, the depression may not resolve for months. Though the cause of the depression is unknown, we do know that some areas of the brain have high iron concentrations; perhaps a reduction in brain iron brings on the depression.[36]

NUTRITIONAL HEALING PLAN: Iron Deficiency

Preparation

ferrous sulfate

Dosage: 300 mg 3 times daily

WARNING

Iron supplementation should be given only under a doctor's supervision.

Magnesium Deficiency

Depression, along with irritability and agitation, may be part of a magnesium deficiency syndrome. Inadequate dietary magnesium is common in industrialized societies, and such factors as stress, illness, and the use of medications can increase the risk of magnesium deficiency.[37,38]

NUTRITIONAL HEALING PLAN: Magnesium Deficiency

Dosage: 600 mg of magnesium daily

Potassium Deficiency

Hypokalemia, that is, a low level of potassium in the fluid portion of the blood, may develop, for example, after repeated episodes of vomiting or diarrhea, or following the use of diuretic drugs. With hypokalemia, people are often depressed, weak, and fatigued. They may also find it difficult to think clearly, and can be confused and disoriented.[9]

When the blood of seriously depressed people has been examined, hypokalemia has rarely been found. Potassium may be low, however, in their blood cells. Also, people who have committed suicide have been found to have a low level of potassium in their brains. Though potassium supplementation will relieve depression in people who are hypokalemic, there is no evidence that potassium supplementation will relieve depression in other people.[40,41]

Because of the complexities of the issue of potassium supplementation, the diagnosis and treatment of low potassium levels should be left to your doctor. However, if you have chronic diarrhea or repeated episodes of vomiting, you can provide yourself with some protection against potassium depletion by making sure that your diet is rich in dietary sources of potassium.

NUTRITIONAL HEALING PLAN: Potassium Deficiency

A high-potassium diet (see Appendix D for a list of high-potassium foods).

Other Deficiencies: Hydrochloric Acid (HCl)

Insufficient gastric acidity may reduce the ability of the gut to absorb many of the nutrients we have discussed. Concerning the members of the vitamin B complex, deficiencies of niacin, riboflavin, thiamine, and vitamin B_{12} may develop, even in people consuming a seemingly adequate diet, if your stomach is deficient in hydrochloric acid.

The efficacy of hydrochloric acid supplementation in treating depression has not been studied scientifically. However, clinicians have reported cases where supplementation with hydrochloric acid along with the vitamin B complex seemed to be effective. We have no idea how often nutrient deficiencies due to insufficient hydrochloric acid may cause depression but, due to the decline in stomach acid production with aging, it is likely to be a more common problem in older people.

The following case illustrates the benefits of hydrochloric acid supplementation for depression:

For 17 years, a person suffered from depression due to an unidentified biological abnormality. A physical examination suggested vitamin deficiencies. Treatment consisted of hydrochloric acid supplements before meals along with vitamin B complex. Relief from the longstanding depression was dramatic.[42]

NUTRITIONAL HEALING PLAN: Hydrochloric Acid (HCl) Deficiency

Preparation

10 gr capsules of betaine or glutamic HCl

Instructions: See Appendix C for detailed instructions.

Botanical Extracts

St. John's Wort (*Hypericum Perforatum*)

Norepinephrine is one of the major brain neurotransmitters involved in mood regulation. Taking *hypericin,* a constituent of a plant named St.

John's Wort, increases the amount of the major breakdown product of brain norepinephrine in the urine, which suggests that this botanical preparation may boost the level of norepinephrine in the brain.[43]

Indeed, the results of a clinical trial are consistent with this hypothesis. Fifteen depressed women were given a standardized extract of hypericin after rating their various complaints. The hypericin extract caused no adverse side effects; when they were asked to rate their complaints again, the repeat scores indicated that they were feeling better.[44]

NUTRITIONAL HEALING PLAN: St. John's Wort

Preparation

extract of St. John's Wort standardized as to hypericin content

Dosage: depends upon the specific preparation.

Example:: solid extract (5:1 or 0.125% hypericin 125–250 mg three times daily

---

CHOOSING A PERSONAL PLAN

Despite your depression, push yourself to follow the principles of the Basic Healing diet and try to eliminate caffeine for a minimum of one week. Also consider trying a food-elimination diet, especially if there are other signs or symptoms that suggest you may be reacting to specific foods.

Precursor therapy could be a natural alternative to antidepressants or, with your doctor's assistance, a natural means of increasing the drugs' efficacy. There is no definitive method for predicting which neurotransmitter may require boosting via precursor therapy; it appears that a combination of serotonin and norepinephrine precursors may be more effective than the use of either alone.[45]

Various vitamin and mineral deficiencies can cause depression, and it is not uncommon for depressed people to have evidence of below average levels of these nutrients. Therefore, as a minimal measure, anyone who is depressed should be on the Basic Healing diet. For some people, this measure is not adequate due to the presence of any number of factors, such as physical illnesses and medications that decrease nutrient absorption. The diagnosis and treatment of relevant nutritional deficiencies can best be done by a physician experienced in nutritional medicine. The alternative would be to try supplementation with a vitamin B complex, vitamin C, and magnesium, as detailed in the above sections, along with high potassium foods.

Administration of St. John's Wort may be worth a trial even though its benefits have yet to be proven by scientific experiments. Finally, a trial of hydrochloric acid supplementation should be considered when there is reason to believe that such supplementation would be beneficial.

ADDITIONAL SUGGESTIONS

Because depression has many causes and even more treatments, do not limit yourself to exploring nutritional medicine unless it becomes clear that nothing further is needed. Not all depression even needs help to heal; it can simply be a normal human emotion. At the other extreme are the severe forms of depression that require psychiatric treatment. However, even a moderate level of depression can respond to antidepressant medication. For psychologically caused depressions, psychotherapy may be indicated.

The value of exercise is often forgotten. For example, when half of a group of people hospitalized for depression did one hour of aerobic exercise three times a week for nine weeks, their depression scores were significantly lower than those of the half of the group who did not exercise.[46]

Sometimes, the best way to overcome depression is to take some time off and get away from your responsibilities. As your mind is freed from its usual duties, your problems may no longer seem so odious and solutions may occur to you.

Diabetes

See also: CATARACTS, HEART DISEASE, OBESITY.

Diabetes mellitus is a disease marked by increased sugar (glucose) in the blood which, if high enough, may spill over into the urine. In addition to the danger of becoming acutely ill from abnormal blood sugar levels, diabetics are predisposed to potentially serious long-term complications affecting blood vessels, nerves, and major body organs.

HELPFUL DEFINITIONS

Before reading this chapter, you will find it helpful to learn a few definitions:

- ▶ **Glucose.** The form of sugar found in the bloodstream.
- ▶ **Glucose tolerance.** The ability of the body to regulate blood sugar levels following the ingestion of sugar or starch (which consists of sugar molecules linked together).
- ▶ **Insulin.** A hormone secreted by the pancreas that regulates the amount of sugar (glucose) in the bloodstream and its utilization by the tissues.
- ▶ **Insulin sensitivity.** The responsiveness of the tissues to insulin.
- ▶ **Type I (juvenile; insulin-dependent) diabetes.** Starts suddenly, usually in childhood, and requires insulin injections.
- ▶ **Type II (adult-maturity) diabetes.** Starts slowly, does not usually require insulin, is increasingly common with age, and is often associated with obesity.

DIETARY FACTORS

Obesity should be avoided or, if present, treated. Current thinking emphasizes a diet that is high in complex carbohydrates (starches) and low in sugar, fat (particularly saturated fat), and cholesterol. Fruits and vegetables that are high in fiber, particularly soluble fiber, should be emphasized, since soluble fiber increases the time it takes for the intestines to absorb glucose. (Examples of soluble fibers are those found in oats, fruits, and vegetables.)[1,2]

The following case illustrates the benefits of such a diet:

A type I diabetic male was admitted to the hospital. After ten days on a traditional diabetic diet, he was switched to a high-carbohydrate, high-fiber, low-cholesterol diet. Although he did not change his weight or activity level, his insulin requirements dropped steadily from 28 units to 16 units per day. After 30 days, his elevated fasting blood sugar had fallen from 204 to 143, his serum cholesterol had dropped from 280 to 131, and his fasting serum triglycerides (blood fats) fell from 1,485 to 306.[3]

A vegetarian diet (which is likely to follow the above guidelines) is preferable. Such a diet can help reduce the risk of developing diabetes and the risk of dying from diabetes-related causes.[4,5]

Fatty-acid supplementation for diabetes must also be considered. The essential fatty acids consist of two groups: the omega-3 and omega-6 families. They are called *essential* because our bodies require them but cannot make them, and thus we must get them from food. Though there is evidence that supplementing the diet with omega-3 fatty acids can be beneficial for good health, there is also evidence that, for diabetics, such supplementation could have adverse effects on cholesterol and sugar regulation. I feel, therefore, that it is premature to recommend them as dietary supplements until further studies are done. In the meantime, I would suggest that diabetics include cold-water fish, which are an excellent source of omega-3 fatty acids, as part of the diet.[6,7]

By contrast, there is much evidence that suggests enriching the diet with omega-6 fatty acids, which consist of linoleic acid and its derivatives, is beneficial for diabetes. For example, five years after a group of newly diagnosed diabetics were placed on a linoleic acid-enriched diet, they had less microangiopathy (small blood vessel disease) and heart ischemia (inadequate blood flow from the coronary arteries) compared to an equal number of similar patients who had been eating a traditional Western diet. Three men eating the Western diet died of heart attacks; there were no deaths due to heart attacks in the group eating the linoleic acid-enriched diet. One reason for this difference is that diabetics placed on a linoleic acid-enriched diet show decreases in both total cholesterol and LDL cholesterol levels, each of which is associated with the development of coronary heart disease.[8,9]

Eating a wide variety of foods may prevent or retard the development of disease of the large blood vessels, a common complication of diabetes. Alcohol consumption is generally not advisable for diabetics because it may worsen their ability to handle sugar.[10,11]

Results of a fascinating study of Australian aborigines underscore the intimate relationship between diabetes and the diet. Until the 1930s, aborigines ate few processed foods. Since meat from wild animals is lean, their diet was high in protein but low in fat. Dietary fiber was high. That diet began to change when missionaries introduced flour and sugar. As urbanization radically changed their life style, they adopted a typical Western diet. Diabetes, which had been virtually unknown, became so common that it was diagnosed in 20 percent of the adult population.

For the study, ten urbanized type II diabetic aborigines agreed to return to the hunter-gatherer existence of their ancestors and to only eat what they could hunt, fish, or collect for seven weeks. All were overweight and rarely exercised. Most ate a diet high in fatty meat and several suffered from hypertension (high blood pressure). Five of the ten drank moderately to heavily.

During the 7 weeks of the study, their activity levels increased, while their food intake was reduced to 1,200 calories per day. All lost weight steadily. Their diabetes improved markedly; both their fasting blood sugar and their blood sugar levels after eating were significantly reduced. In addition, their blood pressures fell toward normal.[12]

THE HEALING DIET

Follow the Basic Healing diet as described in Appendix A. This diet is recommended for both type I and type II diabetics.

NUTRITIONAL HEALING PLANS

Vitamins

Niacin (Vitamin B₃)

Neither a vitamin nor a mineral, *glucose tolerance factor* (GTF) is a nutrient that augments the action of insulin. GTF occurs preformed in certain foods, especially brewer's yeast, and humans have a varying ability to synthesize it from inorganic chromium, niacin, and amino acids.

Since niacin (a form of vitamin B_3) is a component of GTF, a niacin deficiency interferes with GTF synthesis and the body's ability to regulate blood sugar levels. Even assuming that niacin levels are normal, it is possible that additional supplementation could still improve blood sugar regulation.

In one study, part of a group of newly diagnosed type I diabetics received niacinamide while the rest received a placebo. Then, under their doctors' direction, the diabetics gradually reduced their insulin dose. The results were exciting: niacinamide supplementation extended the time they could go without insulin. In fact, even after three years, two of the nine patients taking niacinamide still did not require insulin while, only nine months after the study began, all nine diabetics who received a placebo had to return to their insulin injections.[13]

Results of a study using an animal model of diabetes have suggested another benefit from niacin. When diabetic rats were supplemented with niacinamide, kidney disease (one of the complications of diabetes) developed more slowly than usual. Perhaps niacinamide can do the same for humans.[14]

NUTRITIONAL HEALING PLAN: Niacin

To Reduce Insulin Dosage (Type I Diabetics)

Directions: **Under medical supervision only,** diabetics who have recently started insulin treatment can attempt to wean themselves off insulin by taking 1 g of niacinamide (nicotinamide) 3 times daily.

To Prevent Diabetic Kidney Disease

Dosage: not well established, but 50 mg of niacin or niacinamide daily would be reasonable

---

Thiamine (Vitamin B₁)

As with some of the other B vitamins, diabetics may have lower levels of thiamine (vitamin B_1) in the blood than healthy nondiabetics. A serious deficiency of thiamine may cause a neuropathy (disease of the nerves) that responds to thiamine supplementation. Whether diabetics with a neuropathy and marginal thiamine deficiency respond to thiamine has not been well explored; however, one physician reported that 80 percent of his diabetic patients with sensory neuropathy improved after they took thiamine.[15,16,17]

NUTRITIONAL HEALING PLAN: Thiamine

Suggested Use

diabetic neuropathy

Dosage: not well established, but 50 mg of thiamine daily would be reasonable

Trial Period

two weeks

Vitamin B₆

Elderly, nondiabetic volunteers given a vitamin B_6-deficient diet developed increased fasting blood sugar levels that returned to normal when their deficiency was corrected. Many diabetics are vitamin B_6-deficient, which suggests that they may benefit from supplementation. Although B_6 supplementation failed to improve the glucose tolerance of one group of diabetics with a vitamin B_6 deficiency, supplementation did improve glucose tolerance in a group of vitamin B_6-deficient women who developed diabetes during pregnancy (known as gestational diabetes). More studies are needed to clarify the efficacy of this vitamin for improving glucose tolerance.[18,19,20,21]

Diabetics with a neuropathy may have even lower levels of vitamin B_6 than diabetics in general. In a pilot study, supplementation with pyridoxine, a form of the vitamin, seemed to reduce the symptoms of neuropathy in diabetics who had both neuropathy and evidence of a vitamin B_6 deficiency, although a later double-blind study found pyridoxine supplementation to be ineffective.[22,23,24]

NUTRITIONAL HEALING PLAN: Vitamin B₆

Suggested Use

▶ diabetic neuropathy
▶ gestational diabetes (diabetes of pregnancy)

Preparation

pyridoxine

Dosage: 50 mg twice daily

Trial Period

two weeks

Vitamin B$_{12}$

Vitamin B$_{12}$ is yet another member of the vitamin B complex that can be beneficial in treating diabetic neuropathy. The results of an animal study suggest that, when tissues are deprived of adequate amounts of this vitamin, a neuropathy or other neurologic disorder may develop that responds to injections of the active form of B$_{12}$. In preliminary human trials, injections of vitamin B$_{12}$ gave dramatic relief to diabetics suffering from neuropathy. While it is possible that oral B$_{12}$ is helpful, no such studies have been done, and oral B$_{12}$ is often ineffective for other conditions that respond to B$_{12}$ injections.[25,26]

NUTRITIONAL HEALING PLAN: Vitamin B$_{12}$

Suggested Use

diabetic neuropathy

Route of Administration: intramuscular injection

Dosage: determined by your physician

Trial Period

two weeks for initial benefits

Vitamin C

Diabetes is associated with abnormal vitamin C metabolism, and depressed levels of the vitamin may be found in the blood despite what would seem to be an adequate dietary intake. A deficiency of vitamin C impairs glucose tolerance; conversely, in type II diabetes, vitamin C supplementation may improve glucose tolerance.[27,28,29]

Vitamin C may help protect us from atherosclerosis, a disease that diabetics develop more readily than others. This relationship could be explained by the finding that, when blood sugar is elevated, vitamin C has difficulty getting into blood vessel walls. Moreover, in type II diabetes, vitamin C supplementation has been shown to help normalize the level of elevated blood fats, and elevated blood fats are known to increase the risk of atherosclerosis.[30,31,32]

In addition, older diabetics who find that small blood vessels in the skin are prone to break and leave an ugly discoloration until the blood is absorbed will be pleased to learn that vitamin C supplementation has been shown to increase the strength of these blood vessels in type II diabetics.[33]

NUTRITIONAL HEALING PLAN: Vitamin C

Suggested Use

▶ regulate blood sugar in type II diabetics
▶ prevent disease of the heart and the large blood vessels
▶ decrease small blood vessel fragility

Dosage: 1 gram of vitamin C daily

Trial Period

▶ improve blood sugar regulation: ten days
▶ lower cholesterol and triglycerides: one year
▶ strengthen small blood vessels: two months

Vitamin E

Diabetics appear to have an increased requirement for vitamin E, and those on insulin may find that they need less insulin when they increase their vitamin E intake.[34,35]

Platelets are small disk-shaped particles in the blood that are the building blocks of blood clots. Diabetics' platelets are hyperaggregable (prone to clump together); this is believed to contribute to the tendency for diabetics to develop diseases of both small and large blood vessels. Supplementation with vitamin E has been shown to reduce this abnormal clumping tendency and reduce elevated blood fats. Vitamin E may therefore help to prevent the development of such complications as retinopathy (a disease of the eye's retina) and heart disease.[36]

NUTRITIONAL HEALING PLAN: Vitamin E

Suggested Use

▶ reduce insulin requirements (type I diabetics)
▶ prevent long-term complications

Dosage: 500 IU of vitamin E twice daily

Special Precautions

1. Because vitamin E may reduce insulin requirements, diabetics on insulin should start with no more than 100 IU daily and slowly increase the dosage under their physicians' guidance.
2. Because vitamin E may improve the action of the heart (which may place added strain on a weak heart or require readjustment of heart medications), diabetics with heart disease should start with no more than 100 IU daily and slowly increase the dosage under their physicians' guidance.

Minerals

Chromium

Most, but not all, studies have found chromium to be a necessary component of glucose tolerance factor, and serum chromium levels reflect serum insulin levels. People who are deficient in chromium have difficulty regulating their blood sugar. Supplementation with trivalent chromium, at least in people with sub-optimal chromium status, may improve blood sugar regulation as well as the sensitivity of the tissues to the effects of insulin. Also, a case report suggests that diabetics with neuropathy who are deficient in chromium may find that their neuropathy improves once they begin chromium supplementation.[37,38,39,40,41,42]

The following case illustrates the benefits of chromium supplementation for diabetes:

> When a 51-year-old type I diabetic woman was examined, she had evidence of a number of diabetic complications: disease of the large blood vessels (atherosclerosis), small blood vessel disease (glomerular nephritis, retinitis), peripheral neuropathy, and ulceration of a portion of her left first toe. She became diabetic when she was 27 years old; abnormal findings in her retina were noted when she was 39. At age 46, typical bilateral diabetic sensory neuropathy of the feet and hands began, and subsequently had slowly progressed. At

*age 50, atherosclerosis with discoloration and ulceration of the big
toe was diagnosed.*

*Her dietary history revealed a healthy high-complex-carbohy-
drate diet with adequate protein and limited refined sugar. Hair chromium and manganese levels were depressed, and analysis of her
urine showed evidence of glomerular nephritis.*

*She was placed on trivalent chromium in the form of glucose
tolerance factor and vitamin E. Follow-up visits at three, six, and nine
weeks showed gradual improvement. By 6 months, her insulin requirement had decreased from 140 units to 40 units daily, her glomerular nephritis was in remission, there was a moderate reduction
in her peripheral neuropathy, and her big toe looked entirely normal.*[43]

NUTRITIONAL HEALING PLAN: Chromium

Suggested Use

▶ regulate blood sugar (type II diabetes)
▶ diabetic neuropathy (if chromium-deficient)

Note: A nutritionally trained physician can evaluate you.

Dosage: 200 micrograms daily

Trial Period

▶ regulate blood sugar: three months
▶ diabetic neuropathy: two months

Copper Deficiency

Copper deficiency is associated with difficulty regulating blood sugar.
Also, when a person with a copper deficiency eats sugar, a substance
called *sorbitol,* which is derived from glucose, may accumulate in the
tissues. Intracellular sorbitol fosters the development of cataracts, retinopathy, neuropathy, and other complications of diabetes by drawing water
into the cells and forcing important small molecules out.[44,45,46]

NUTRITIONAL HEALING PLAN: Copper Deficiency

Suggested Use

prevent long-term diabetic complications (if deficient)

WARNING

Not recommended unless copper deficiency is found on testing.

Dosage: 2–4 mg of copper daily

Magnesium

Magnesium is frequently low in diabetics, and is especially low in diabetics who have coronary heart disease or disease of the retina of the eye. Since experimental magnesium deficiency causes disease in the small coronary arteries of the heart, it is quite possible that low magnesium levels contribute to disease of the heart and blood vessels. Unfortunately, it is not known whether magnesium supplementation prevents or treats these complications, although it does appear to be worth trying.[47,48,49,50]

Magnesium also relates closely to insulin and blood sugar regulation. In type II diabetics, magnesium supplementation has been shown to improve both the production of insulin in response to dietary sugar and the action of insulin in regulating blood sugar levels.[51]

NUTRITIONAL HEALING PLAN: Magnesium

Suggested Use

▶ improve blood sugar regulation (type II diabetics)
▶ prevent disease of the heart and blood vessels (if deficient)

Note: A nutritionally trained physician can evaluate you.

Dosage: not well established, but 400 mg of magnesium daily is reasonably safe; higher dosages should be supervised by your physician

---

Manganese Deficiency

Manganese, another mineral whose blood levels in diabetics are depressed, is necessary to activate the key enzymes involved in the body's ability to use sugar for energy. Animals who are made manganese-deficient have reduced insulin activity.[52,53,54]

Though routine manganese supplementation is inadvisable, type I diabetics with depressed manganese levels may find their insulin needs reduced following supplementation.[55]

NUTRITIONAL HEALING PLAN: Manganese Deficiency

Suggested Use

improve blood sugar regulation in type I diabetics

Dosage: 3–5 mg of manganese daily

WARNING

Because insulin requirements may decrease, supplementation must be closely monitored by a physician.

Phosphorus

When a person is phosphorus-deficient, the body fails to respond normally to insulin. Moreover, the red blood cells in type I diabetics have difficulty properly releasing their oxygen to tissues; this impairment is related to the level of phosphorus (as inorganic phosphate) in the blood. Theoretically, an increase in plasma inorganic phosphate levels should make more oxygen available to the tissues. This would help prevent diabetic angiopathy (blood vessel disease) and improve energy.[56,57]

In a pilot study, type I diabetics without kidney disease received inorganic phosphate salts. They reported feeling less tired and their diabetes was more easily controlled; in some of the diabetics, insulin requirements were slightly decreased.[58]

NUTRITIONAL HEALING PLAN: Phosphorus

Suggested Use

In type I diabetes:

▶ improve energy
▶ improve blood sugar regulation
▶ prevent vascular complications

Preparation

dibasic calcium phosphate

Dosage: 2 g 3 times daily with meals

WARNING

Phosphorus must be taken under the direction of a nutritionally trained physician.

Other Nutritional Factors

Inositol

Though inositol is low in the blood of diabetics, it is extremely high in the nerves, suggesting that this member of the vitamin B complex may play a role in nerve functioning. Indeed, nerves affected by diabetic neuropathy may have lower levels of inositol. Though pilot studies have reported improved nerve function after inositol supplementation, other studies, including a double-blind study, have failed to confirm these findings. Thus, at present, the benefit of inositol supplementation remains unclear.[59,60,61]

NUTRITIONAL HEALING PLAN: Inositol

Suggested Use

diabetic neuropathy

Dosage: 2 g of inositol daily

Trial Period

one month

Botanical Factors

Bioflavonoids

In the discussion about copper, I mentioned that sorbitol accumulation in cells is associated with various complications of diabetes. Avoiding a copper deficiency may not be the only natural way of preventing sorbitol accumulation. Certain bioflavonoids, such as naringin (from the flowers, fruit, and rind of grapefruit) and quercetin (from fruit rinds and tree bark), inhibit the action of *aldose reductase,* an enzyme needed for the synthesis of sorbitol from glucose. Though studies have yet to be done to ascertain whether bioflavonoids can prevent or treat diabetic complications in humans, sorbinil, a drug known to be a potent aldose reductase inhibitor, has been shown to benefit neuropathy and amyopathy (muscle wasting).[62,63]

Disease of the capillaries (the smallest blood vessels) appears to be responsible for some of the complications of diabetes. Though scientific studies are lacking, it appears that bioflavonoids may protect capillaries in diabetics from damage because they strengthen capillary walls; in addition, in the small intestines they prevent vitamin C from being changed (oxidized) to a compound that damages the inner lining of capillaries. Moreover, one bioflavonoid (daflon) has been shown to improve blood flow through diabetic capillaries by reducing the thickness of the blood.[64,65,66]

NUTRITIONAL HEALING PLAN: Bioflavonoids

Suggested Use

prevent long-term complications

Preparation

citrus bioflavonoids

   Dosage: not well established, but 2 g daily would be
   reasonable

Omega-6 Fatty Acids

In the discussion of dietary factors in diabetes, I recommended that oils rich in linoleic acid, an omega-6 fatty acid, be part of the diabetic diet. The oil from the evening primrose plant is a particularly rich source of *gamma-linolenic acid* (GLA), which is derived from linoleic acid. This oil has been shown to actually reverse the nerve damage to peripheral nerves due to diabetic neuropathy.[67]

Since GLA is derived from linoleic acid, it is possible that a linoleic-acid enriched diet also improves diabetic neuropathy. However, sometimes the enzyme needed to convert linoleic acid to GLA does not function properly, so we cannot assume that linoleic acid supplementation would be as effective.

NUTRITIONAL HEALING PLANS: Omega-6 Fatty Acids

Suggested Use

treatment of diabetic neuropathy

Preparation

evening primrose oil

Dosage: 1 g 4 times daily

Other Factors: Brewer's Yeast

Supplementation with brewer's yeast, an excellent source of glucose tolerance factor (GTF), has been shown to improve the glucose tolerance of type II diabetics, increase their sensitivity to insulin, and lower their level of blood fats. There are many commercial GTF products on the market; however their actual GTF activity is variable and largely unproven. Therefore, I suggest that, unless you can find out how potent a particular GTF supplement is, you get your GTF from brewer's yeast.[68]

NUTRITIONAL HEALING PLAN: Brewer's Yeast

Suggested Use

improve glucose tolerance (type II diabetics)

Dosage: 9 g of brewer's yeast daily

Trial Period

eight weeks

CHOOSING A PERSONAL PLAN

All diabetics should benefit from the Basic Healing diet, which I highly recommend. I also suggest considering the Nutritional Healing plans listed in the following chart to help combat the development of medical complications.

NUTRITIONAL HEALING PLANS TO COMBAT
MEDICAL COMPLICATIONS

niacin
thiamine
vitamin B_6
vitamin B_{12}
vitamin C
vitamin E
chromium (if deficient)
copper (if deficient)
magnesium (if deficient)
phosphorus (type I diabetics)
inositol
bioflavonoids
evening primrose oil

Finally, consider the appropriate Nutritional Healing plan(s) to improve your blood sugar regulation, as shown in the following chart.

TO REDUCE INSULIN DOSAGE IN TYPE I DIABETES

niacin
vitamin E
manganese (if deficient)
phosphorus

TO IMPROVE BLOOD SUGAR REGULATION IN
TYPE II DIABETES

vitamin C
chromium
magnesium
brewer's yeast

TO IMPROVE BLOOD SUGAR REGULATION IN GESTATIONAL
DIABETES

vitamin B_6 (if deficient)

Eczema

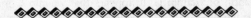

Eczema is a disorder causing skin changes in characteristic locations. Changes initially consist of redness, swelling, little breaks in the skin, and weeping of the skin; later the skin develops scaling, thickening, extra pigmentation, and cracks. Eczema is usually the earliest major allergic disorder to cause symptoms. At least a third of affected children continue to be affected after reaching adulthood.

DIETARY FACTORS

Reactions to foods have been shown to provoke rashes in about one out of two people with a history of eczema, and evidence of increased absorption of foods through the gut wall has been found. Milk and egg are two of the biggest offenders, as the following case shows, but many other foods have been implicated.[1,2]

> *Since birth, a seven-year-old boy had suffered from severe eczema that required several hospitalizations. He was placed on a milk- and egg-free diet and his eczema cleared. Reintroduction of milk, but not egg, produced an exacerbation, although he was able to tolerate reasonable quantities of condensed milk without symptoms.*[3]

THE HEALING DIET

Avoid foods found on testing to provoke rashes. *See Appendix B for information about diagnosing food sensitivities.*

NUTRITIONAL HEALING PLANS

Vitamins

Vitamin C

A double-blind crossover study proved that the symptoms of a group of ten young people with severe eczema were significantly improved with supplementation of vitamin C. It appears that vitamin C may work by boosting the immune response; people treated with vitamin C needed only half as many courses of antibiotics for treating skin infections as people receiving placebos.[4]

NUTRITIONAL HEALING PLAN: Vitamin C

Dosage: 3.5–5 g of vitamin C daily

Trial Period

three months

Minerals

Zinc

Some people with eczema are deficient in zinc. Since zinc, like vitamin C, is important for the proper functioning of the immune system, it is not surprising that zinc deficiency in eczema appears to be related to a tendency toward recurrent skin infection.[5]

Dr. Jonathan Wright reports that eczema disappeared in 39 out of 40 people he treated with zinc supplementation along with other dietary and nutritional measures. (One person with extensive skin involvement showed only a partial improvement.) However, controlled studies proving the efficacy of zinc alone have yet to be reported.[6]

NUTRITIONAL HEALING PLAN: Zinc

Dosage: 50 mg 3 times daily

Instructions

1. Take zinc with 2 mg of copper amino acid chelate daily.
2. Attempt to gradually reduce the dosage once satisfactory improvement has occurred.

WARNING

Take under medical supervision.

Trial Period

six weeks

Omega-3 Fatty Acids

These essential fatty acids are known to have beneficial effects on inflammation and the immune response. When people suffering from eczema were supplemented with a fish oil extract high in the omega-3 fatty acids, they had less itching and scaling of their skin, and overall their skin problems were fewer, as compared to others who received placebos.[7]

NUTRITIONAL HEALING PLAN: Omega-3 Fatty Acids

Preparation

fish oil extract (cholesterol-free)
    Example: MaxEPA™

Dosage: 5 g twice daily

WARNING

Take under medical supervision.

Trial Period

three months

Omega-6 Fatty Acids

The omega-6 essential fatty acids work closely with their partners, the omega-3 essential fatty acids, and also play an important role in regulating inflammation and the immune response. Evening primrose oil is a particularly rich source of GLA, an important omega-6 fatty acid. The results of administering primrose oil to people with eczema have been reported in nine double-blind studies. The results of these studies were recently analyzed together. Primrose oil was found to be an effective treatment, and it was found to be particularly effective in reducing itching.[8]

NUTRITIONAL HEALING PLAN: Omega-6 Fatty Acids

Preparation

evening primrose oil

Dosage: 1–2 g 3 times daily

Trial Period

four weeks

Other Factors: Hydrochloric Acid (HCl) Deficiency

The majority of people with eczema have low levels of hydrochloric acid (HCl) in their stomachs. Moreover, the lower the acid level, the worse their skin problems, and the more likely they are to complain of gastrointestinal symptoms.[9,10]

People with both eczema and hydrochloric acid deficiency may find that their eczema improves when they are supplemented with HCl, although double-blind studies have yet to be reported:

A 52-year-old person had suffered from eczema for the past 46 years and, for at least one year, complained of gas in the stomach and bowels. Analysis of the stomach contents before and after eating showed a total absence of free hydrochloric acid. Treatment with dilute hydrochloric acid was dramatically effective and, after almost one year of follow-up, the skin condition remained practically normal.[11]

NUTRITIONAL HEALING PLAN: Hydrochloric Acid (HCl) Deficiency

Preparations

10-gr capsules of betaine or glutamic HCl

Instructions: See Appendix C for detailed instructions.

Special Consideration

Especially consider HCl supplementation if you have gas, cramps, or bloating after meals.

CHOOSING A PERSONAL PLAN

Definitely give a food-elimination diet an adequate trial. If you wish to try the Nutritional Healing plans one at a time, you may wish to start with evening primrose oil because it is the plan with the best documented benefits.

Preferably, the decision to try hydrochloric acid supplementation should be made on the basis of an examination of your stomach's acid production. The presence of gas, cramps, or bloating after eating should increase your suspicion that your level of stomach acid may be low.

There is no reason why the Nutritional Healing plans cannot be combined, although I would recommend against trying them together with a food-elimination diet because, if your rash fades, it would interfere with interpreting the results. The following case illustrates the successful combination of nutritional supplements:

A 44-year-old man developed itchy red patches on his arms and legs that were diagnosed as eczema. He was found to have a very low level of sweat zinc and was treated with zinc together with evening primrose oil and multivitamins. His intense itching improved markedly over the next four weeks, and disappeared almost completely after eight weeks.[12]

Epilepsy

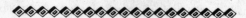

Epilepsy refers to recurrent attacks of *seizures* (convulsions), unconsciousness, or both. These attacks often begin during childhood and adolescence; about half of all cases start before the age of twenty. They result from a combination of heredity, which determines how vulnerable a person is to seizures, and events such as injuries, which cause the seizures to begin to occur.

DIETARY FACTORS

Healthy, nutritionally well-balanced meals eaten at regular intervals are recommended. A seizure could be provoked in an epileptic by eating a very large meal or by consuming excessive water.[1]

Regular alcohol consumption can cause recurring seizures in otherwise normal people, usually once or twice yearly. The degree of risk is directly related to the amount of alcohol consumption and returns to normal once a person gives up alcohol. Alcohol withdrawal can also trigger seizures that are often multiple and occur 10 to 48 hours after discontinuing or reducing alcohol intake.[2]

Caffeine, a stimulant, also makes it easier for a seizure to occur. Therefore caffeine-containing beverages can increase the occurrence of seizures in epileptics.[3]

The *ketogenic diet* is a very specialized low-carbohydrate, high-fat diet that has been proven effective for treating certain types of childhood seizures that fail to respond to medications. Since this diet is unhealthy for growing children and needs to be introduced by highly trained personnel during a hospitalization, it should be attempted only under close medical supervision.[4,5]

Reactions to specific foods have been proven to cause seizures, especially in people who have other symptoms due to food sensitivities. In one study, 45 epileptic children who also suffered from recurrent headaches, stomach symptoms, or hyperactive behavior were placed on a food-exclusion diet. When foods were reintroduced singly, some caused reactions. The same testing was performed with another 18 epileptic children who did not have additional symptoms, and they had no reactions when foods were reintroduced.

Foods found to provoke seizures or other symptoms in the first group of children were removed, and 36 of the children (80 percent) recovered or improved. In order to be sure that the children were not reacting only because they believed the foods bothered them, 16 of these 36 children were then retested by being given either foods that had caused them reactions before or a placebo in such a way that neither the child nor the researcher knew which was being given. All but one child had a recurrence of symptoms when supposedly reactive foods were tested, while none had symptoms when a placebo was given.[6]

The following case illustrates the benefits of a food-elimination diet for epilepsy:

A 19-year-old woman had developed grand mal (generalized) seizures 2 years earlier that were treated unsuccessfully with standard medications. Her EEG (brain wave) tracing showed a typical abnormality seen in epileptics. She reported that several of the seizures followed food ingestion by one to two hours.

After a four-day elimination diet, individual foods were tested, and she showed strong reactions (seizures, rapid heartbeat, and body coldness) when given beef or substances derived from beef and several other foods. Because chicken was one of the "safe" foods, she was retested for beef and chicken (which were chopped up and placed in gelatin capsules) by being given each of the two foods and a placebo without either her or the person giving them to her knowing the order in which they were given. Beef, but not chicken, caused seizures, even though her EEG failed to show clear evidence of seizure activity.[7]

THE HEALING DIET

1. Follow the Basic Healing diet, as described in Appendix A, with regular meals of average size.
2. Avoid foods found on testing to provoke seizures. *See Appendix B for information about diagnosing food sensitivities.*

Note: Testing should be done only under medical supervision.

NUTRITIONAL HEALING PLANS

WARNING
Because dosages of anticonvulsant medications may need to be readjusted, nutritional supplementation to improve seizure control should be tried only under medical supervision.

Vitamins

Folic Acid (Folate)

Though folic acid (folate) appears to be closely involved with epileptic seizures, studies of its effect on epilepsy have had mixed results, with the results of some pilot studies even suggesting that it may worsen seizures. It is probably best not to try folate supplementation until there is more evidence of its safety and efficacy.[8]

There is, however, another way in which folic acid can help some epileptics. Phenytoin (Dilantin) is a commonly used anticonvulsant drug that has the disquieting side effect of causing the gums around the teeth to overgrow. Used regularly, a folic acid mouthwash can help prevent this side effect from developing.[9]

NUTRITIONAL HEALING PLAN: Folic Acid Mouthwash

Formula: Make a mouthwash by adding 5 mg of folic acid to 5 ml (a little more than a tsp) of water.

Instructions: Use the mouthwash for two minutes twice daily.

Niacin (Vitamin B₃)

Supplementary niacin (a form of vitamin B_3) has a weak anticonvulsant effect. Though it does not appear to be powerful enough to be used alone, it may make anticonvulsant drugs more effective without increasing their toxicity. By permitting drug dosages to be lowered, it may reduce the unpleasant and sometimes intolerable side effects frequently associated with anticonvulsant therapy.[10,11]

NUTRITIONAL HEALING PLAN: Niacin

Dosage: 1 g of niacin 3 times daily

WARNING

Take under medical supervision.

Vitamin B₆ Deficiency

Infants with recurrent seizures may be suffering from insufficient vitamin B_6. The enzyme that converts glutamic acid to *gamma-aminobutyric acid* (GABA), an important inhibitory (brain-calming) neurotransmitter, is activated when vitamin B_6 binds itself to it. In some infants, seizures are due to a defect in the enzyme, which makes it difficult for vitamin B_6 to properly bind to it. The result is that GABA levels are reduced, making it abnormally easy for seizures to occur.[12]

Epilepsy in these infants can be cured if they are simply given a high enough dosage of vitamin B_6 so that, despite the binding problem, enough of the vitamin will succeed in binding to the enzyme to permit it to operate normally. This is a classic example of a *vitamin dependency,* that is, a need for an unusually high amount of a vitamin in order to overcome a genetic defect.[13] The following case is such an example:

> At age six months, Jason began to have three or four series of grand mal seizures starting shortly after awakening, which left him irritable and tired and caused his mental development to regress. He was placed on a daily dosage of 2 tbsp of brewer's yeast, which is rich in vitamin B_6. Within five days he began to improve, and soon he was going for days without a seizure. He was then switched to 10 mg of pyridoxine, a form of vitamin B_6, daily. Immediately he stopped twitching at night, perked up mentally, became energetic, regained what he had forgotten, and began to learn again. Since then, the only signs of seizure activity were two episodes during which his eyes watered and he blinked.[14]

Though less common, vitamin B_6 dependency has also been reported in adults. The value of B_6 supplementation for adult epileptics is unproven, although it is possible that it may be of value to adults who are vitamin B_6-deficient. (Your doctor can evaluate whether you are deficient in this vitamin.)[15]

NUTRITIONAL HEALING PLAN: Vitamin B$_6$ Deficiency

To Treat Vitamin B$_6$-Dependent Infantile Seizures

Preparation

pyridoxine

Dosage: 20–50 mg/kg in divided doses

(Your doctor will calculate the correct dosage for your infant.)

To Treat Vitamin B$_6$ Deficiency

Preparation

pyridoxine

Dosage: 40 mg daily

Vitamin E

Epileptic children receiving anticonvulsants may have reduced levels of vitamin E in their blood. Although its efficacy as an anticonvulsant when used alone is unknown, several studies have shown that vitamin E supplementation may reduce seizures when added to anticonvulsant therapy.[16]

For example, in a double-blind study, half of a group of 24 epileptic children whose seizures could not be controlled by medication received vitamin E supplementation in addition to their regular medication, while the other half received placebos. Three months later, 83 percent of the treated children had a greater than 60 percent reduction in seizures (and half of these children had a 90 to 100 percent reduction) compared to none of the children given placebo. When the children who received placebo were switched to vitamin E, the frequency of seizures was reduced 70 to 100 percent in all of them.[17]

NUTRITIONAL HEALING PLAN: Vitamin E

Preparation

D-alpha tocopherol acetate

Dosage: 400 IU daily

Minerals

Copper Deficiency

A deficiency of copper, which occasionally results from a hereditary defect, can cause seizures. Supplementary copper does not appear to be beneficial unless a deficiency exists. (Your physician can evaluate you for copper deficiency.)[18]

The following case illustrates how a copper deficiency can cause seizures:

> A 21-month-old boy was admitted to the hospital because of repeated seizures and failure to thrive. His mother and maternal uncle had copper deficiency with mild symptoms. Because his blood copper level was low, oral copper supplementation was given and was followed by general improvement. As soon as the copper was reduced or stopped, however, his blood copper levels fell and his seizures resumed.[19]

NUTRITIONAL HEALING PLAN: Copper Deficiency

Preparation

copper amino acid chelate

Dosage: 2 mg daily

Magnesium Deficiency

Seizures can be caused by a magnesium deficiency. Among epileptics, not only are blood magnesium levels reduced, but the lower the blood magnesium, the worse the severity of the epilepsy.[20,21]

Magnesium supplementation to correct a gross magnesium deficiency is definitely indicated. Less certain is the value of magnesium supplementation when blood magnesium levels are at the low end of the normal range, although evidence is accumulating that it may well be worth a trial.[22,23]

NUTRITIONAL HEALING PLAN: Magnesium Deficiency

Dosage: 450 mg of magnesium daily

Manganese Deficiency

Both hair and blood manganese may be reduced in epileptics, most likely as the result somehow of the presence of the seizure disorder. Early reports suggest that manganese supplementation may be beneficial, especially when manganese levels are very low, but controlled trials have not been done to confirm its value.[24,26]

The possible benefits of manganese supplementation for seizures is shown by the following case from my own practice:

A middle-aged woman developed increasing shoulder pain. X-rays suggested that the pain was caused by osteoarthritis and she was placed on a nonsteroidal anti-inflammatory drug. The pain gradually worsened until it became severe, and she developed frequent grand mal seizures. Hair mineral analysis revealed a markedly low manganese level. Manganese supplementation was started and the seizures rapidly disappeared. Repeat radiographic studies then showed evidence of a Pancoast tumor (a cancer at the top of her lung) as the actual cause of her pain.

NUTRITIONAL HEALING PLAN: Manganese Deficiency

Dosage: 20 mg of manganese daily

Zinc

Blood zinc levels are reduced in epileptics, most likely because of the disorder, although certain anticonvulsants can cause a zinc deficiency. Due to inadequate zinc in their diets, chronic alcoholics may develop seizures that respond to zinc supplementation.[27,28,29]

Whether zinc supplementation is beneficial in other situations is unproven. However, zinc supplementation has been shown to protect against the development of seizures in various experimental animal models of epilepsy, suggesting that it may have a natural anticonvulsant effect. If your doctor finds evidence of zinc deficiency, supplementation should be tried; otherwise the value of supplementary zinc is uncertain.[30]

NUTRITIONAL HEALING PLAN: Zinc

Dosage: 100 mg of zinc daily

Other Nutritional Factors

Dimethylglycine (DMG)

In the body, the substance dimethylglycine (DMG) is converted to glycine, a neuroinhibitory (brain-calming) amino acid. There is preliminary evidence that supplementation with DMG may occasionally reduce the frequency of seizures in people who respond poorly to anticonvulsant medications. Further studies are needed to determine more clearly if and when it is effective.[31]

NUTRITIONAL HEALING PLAN: Dimethylglycine

Dosage: 100 mg of dimethylglycine twice daily

Omega-6 Fatty Acids

WARNING

Supplementation with omega-6 fatty acids may worsen temporal-lobe epilepsy and therefore should be avoided.[32]

CHOOSING A PERSONAL PLAN

All epileptics should be on the Basic Healing diet and eat their meals at regular intervals. If seizures are easily provoked, large meals and excessive water consumption should be avoided. Alcohol and caffeine ingestion should be minimal.

If there are other symptoms that are typical of food sensitivities, consider trying a food-elimination diet. The ketogenic diet should not be tried except under medical supervision.

Best proven, and best understood, of the Nutritional Healing plans is the use of supplementary vitamin B_6 for the treatment of infantile seizures. If Vitamin B_6 dependency is suspected, a trial of supplementation is mandatory.

Deficiencies of several nutrients—including folic acid, vitamin B_6, copper, magnesium, manganese, and zinc—can cause seizures, and anticonvulsant medications can cause nutritional deficiencies. I would therefore suggest that epileptics, especially those on anticonvulsants, and most particularly those for whom the anticonvulsants are less than fully effective, be evaluated for vitamin and mineral deficiencies.

Even if you are not nutritionally deficient, several nutrients may be worth trying for a limited period of time to see if they reduce seizures. Though none of the following has been well proven, they are reasonably safe to try as long as your doctor agrees. Vitamin E is the best proven of the group, so vitamin E supplements would be the best way to start. Niacin, magnesium, zinc, and DMG may also be worth a try.

At the recommended dosages, it would be reasonable to try all the plans at once if you prefer. Then, if you are successful in reducing your seizures, try stopping one every two months to discover which nutrient(s) are responsible for your progress. Be sure to coordinate your experimentation with your physician so that anticonvulsant dosages can be adjusted accordingly.

ADDITIONAL SUGGESTIONS

In recent years, we have begun to recognize that, to some extent, people can achieve control over their seizures with mind control techniques. These include mental imagery, relaxation, and biofeedback training. Emotions can have an important role in precipitating seizures, so learning to deal more effectively with your emotions can also lead to improved seizure control.

Fatigue

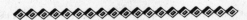

See also: Depression, Insomnia.

At least 50 percent of adults seeking medical treatment complain of fatigue. It may be constant, beginning in the morning after a full night's sleep, or it may build rapidly during the day until by nightfall the sufferer feels utterly exhausted. Though fatigue may be due to an underlying illness, often no evidence of another illness can be found.

DIETARY FACTORS

Food sensitivities have been accused of causing an "allergic tension-fatigue syndrome" consisting of hyperactivity and/or fatigue along with more classical allergy symptoms, such as bronchial asthma or a runny nose. Published reports of this syndrome go back half a century, although very little scientific investigation has been done to prove that these symptoms are caused by foods.

An example of food sensitivities causing fatigue is shown by the following case:

A 13-year-old boy with severe, poorly controlled bronchial asthma was strikingly pale with dark circles under his eyes. He was morose, listless, and lethargic and complained of headaches and pain in his muscles, joints, and belly. Every day he drank two pints of milk and ate chocolate or drank a cola-type beverage.

He was asked to avoid all dairy products and chocolate. Within 48 hours of stopping these foods, his facial pallor and the dark circles under his eyes almost completely disappeared. Most remarkable was the improvement in his mood and behavior. He became alert, cheer-

*ful, and interested in his surroundings. His physical complaints
ceased and his asthma became easy to control with medications.
   After three weeks, milk was added back to his diet. Within a week
his pallor and the dark circles under his eyes returned and he again
became morose, listless, and lethargic and behaved badly. He was
then returned to the therapeutic diet; his subsequent improvement
was as dramatic as before.[1]*

A poor diet may provide you with enough fuel as calories though fail
to provide you with adequate nutrients to take care of your metabolic
needs. If fact, you can even be overweight and still suffer from malnutrition
if much of your diet consists of foods that are low in nutrients.

Although caffeine can quickly relieve fatigue and increase endurance,
chronic caffeine use, at least at higher levels of ingestion, is a hidden cause
of fatigue. In a survey of a group of hospitalized psychiatric patients, 61
percent of those ingesting at least 750 mg of caffeine (at least 5 cups of
coffee) daily complained of tiring easily, compared to 54 percent of those
ingesting 250 to 749 mg daily, and only 24 percent of those ingesting less
than 250 mg daily.[2,3]

Evidence that chronic heavy caffeine use may cause fatigue comes from
an animal study that examined the effects of caffeine on the ability of mice
to swim. In contrast to a single dose of caffeine, six weeks' treatment with
caffeine greatly reduced their swimming capacity. The investigators' findings suggested that chronic caffeine ingestion may interfere with the ability
of muscles to utilize their available sources of energy.[4]

Since caffeine gives an initial energy boost but fatigue is a symptom of
caffeine withdrawal, a vicious cycle can be created in which a person
drinks increasing amounts of caffeine to prevent withdrawal fatigue.[5] This
can be seen in the following case:

*A middle-aged physician complained of constant fatigue and diffi-
culty falling asleep. Physical examination and laboratory testing
were normal. He was found to be drinking 15 cups of coffee daily
while in the hospital to "perk him up." Once weaned away from
coffee, he was soon feeling fine.[6]*

Like caffeine, refined sugar has long been suspected of acutely increasing energy but promoting fatigue when consumed at chronically high
levels. In one study, 16 people complaining of such symptoms as fatigue,
depression, headaches, and moodiness were placed on a diet free of
caffeine and refined sugar for up to 2 weeks. Those who improved were
given caffeine, a cellulose placebo, sugar-sweetened Kool-Aid, and aspar-
tame-sweetened Kool-Aid (fake sugar) to add to their diet regularly, one
at a time for six days each. Neither the researchers nor their subjects knew
when they were ingesting caffeine or sugar. When caffeine or sugar was

returned to their diets, but not when they were taking a placebo, 7 out of the 16 subjects (44 percent) reported that their symptoms and mood disturbances returned.[7]

Since carbohydrates promote the synthesis of serotonin, a calming neurotransmitter, a meal that consists primarily of carbohydrates (such as vegetarian pasta) can temporarily worsen fatigue. Carbohydrates are important for good nutrition, so this effect is no reason to avoid them. Be aware, however, that your energy level may be lower after eating a high-carbohydrate meal.[8]

THE HEALING DIET

1. Follow the Basic Healing diet as described in Appendix A.
2. Minimize regular consumption of caffeine.
3. Avoid foods found on testing to provoke fatigue. *See Appendix B for information about diagnosing food sensitivities.*

NUTRITIONAL HEALING PLANS

Vitamins

Folic Acid (Folate) Deficiency

Folic acid (folate) is the most common vitamin deficiency. A major survey found the average dietary folate of American adults to be only 61 percent of the U.S. RDA *(see Appendix E for an explanation of the U.S. RDA).* Adolescent and pregnant women, the elderly, and people with malabsorption are particularly prone to becoming folate-deficient. Folate deficiency is often easily diagnosed because it is commonly associated with anemia and neurological problems; however, the anemia may be absent and the neurological problems may be so minor that they are missed in a medical evaluation. When folate deficiency is associated with only minor neurological signs, fatigue is a prominent symptom along with depression and lassitude.[9,10]

A nutritionally trained physician can evaluate you for a folate deficiency. Since high-dose folic acid supplementation may cure the anemia of pernicious anemia (caused by a vitamin B_{12} deficiency) without preventing further damage to the nervous system, it is not recommended except under medical supervision.

The following case provides an example of a folate deficiency causing fatigue:

*An 81-year-old man ate poorly after the death of his wife. Initially
depressed by his wife's death, he seemed cheerful and was making
plans several months later. Gradually, however, he became increasingly apathetic and confused and began to complain of sharp, stab-
bing leg pains, easily tiring, blurred vision, and weakness. His bowel
movements were infrequent. Oral supplementation with a vitamin B
complex was ineffective.*

*The results of laboratory testing were consistent with folate defi-
ciency, and he was started on folic acid supplementation. After two
months, his folic acid levels normalized, and by the end of the second
month his symptoms had cleared.*[11]

Vitamin B_{12}

Vitamin B_{12} injections have long been used for the treatment of fatigue in
people with no evidence of vitamin B_{12} deficiency. The only scientific
proof of its efficacy comes from a study in which 28 people who complained of tiredness but had normal serum B_{12} levels and no physical
findings were given injections of either vitamin B_{12} or a placebo twice daily
for 2 weeks. Then, after a two-week rest period, they received the other
treatment for two weeks.

Those who received placebos first felt significantly better during the
second period when they received vitamin B_{12}. However, those who initially received vitamin B_{12} noted no differences between vitamin B_{12} and
the placebo. To explain these results, the investigators suggested that the
effects of the vitamin may persist for at least four weeks; thus people who
received vitamin B_{12} first were still feeling the effects of the vitamin while
they were receiving the placebo.[12]

In the absence of evidence of a marginal vitamin B_{12} deficiency, a
response to vitamin B_{12} does not prove that you are deficient in the
vitamin. As with most of the other applications for vitamin B_{12}, supplementation with this vitamin appears to reduce tiredness only when it is
given by injection. Your physician could start you off on a trial of B_{12}
injections and, if they appear to be effective, teach you to give them to
yourself.

The following case illustrates the benefits of vitamin B_{12} injections for
relieving fatigue:

*A 44-year-old male university professor complained of an inadequate
energy level. A thorough work-up had failed to find any abnormality.
He exercised regularly and ate a healthy diet. There was no evidence
of depression. He took 300 mcg injections of vitamin B_{12} 3 times a
week for 2 weeks and his tiredness vanished. Two or three weeks
after stopping the injections, however, his energy level lowered
again. He repeated the trial. Since the results were identical, he decided to continue to take the injections on a regular schedule.*[13]

NUTRITIONAL HEALING PLAN: Vitamin B$_{12}$

Dosage: 1000 mcg of vitamin B$_{12}$ every 1 to 4 weeks, as needed, by intramuscular injection

---

Vitamin C Deficiency

A survey of vitamin C intake among 411 dentists and their wives found that the average number of fatigue-related symptoms among the low-vitamin C users was double that among the relatively high users of the vitamin. These results are consistent with our knowledge that a marginal vitamin C deficiency impairs a person's ability to work, and that the performance deficit usually disappears following supplementation. They suggest that fatigue due to a vitamin C deficiency may be fairly common.[14,15]

It is not known whether vitamin C supplementation reduces chronic fatigue when it is not at least marginally deficient. However, since vitamin C is generally quite safe, a trial may be worthwhile even without laboratory testing to determine if you are marginally deficient.

NUTRITIONAL HEALING PLAN: Vitamin C Deficiency

Dosage: 1000 mg of vitamin C daily

Minerals

Iron Deficiency

Iron deficiency has been shown to be associated with both fatigue and a diminished work capacity even in the absence of an iron-deficiency anemia. In a double-blind study, about two-thirds of a group of chronically fatigued women improved following iron supplementation, even though they were not anemic.[16,17]

Iron should not be supplemented unless blood tests show evidence of a deficiency; too much iron may even be a cause of disabling fatigue. For example, fatigue is the most common symptom in hereditary hemo-chromatosis, a genetic disorder in which too much iron accumulates in the body.[18]

The benefits of iron supplementation for fatigue are shown by the following case:

A 34-year-old woman with constant tiredness for 20 years had no evidence of iron-deficiency anemia, but her serum ferritin (an iron-

*protein complex) was very low. She was started on iron supple-
ments. Four months later, her ferritin had risen into the normal range
and she no longer felt tired.*[19]

Potassium Deficiency

Along with muscle weakness, malaise is the most common symptom of
chronic potassium deficiency. The elderly, who are often potassium-deficient, have been shown to suffer from muscle weakness when they fail to
ingest adequate potassium in their diets. Your doctor can perform laboratory tests to determine whether you are potassium-deficient. Eating more
high-potassium foods should restore your strength and energy *(see Appendix D for a list of high-potassium foods)*.

The following case illustrates the benefits of a potassium-rich diet for
muscle weakness:

*A 78-year-old man complaining of increasing generalized muscle
weakness and rapid fatigue had a low level of whole blood potassium. Three months after the addition of fresh fruit and vegetable
juices to his diet, his energy and muscle strength had returned to
normal.*[23]

Sometimes a potassium deficiency cannot be corrected because there
is also a magnesium deficiency. Magnesium deficiency is common when
potassium is deficient, and must be corrected before potassium can be
normalized. Thus, if you are found to have a potassium deficiency, make
sure that your doctor also evaluates your magnesium levels.[24]

Zinc Deficiency

Perhaps half of the population of industrialized societies consumes less
than the U.S. RDA for zinc *(see Appendix E for an explanation of the U.S.
RDA)*. A marginal zinc deficiency can be associated with decreased muscle
strength and endurance and mental lethargy. Leukonychia (white spots on
the fingernails), believed to be an indicator of a lack of zinc, is said to
disappear within a few months after starting zinc supplementation.[25,26,27]

In a study of college students, 74 percent of 28 students who reported
themselves to be "very often drowsy" had leukonychia compared to only
46 percent of 11 students who reported themselves as "never drowsy."
Moreover, students with leukonychia were significantly more likely to
report longer sleep times.[28]

Laboratory testing will show if zinc is deficient. However, if you suffer
from chronic fatigue and have leukonychia, it would be reasonable to
undertake a trial of zinc supplementation.

NUTRITIONAL HEALING PLAN: Zinc Deficiency

Dosage: 100 mg of zinc daily

Other Nutritional Factors

Aspartic Acid

In addition to playing an important role in energy production, *aspartic acid* transports potassium and magnesium into the cell. The value of supplementation with potassium/magnesium aspartate for treating fatigue has been investigated in several double-blind studies. The results showed that between 75 and 91 percent of people treated with the aspartate salt experienced pronounced relief of fatigue compared to only 5 to 25 percent of people given placebos. Side effects, which were mild and uncommon, included mild gastrointestinal distress and dryness of the mouth.[29]

NUTRITIONAL HEALING PLAN: Aspartic Acid

Preparation

potassium/magnesium aspartate

Dosage: 1 g twice daily

Trial Period

ten days

Instructions: Supplementation can often be stopped after four to six weeks.

CHOOSING A PERSONAL PLAN

Follow the principles of the Basic Healing diet to ensure that you are meeting your fundamental nutritional needs. If you have a fairly high intake of caffeine, try avoiding it for at least two weeks. If you have reason to be suspicious of food sensitivities, go on a food-elimination diet and see if you feel more energetic.

Be particularly suspicious of one or more nutritional deficiencies causing your fatigue if you eat a "junk food" diet, have a problem absorbing nutrients, or are elderly. Consider having laboratory tests done to evaluate whether you have a marginal deficiency of folic acid, vitamin C, iron, potassium, or zinc. You may even wish to try increasing vitamin C, potassium, and zinc without first having laboratory testing.

If foods are not causing your fatigue, and you have no relevant nutritional deficiencies, potassium/magnesium aspartate is worth a trial. Vitamin B$_{12}$ is also worth trying; however, since it has to be taken by injection, you may wish to leave it for last.

Gallstones

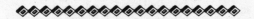

Bile, made by the liver, is stored in the gallbladder; from there it is eventually transferred into the intestines so that it can assist in the process of digestion. *Gallstones* are little rocklike balls, usually composed chiefly of cholesterol crystals, that can develop in the gallbladder. Gallstones can block the route of bile from the liver to the intestines, and can irritate the lining of the gallbladder, causing inflammation (cholecystitis). In industrialized countries, they are found in about 10 percent of the population.

DIETARY FACTORS

Diet appears to have a major influence on the development of gallstones. Both obesity and a high-fat diet are known to be risk factors, while losing excess weight appears to help reverse their course:[1]

> *A 41-year-old woman who was 55 pounds overweight had a large gallstone. She went on a 1000 calorie diet. After 15 months, she had lost 42 pounds and her gallstone had disappeared. Four months later, she was down to her ideal weight and her gallbladder was functioning normally.*[2]

Though the risk of gallstones is increased by the consumption of animal products, fiber intake decreases the risk. These relationships help to explain why a vegetarian diet has been repeatedly shown to be beneficial. Breakfast each morning also reduces the risk of gallstones, whereas overconsumption of carbohydrates, particularly of sugar, fosters their development.[3,4,5,6,7]

Surprisingly, both alcohol and caffeine decrease the risk of developing gallstones. I would still advise you to consume them in moderation, however, because of their adverse effects on health at higher levels of intake. Also, coffee, regardless of its caffeine content, may cause painful gallbladder spasms in people with gallbladder disease.[8,9,10]

If you have gallstones, consumption of fat in any form may bring on a wave of gallbladder spasms. The more solid a fat is at room temperature, the more it stimulates the gallbladder to contract.[11,12]

Food sensitivities are often an unrecognized cause of gallbladder symptoms. When 69 people with gallbladder symptoms were placed on an elimination diet consisting of beef, rye, soy, rice, cherry, peach, apricot, beet, and spinach, **all** of them were relieved of their symptoms. Improvements usually occurred in three to five days.

After a week on the diet, one food that had been eliminated from their diets was added every few days. If it produced symptoms, it was retested several times. Eggs were by far the most frequent offenders; 93 percent of the people studied developed gallbladder symptoms after eating it. Pork was the next most frequent, (64 percent), followed by onions (52 percent).[13]

The following case illustrates how food sensitivities can cause gallbladder pain:

A woman had a ten-year history of indigestion after some meals. The indigestion gradually worsened until she was having pain under her right ribs. Reducing her fat intake helped slightly. Two years prior to her medical evaluation, she had awoken in the middle of the night after an unusually large meal with intense pain that was diagnosed as cholecystitis (inflammation of the gallbladder). The symptoms continued to worsen until she was bedridden four to five days each month. She eliminated all fats, oils, and spices from her diet without improvement. X-rays revealed two gallbladder stones.

She began a food-elimination diet that restricted her to beef, rye, soy, rice, cherry, peach, apricot, beet, and spinach. One week later, she reported that she had had no pain for three days. She was told to reintroduce foods singly and found that ingestion of eggs, chicken, coffee, peanuts, onions, carrots, and wheat provoked gallbladder pain. Two years later, she reported that she had remained fully asymptomatic.[14]

THE HEALING DIET

1. Eat a low-fat, low-sugar, high-fiber diet as described in Appendix A.
2. If you find a vegetarian diet too restrictive, follow the Basic Healing diet *(see Appendix A for detailed information).*

3. If you are overweight, modify your diet so as to gradually achieve your ideal weight *(see the chapter on obesity for specific dietary information)*.
4. Eat breakfast daily.
5. Avoid foods found on testing to provoke gallbladder symptoms. *See Appendix B for information about diagnosing food sensitivities.*
6. Avoid coffee if it provokes gallbladder symptoms.

NUTRITIONAL HEALING PLANS

Vitamins

Vitamin C Deficiency

When given a high-cholesterol diet, animals made deficient in vitamin C are prone to developing gallstones. This appears to be the result of the combination of decreased bile acids and increased cholesterol in their blood and livers.[15]

Vitamin C supplementation failed to change the fat composition of the bile of normal volunteers, which suggests that, if it does help to prevent gallstones, it may do so only in people who are marginally deficient in vitamin C.[16]

NUTRITIONAL HEALING PLAN: Vitamin C Deficiency

Dosage: not well established, but 1000 mg of vitamin C daily would be reasonable

---

Vitamin E

Like vitamin C, a deficiency of vitamin E is associated, at least in animals, with gallstone formation. Adequate vitamin E nutrition protects against the formation of gallstones in animals given large amounts of cholesterol or fat, whereas vitamin E-deficient animals develop cholesterol stones even while on a fat-free, cholesterol-free diet. These findings suggest that the adequacy of vitamin E in the diet is more important than the amount of fat or cholesterol.[17,18]

Results of another animal study suggest how effective vitamin E supplementation might be if a person with gallstones who was deficient in vitamin E received the vitamin. In these animals, vitamin E supplementation actually dissolved their gallstones.[19]

A pilot study gave five people with cholesterol gallstones who were not known to be deficient in vitamin E a high dosage of the vitamin to see what would happen. Though their gallstones did not dissolve, their tendency to form gallstones was reduced.[20]

NUTRITIONAL HEALING PLAN: Vitamin E

Preparation

D-alpha tocopherol

Dosage: 200 mg (300 IU) 3 times daily

Other Nutritional Factors

Taurine

The amino acid *taurine* is no stranger to the bile, since bile acids are often chemically linked to taurine. When animals are given a diet that encourages cholesterol gallstone formation, taurine supplementation inhibits the formation of gallstones by increasing the formation of bile acids.[21,22]

In humans, taurine supplementation has been shown under controlled conditions to reduce the risk of gallstones. In theory, women are better candidates for taurine supplementation, since they are more prone to gallstones, have lower levels of the enzymes needed to make taurine, and may be more affected by dietary taurine deficiency.[23]

NUTRITIONAL HEALING PLAN: Taurine

Dosage: not well established, but 1000 mg of taurine daily would be reasonable

---

Other Factors: Hydrochloric Acid (HCl) Deficiency

The formation of gallstones appears to be associated with the backward movement of bile and pancreatic juices into the stomach. These juices can destroy the gastric acid-producing cells, causing flatulent dyspepsia (gas and indigestion) as well as other symptoms of hydrochloric acid (HCl) deficiency. About half of all people with gallstones are deficient in HCl.[24]

In a pilot study, people who were deficient in HCl were occasionally relieved of symptoms of gas, abdominal fullness and burning, diarrhea, and hives with HCl supplementation. Supplementation had no effect, however, on food sensitivities or such symptoms as nausea, abdominal pain, constipation, bad breath, burning tongue, or metallic taste.[25]

Stomach acid is necessary for the ability of the body to properly utilize nutrients. Also, a deficiency increases both the susceptibility to and the severity of bacterial infections of the intestines. Therefore, in addition to its possible value in reducing symptoms, HCl supplementation is suggested for anyone who is found on testing to be deficient.

NUTRITIONAL HEALING PLAN: Hydrochloric Acid (HCl) Deficiency

Preparation

10-gr capsules of betaine or glutamic HCl

Instructions: See Appendix C for detailed instructions.

CHOOSING A PERSONAL PLAN

If you are prone to developing gallstones, follow the principles of the Basic Healing diet, and consider becoming a vegetarian. Plan a trial of a food-elimination diet to discover whether you are food sensitive.

Though dietary changes make good sense, the value of supplementation is much less clear. I would suggest that you see a nutritionally trained physician in order to rule out deficiencies of vitamin C and hydrochloric acid. If either deficiency is found, supplementation is clearly indicated to correct it.

Further studies are needed to clarify the efficacy of vitamin E and taurine supplementation in combating the development of gallstones. Since these supplements appear to be reasonably safe, and their results appear promising, they may be worth taking, with the approval of your doctor.

Glaucoma

Glaucoma, a condition in which there is increased pressure within the eyeball, is the second leading cause of blindness in the industrialized nations. In its most common form, it develops slowly and without warning, first causing halos to appear around lights, a narrowing of the visual field, intermittent blurred vision, watering of the eye, and vague headaches or eyestrain. Medications and surgery can often control glaucoma but do not always keep the disease from progressing.

DIETARY FACTORS

Food sensitivities, as well as classical allergic reactions, may increase eyeball tension in some people with chronic simple glaucoma.[1,2]

A 46-year-old woman had been treated for 4 years for glaucoma of her right eye. She complained of sharp pain over that eye as well as of severe gastrointestinal distress and chronic constipation. Her right eyelids were swollen and red, and the white of the eye looked pink from congestion with blood. Eyeball tension was 30 mm Hg in the right eye compared to 12 mm Hg in the normal left eye. There was also evidence of sinus inflammation.

Drug treatment was unsuccessful and surgical procedures only reduced her intraocular tension, which rose at times to 60 mm Hg. After almost two years, her tension began to rise again, this time in both eyes. She was tested for food sensitivities and eliminated reactive foods. Two weeks later, while continuing on the same dose of pilocarpine (a medication to reduce the tension), her intraocular tension had reduced to the normal range and her gastrointestinal symp-

*toms had disappeared for the first time in her memory. One year after
starting the diet, despite stopping pilocarpine two months earlier,
her tension was still lower.*[5]

Ninety minutes after ingestion, caffeine has been shown to increase
eyeball tension in people with glaucoma. Until more studies are completed, we will not know whether this temporary increase in tension
affects the course of the illness; in the meantime, caffeine avoidance appears worthwhile.[4]

Although not directly studied, there are reasons to believe that it may
be beneficial to include plenty of vegetables in your diet. For example,
rutin, which is commonly found in vegetables, has been shown to reduce
eyeball tension in people with glaucoma. Also, one scientist was unable
to find cases of glaucoma among a racial group who were mainly vegetarians and fish eaters, suggesting that something in their diet was protective.[4]

THE HEALING DIET

1. Avoid foods found to increase eyeball tension. *See Appendix B for
   information about diagnosing food sensitivities.*
2. Avoid caffeine.
3. Eat plenty of vegetables.

NUTRITIONAL HEALING PLANS

Vitamins

Thiamine (Vitamin B₁) Deficiency

Though not well proven, a thiamine (vitamin B_1) deficiency may contribute to the development of glaucoma. This possibility is strongest in regard
to degeneration of the optic nerve—a common finding in glaucoma.
There is preliminary evidence that people with chronic open-angle glaucoma may not be able to absorb thiamine normally. Thus, even if their
dietary intake of thiamine is normal, their blood thiamine level may be
relatively low.[5]

When thiamine deficiency is corrected by supplementation, some recovery appears to be possible. There is, however, no evidence that thiamine supplementation is helpful unless it is deficient.[6] (Your doctor can
determine if you have adequate thiamine.)

NUTRITIONAL HEALING PLAN: Thiamine Deficiency

Dosage: 100 mg of thiamine daily

Instructions: Take by intramuscular injection for ten days.
Then take oral supplementation as needed to maintain a
normal blood thiamine level.

Vitamin C

Though thiamine supplementation appears helpful only when there is
deficiency of the vitamin, vitamin C may be helpful even though people
with glaucoma usually have normal levels of this vitamin in both the
bloodstream and the eye. Clinical trials have shown that oral vitamin C
supplementation can lower eyeball pressure, and one study has found
vitamin C to be effective when applied as eyedrops. However, for unexplained reasons, other studies have found no improvement in eyeball
pressure following supplementation with the vitamin.[7,8,9,10,11]

NUTRITIONAL HEALING PLAN: Vitamin C

Dosage: not well established, but 500 mg 4 times daily
would be reasonable

Trial Period

six weeks

Botanical Extracts: Rutin

In a pilot study, the administration of rutin, a common plant constituent,
for 4 or more weeks reduced eyeball pressure at least 15 percent in the
majority of people with primary glaucoma. Further studies are needed to
confirm this finding.[12]

NUTRITIONAL HEALING PLAN: Rutin

Dosage:
20 mg three times daily

CHOOSING A PERSONAL PLAN

We do not know how frequently food sensitivities raise eyeball pressure, but this possibility is greatest if you have other symptoms that are suggestive of food sensitivities. Unless your glaucoma is producing pain, swelling of the eyelids, or other obvious symptoms, you will need to have your eyeball pressure checked both before and after you go on a food-elimination diet in order to discover whether food sensitivities are affecting your glaucoma.

There is also little evidence to prove the value of eating plenty of vegetables and eliminating caffeine. However, these are safe and simple measures to take that are certainly worth trying.

Your doctor can evaluate you for a marginal thiamine deficiency to determine whether thiamine supplementation may be of value. Everyone, by contrast, should give vitamin C supplementation a trial. If rutin is available, it may also be worth trying, perhaps in combination with vitamin C.

Heartburn

See also: PEPTIC ULCERS.

Heartburn is a burning pain caused by the return of stomach contents back into the esophagus. The pain rises from the midline of the chest and can extend into the neck, throat, or face. It usually occurs after eating, especially when lying down.

DIETARY FACTORS

Normally, once food has traveled down the esophagus and entered the stomach, a valve (the lower esophageal sphincter) closes to prevent the mixture of food and stomach acid from re-entering the esophagus, which is unprotected from the irritating effects of the acid mixture. Starting about half an hour after they are consumed, certain foods relax the valve. For most people, this action is harmless. People who tend to experience heartburn, however, may develop symptoms after eating these foods, especially if their heartburn is due to the valve's failure to close tightly.[1]

Once heartburn has become chronic, other foods may increase the pain and inflammation by directly irritating the inflamed lining of the lower esophagus on their way to the stomach. (This is probably the reason why certain spicy foods cause heartburn.) Foods may also worsen symptoms by decreasing the force of the wave of muscle contractions that propel foods into the stomach (peristalsis) or by stimulating production of extra stomach acid.[2]

The Healing Diet

1. The foods listed in the following chart contribute to heartburn, so try to avoid them if you are symptomatic.[3,4,5,6,7,8,9,10]

FOODS THAT CAN CAUSE HEARTBURN

alcohol
chocolate
coffee
fats (fatty meals)
milk
orange juice
peppermint
spearmint
spicy foods
sugar
tea
tomato juice and products

---

2. If you tend to suffer from heartburn, drink plenty of water, especially after meals. Water soothes the irritated esophageal lining by flushing the mixture of food and stomach acid back into the stomach.
3. Keep your meals small because large meals distend the stomach, causing strain on the esophageal muscle.
4. Excess weight increases the pressure in the abdomen. This increases the tendency for the stomach contents to be pushed back up into the esophagus. Therefore, if you are overweight, plan to lose your extra pounds.

NUTRITIONAL HEALING PLANS

Certain minerals can reduce heartburn by neutralizing stomach acid. See the chapter on peptic ulcers for detailed information.

ADDITIONAL SUGGESTIONS

Though vigorous exercise like running, tennis, or weight lifting may worsen heartburn by increasing abdominal pressure, moderate exercise, like brisk walking, may help to prevent it.

Emotional distress increases stomach-acid secretion, so it is important to learn to keep calm, especially during and after meals.

Use gravity to reduce symptoms. When heartburn occurs, try to stand up rather than lie down so that gravity can encourage stomach acid to flow back into the stomach. Don't lie down for three hours after eating, and don't eat just before going to bed. Lift the head of your bed up on six-inch blocks to keep your esophagus higher than your stomach while you sleep.

Heart Disease

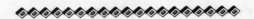

See also: CATARACTS, DIABETES, OBESITY.

Coronary heart disease resulting from *atherosclerosis* is the most common cause of death among adults in industrialized societies. Heart disease develops as the coronary arteries, which provide oxygen and nutrients to the heart muscle, become clogged as the result of the complex process called atherosclerosis. As it becomes progressively less able to obtain vital supplies, the heart muscle's ability to pump blood is increasingly threatened.

HELPFUL DEFINITIONS

Before reading this chapter, you will find it helpful to learn a few definitions:

▶ **Angina pectoris.** Pain, usually a crushing pain, especially in the left chest, resulting from inadequate blood flow to the heart.

▶ **Atherosclerosis.** Hardening of the arteries associated with irregularly distributed fat deposits in their inner linings.

▶ **Cholesterol.** The most abundant steroid in animal tissues, especially in the bile. Elevated levels are associated with the development of atherosclerosis.

▶ **LDL cholesterol.** Low-density lipoprotein cholesterol; the "bad" cholesterol. The higher it is, the greater the risk of atherosclerosis.

▶ **HDL cholesterol.** High-density lipoprotein cholesterol; the "good" cholesterol. The higher it is, the less the risk of atherosclerosis.

▶ **Fatty acids.** Components of fats, some of which affect the risk of atherosclerosis.

▶ **Lipids.** Substances that are soluble in fat rather than in water. Includes cholesterol and triglycerides.

▶ **Thrombosis.** Clotting within a blood vessel. If a thrombosis occurs in a coronary artery, it may cause a heart attack by reducing the blood supply to the heart.

▶ **Triglycerides.** Blood fats. Composed of glycerol attached to three fatty acids. Nutritional factors are now known to play a major role in the development of atherosclerosis, and we are gradually learning how to manipulate these factors to affect the course of the disease. For example, cholesterol levels in the blood serum, which tend to respond to nutritional factors, are closely related to heart disease risk; for every 1 percent rise in serum cholesterol, the risk of developing heart disease increases by almost 3 percent. In fact, it may be possible to slowly **reverse** the process, especially if serum cholesterol levels are lowered far enough.

DIETARY FACTORS

Obesity

Obesity, defined as a body weight 20 to 30 percent above the ideal weight, contributes to elevated levels of blood fats. If you are obese and have an elevated serum cholesterol, weight loss may significantly reduce your cholesterol levels and your risk of developing heart disease.[1]

Fat and Cholesterol

Generally, the more fat there is in your diet, the higher the cholesterol level will be in your blood. No more than 30 percent of your calories should come from fat. Some experts suggest that limiting fat to 10 percent of calories is ideal, but many people are unable or unwilling to make the sacrifices that such a strict diet requires.[2]

Not all dietary fats have the same effects, however, and the picture has become increasingly complicated as the effects of individual fatty acids, which determine the differences between fats, have been examined. Saturated fats bear much of the responsibility for the adverse effects of fats because they promote not only atherosclerosis but also the development of clots within the blood vessels. Moreover, saturated fat brings down the HDL cholesterol level.[3,4]

Saturating an unsaturated vegetable oil by hydrogenation to make it solid at room temperature or to increase its shelf life, as is done with margarine, makes the oil less desirable for the health of your arteries. Despite the massive advertising campaign for margarine as a butter substitute, whether it is better than butter is an unsettled question; there is even reason to believe that it may be worse.[5,6]

Generally, polyunsaturated fats are half as powerful in lowering total serum cholesterol levels as saturated fats are in raising them. While polyunsaturates lower LDL cholesterol levels, HDL cholesterol levels are unaffected or may even be lowered. Oleic acid, a monounsaturate that is abundant in olive oil, has also been found to lower LDL cholesterol.[7,8,9]

Most people do not realize that serum cholesterol levels are considerably more sensitive to saturated fat in the diet than to dietary cholesterol; reducing dietary cholesterol to low levels may thus be of no value for people following a low-fat, high-fiber diet. People with elevated cholesterol levels can benefit by minimizing cholesterol in their diets; most people with normal cholesterol levels probably do not need to limit cholesterol to less than average levels of intake.[10,11,12]

In summary, a heart-protective diet must be low in total fat. What fat is eaten should come primarily from polyunsaturates and monounsaturates. Cholesterol intake may be moderate as long as the diet is also high in soluble fiber and serum cholesterol is not elevated.

Vegetables

Any diet designed to combat atherosclerosis should emphasize the consumption of vegetables. Low in saturated fatty acids and cholesterol-free, vegetables are high in dietary fiber. Water-soluble fibers, such as oat bran, pectin, psyllium, and guar gum, help to keep serum cholesterol low by binding cholesterol in the gut to prevent its absorption into the bloodstream; water-insoluble fibers, such as wheat bran, are less effective. With their high-fiber content, just two carrots a day may lower elevated serum cholesterol levels by 10 to 20 percent.[13,14,15]

Several vegetables have been investigated for their specific benefits. Common beans—such as pinto, navy, and kidney beans—and alfalfa seeds have been shown to lower total serum cholesterol levels. Garlic and onions may protect against thrombosis (blood clots) while helping to normalize blood lipids. Ginger may be as effective as aspirin in protecting against thrombosis; in one study, it was more effective than garlic or onions.[16,17,18,19]

Not surprisingly, when serum cholesterol levels are compared, vegans (who avoid all animal products) have the lowest total and LDL cholesterol levels and meat eaters have the highest; vegetarians and fish eaters who avoid meat have values that are in between. HDL cholesterol, which is protective, is highest in fish eaters.[20]

Dairy Products

The effect of cow's milk on cholesterol depends upon its butterfat content. Whole milk is only 4 percent fat by weight; however, 48 percent of its calories come from fat. Though it raises HDL cholesterol, it raises LDL cholesterol about three times as much. "Low-fat" milk (2 percent fat by weight, but with 31 percent of calories from fat, making it a high-fat food) has a slight total cholesterol-lowering effect, while skim or nonfat milk (3 percent of calories from fat) lowers elevated total cholesterol levels.[21,22,23]

Yogurt, even without reduction of its fat content, tends to reduce total cholesterol. Although it remains to be studied, reducing the fat content of yogurt most likely increases its efficacy in lowering elevated cholesterol levels.[24]

Sugar

Long-term consumption of excessive sugar increases the risk of coronary heart disease. Associations have been found between sugar intake and increased total cholesterol and triglycerides, as well as decreased HDL cholesterol. In addition, urinary chromium loss is increased, and chromium deficiency is a risk factor for coronary heart disease. A reasonable goal would be to restrict your consumption of sugar to fewer than 10 percent of your total calories.[25,26,27,28]

Alcohol

Although heavy alcohol consumption is clearly detrimental to your health, there is some evidence that moderate alcohol consumption (up to two drinks per day) can reduce the risk of coronary heart disease and its complications. However, as there is also evidence that even moderate alcohol consumption can promote coronary heart disease as well as breast cancer, stroke, and other diseases, consumption of even moderate amounts of alcohol cannot be recommended.[29,30]

Coffee

Coffee consumption appears to raise total cholesterol levels, and abstention has reduced cholesterol in men with elevated cholesterol levels, yet certain issues about this apparent relationship, including the role of caffeine, are unresolved. Even studies exploring the relationship between coffee ingestion and the risk of coronary heart disease have had contradictory results. Differences in brewing methods may be relevant. In one study, for example, consumption of boiled (but not filtered or instant) coffee was the main explanation for the strong association between coffee and cholesterol levels. Since there is evidence that heavy coffee drinkers eat much more saturated fat than those that don't drink coffee, it may be that we are merely looking again at the relationship between saturated fat and atherosclerosis.[31,32,33,34]

THE HEALING DIET

1. Follow the Basic Healing diet as described in Appendix A.
2. Minimize coffee consumption.

NUTRITIONAL HEALING PLANS

The Homocysteine Theory of Atherosclerosis

The causes of atherosclerosis are still not well understood and, as with other degenerative diseases, appear to be a combination of hereditary and environmental factors. The *homocysteine theory* was formulated by Kilmer McCully, professor of pathology at Harvard Medical School, who theorized that the initial damage to blood vessels that eventually leads to the development of atherosclerosis is caused by the accumulation of the toxic amino acid *homocysteine*. For example, homocysteine infused directly into the veins of baboons has been shown to produce clogging of their arteries.[35,36]

Homocystinuria (the removal of excessive homocysteine in the urine) in adequately nourished people is a genetic disorder characterized by a deficiency in the enzyme needed to break down homocysteine. Homozygous homocystinuria, which is inherited from both parents, is very rare. However, roughly 1 out of 70 people have heterozygous homocystinuria (that is, they have inherited the defective gene from one parent); these people are predisposed to developing coronary heart disease unless they are treated with especially high amounts of folic acid, vitamin B_6, and vitamin B_{12}—the nutrients needed to break down homocysteine. Even more important, inadequate supplies of these three vitamins may promote coronary heart disease in the general population by fostering homocysteine accumulation.[37]

Dr. McCully blames the Western diet for promoting homocysteine accumulation and its consequences. He points out that not only does modern food processing destroy vitamin B_6, but animal protein has two to three times as much methionine as plant protein by weight (homocysteine comes from methionine) and is lower in B_6. (This may be another reason why vegetarian diets are associated with a decreased risk of coronary heart disease.)[38]

If your physician's laboratory can measure plasma and urine homocysteine levels, you can discover whether your levels are elevated; if so, you could benefit from a nutritional program designed to lower those levels. After following the program for several weeks, a repeat study would assess your progress.

Vitamins

Folic Acid (Folate)

With the aid of folic acid (folate), toxic homocysteine can be converted back to methionine, an amino acid that does not foster arterial damage. The lower the level of folic acid in the blood, the higher the level of homocysteine. In fact, homocysteine levels can be reduced by supplementation with folic acid, even in people whose blood folic acid levels are normal.[39,40]

NUTRITIONAL HEALING PLAN: Folic Acid

Suggested Use

reduce elevated homocysteine levels

Dosage: **5 mg of folic acid daily**

WARNING

Folic acid, at this high a dosage, should be taken under medical supervision.

Niacin (Vitamin B₃)

Niacin (a form of vitamin B_3) is so well established as being effective for lowering elevated LDL cholesterol levels that it has been recommended as the "first drug to be used" when dietary intervention is inadequate. It has also been shown to be effective in raising HDL cholesterol and in lowering triglycerides.[41,42]

In one long-term study, men with a previous heart attack who took niacin daily for an average of six years were less likely to suffer from another, nonfatal heart attack than men with a similar history who didn't take niacin. Moreover, even 15 years after the study began, they continued to have a lower death rate than the men who didn't take niacin.[43]

Unfortunately, at the high doses needed to be effective, niacin can have significant side effects. Most common is a flush due to the release of histamine into the body; it starts about 20 minutes after taking niacin and can last for one and a half hours. The flush usually is reduced after three days on niacin supplementation and may later disappear. It can be minimized by taking niacin with meals, raising the dosage gradually, and, if necessary, by temporarily taking 300 mg of aspirin 15 to 30 minutes before taking the niacin.

Both flushing and itching, another niacin side effect, are harmless. Other potential side effects, however, although rare, are more worrisome. These include elevated uric acid, liver inflammation, skin pigmentation, and diabetes. Because of these dangers, and because you need your doctor to monitor your blood lipid levels, high-dose niacin supplementation should be taken under medical supervision.

NUTRITIONAL HEALING PLAN: Niacin

Suggested Use

normalize blood lipids

> *Dosage:* Start with 100 mg of niacin 3 times daily with meals.

Increase by 100 mg 3 times daily each week to a maximum of 1 g 3 times daily if needed to achieve adequate results.

WARNING

Take under medical supervision.

Vitamin B₆

Investigators have repeatedly shown that animals given a vitamin B_6-deficient diet develop widespread atherosclerosis. The reasons for this important finding are only gradually becoming understood. We have already listed vitamin B_6 as one of the nutrients needed to reduce the level of the toxic amino acid homocysteine. Later, we will discuss its role in regulating essential fatty acids. There is also early evidence that vitamin B_6 may help to protect you from a heart attack that results from a clot forming in a damaged coronary artery. Finally, though more evidence is needed, it is suspected that vitamin B$_6$ may play a role in regulating the level of fats in the blood.[44]

NUTRITIONAL HEALING PLAN: Vitamin B$_6$

Suggested Use

▸ combat the development of atherosclerosis (if deficient)
▸ reduce the risk of clots in the coronary arteries
▸ normalize blood lipids
▸ reduce elevated homocysteine levels

Preparation

pyridoxine

Dosage: 40 mg daily

Pantethine

Pantethine is the active form of pantothenic acid, one of the vitamins in the vitamin B complex. In several studies, supplementation with pantethine decreased elevated cholesterol and triglyceride levels. When pantethine was compared to a standard cholesterol-lowering drug (fenofibrate), it was just as effective, but without the side effects of the drug.[45,46]

NUTRITIONAL HEALING PLAN: Pantethine

Suggested Use

normalize blood lipids

Dosage: 300 mg of pantethine 2 to 4 times daily with food

Vitamin C

There are at least three reasons why a marginal vitamin C deficiency can contribute to atherosclerosis:

1. **Fat metabolism.** Vitamin C stimulates the enzyme that breaks down triglycerides (blood fats).
2. **Cholesterol metabolism.** Vitamin C stimulates the enzyme that converts cholesterol into bile acids.
3. **Arterial wall integrity.** Vitamin C is required for the formation of collagen, which provides strength to the vessel walls.

In coronary heart disease, the level of vitamin C, or *ascorbic acid,* in the white blood cells is significantly decreased. The level of ascorbic acid in the plasma (the fluid portion of the blood) correlates with the HDL cholesterol level; when both are low, supplementation with vitamin C may raise HDL cholesterol while also decreasing LDL cholesterol. Even if vitamin C levels are normal, supplementation may lower total cholesterol and diminish the tendency toward thrombosis.[47,48,49,50]

NUTRITIONAL HEALING PLAN: Vitamin C

Suggested Use

▶ normalize blood lipids
▶ reduce the risk of thrombosis
   Dosage: 1 g of vitamin C 3 times daily

Vitamin D Excess

Although increasing the intake of a number of nutrients appears to be beneficial, the intake of vitamin D can at times be too high, and should not exceed the U.S. RDA for adults *(see Appendix E for RDA values).* Elevated cholesterol levels may be associated with a high daily intake of vitamin D, and studies of pigs suggest that too much vitamin D may weaken arteries.[51,52]

There is still no proof that excess vitamin D accelerates atherosclerosis in humans; it seems prudent, however, to guard against excessive vitamin D intake. With so many foods fortified with vitamin D, multivitamins that include vitamin D, and livestock that have been fed high levels of vitamin D prior to slaughter, the possibility of vitamin D toxicity should not be overlooked.

Vitamin E

Vitamin E is known to protect against tissue damage resulting from a destructive process called lipid peroxidation, and there is evidence that the vitamin is involved in the growth and repair of the inner lining of the arterial walls. The higher the vitamin E levels of a group of middle-aged men, the lower their risk of dying from coronary heart disease.[53,54]

Even when your body is not low in vitamin E, supplementation can help. Several studies have found HDL cholesterol levels to rise with vitamin E supplementation, and there is some evidence that vitamin E may reduce the tendency for thrombosis.[55,56,57]

NUTRITIONAL HEALING PLAN: Vitamin E

Suggested Use

▶ protect the coronary arteries (if deficient)
▶ increase HDL cholesterol
▶ prevent coronary thrombosis

Dosage: 600 IU of vitamin E daily

WARNING

Because vitamin E strengthens the heartbeat, people with heart disease or high blood pressure should take no more than 100 IU daily except under medical supervision.

Minerals

Calcium

The intake of calcium in Western diets is often inadequate, yet adequate calcium can help to protect us against atherosclerosis. Calcium supplementation has been proven to decrease elevated cholesterol levels in humans.[58,59]

One animal study produced intriguing preliminary findings. Like humans, rabbits can develop atherosclerosis. In fact, when they are fed the same type of diet that promotes atherosclerosis in humans, they readily develop the disease. In this particular study, rabbits that were fed an atherosclerosis-promoting diet that was also low in calcium developed pronounced atherosclerosis. However, when other rabbits were fed the same diet but were supplemented with calcium, two out of three failed to develop evidence of the disease. Moreover, when the arteries of the calcium-supplemented rabbits were compared to those of the low-calcium rabbits, the amount of cholesterol deposited in their arteries was greatly reduced.[60]

NUTRITIONAL HEALING PLAN: Calcium

Suggested Use

▶ normalize blood lipids
▶ protect against atherosclerosis

Preparation

calcium citrate

Dosage: 500 mg daily

Chromium

Our dietary intake of chromium is often marginal, yet studies suggest that low chromium levels increase the risk of atherosclerosis. Supplementation with the better-absorbed organic forms of chromium (such as that found in brewer's yeast) appears to lower serum triglycerides and LDL cholesterol while raising HDL cholesterol.[61,62]

NUTRITIONAL HEALING PLAN: Chromium

Suggested Use

▶ protect against atherosclerosis
▶ normalize blood lipids

Preparations and Dosages

200 mcg of chromium daily, **or**
20 g (2 tbsp) of brewer's yeast daily

Magnesium

Magnesium is another mineral whose intake is often inadequate. In many people experiencing heart attacks, the amount of magnesium in the body tissues is not only depressed but actually deficient. In fact, magnesium deficiency is associated with an increased risk of coronary artery disease, heart attacks, irregular heartbeats, and sudden cardiac death. In addition to the direct effects of magnesium deficiency, when the heart muscle is magnesium-deficient it is unable to retain potassium, so it also suffers from the effects of potassium deficiency.[63,64,65]

Magnesium supplementation has been shown to combat the development of atherosclerosis and reduce the risk of irregular heartbeats, angina due to the spasm of the coronary arteries, and death following a heart attack. It may also reduce total blood cholesterol levels while raising HDL cholesterol.[66,67]

Water hardness usually results from the presence of calcium and magnesium salts. Since dietary intakes of calcium and magnesium may often be too low, hard water is preferable to soft water for drinking, as shown by both human and animal studies.[68]

NUTRITIONAL HEALING PLAN: Magnesium

Suggested Use

▶ reduce the risk of angina due to coronary artery spasm
▶ reduce the risk of death following a heart attack
▶ normalize blood lipids
▶ reduce the risk of coronary artery thrombosis
▶ protect the coronary arteries

Dosage: 400 mg of magnesium daily

Selenium

As with calcium, chromium, and magnesium, many Western diets are inadequate in selenium. A low level of selenium in the body increases the risk of having a heart attack, whereas selenium supplementation may reduce the risk.[69,70,71]

NUTRITIONAL HEALING PLAN: Selenium

Suggested Use

reduce the risk of a heart attack

Dosage: 200 mcg of selenium daily

Other Nutritional Factors

Carnitine

A naturally occurring amino acid found in all living tissue, *carnitine* is ingested preformed in foods—animal foods are its primary dietary source—or synthesized in the liver. Because it is required to transport long-chain fatty acids within cells, depletion can cause these fatty acids to accumulate rather than being burned up to create energy.

If the heart is suffering from inadequate oxygen due to a reduced blood supply from the coronary arteries, supplementation with carnitine appears to allow the heart to function longer before symptoms develop. It has been proven effective for the treatment of angina pectoris in several studies. In addition, carnitine supplementation may reduce total cholesterol and triglycerides and increase HDL cholesterol:[72,73,74,75]

A 50-year-old man began to note mild chest pain with exercise at age forty-seven. His cholesterol and triglycerides were elevated, and exercise testing revealed EKG abnormalities. He was told by his cardiologist to enroll in a medically supervised exercise program and was prescribed nitroglycerin for pain as well as other medications.

He failed to improve, so three years prior to evaluation he began his own nutritional program. He avoided red meat, caffeine, sugar, and white flour, reduced animal protein, restricted alcohol, and took a multivitamin along with vitamin C, vitamin E, selenium, zinc, lecithin, dolomite, garlic oil, sunflower or safflower oil, and brewer's yeast.

Over the next two years his total cholesterol dropped from 388 to 255, his triglycerides went from 417 to 165, and his angina improved "80 percent," although he continued to show exercise-related EKG changes. His cardiologist was able to slowly discontinue his medications. By the time he was seen for a nutritional consultation he required nitroglycerin only occasionally but had made no further progress in the preceding year.

Carnitine was then added to his own program. Six months later his angina was gone, even with maximal exertion, and the exercise-related EKG changes were almost nonexistent. His triglycerides were further reduced to 114, and his total cholesterol had dropped to 195.[76]

NUTRITIONAL HEALING PLAN: Carnitine

Suggested Use

▶ prevent and reduce angina pectoris
▶ normalize blood lipids

Preparation

L-carnitine

Dosage: 750 mg twice daily

Coenzyme Q_{10} (CoQ$_{10}$)

Coenzyme Q_{10} is a vitaminlike substance found primarily in the heart muscle. Like all muscles, the heart muscle needs adequate energy to contract, and CoQ$_{10}$ facilitates the production of that energy. In people with coronary heart disease, supplementation reduces the frequency of anginal episodes and increases the amount of physical exercise that a person can perform before developing anginal pain.[77]

NUTRITIONAL HEALING PLAN: Coenzyme Q$_{10}$

Suggested Use

reduce angina pectoris

Dosage: 30 mg once or twice daily

Glycosaminoglycans

Substances found in arterial walls known as *glycosaminoglycans,* especially chondroitin sulfate, appear to be involved in the development of coronary atherosclerosis and thrombosis. Supplementation with glycosaminoglycans has been shown to improve the blood lipid profile. By increasing the time it takes for the blood to clot, glycosaminoglycans may reduce the risk of coronary thrombosis. Most exciting is the evidence that, among people with coronary heart disease, glycosaminoglycans may greatly reduce the risk of having a heart attack.[78,79]

NUTRITIONAL HEALING PLAN: Glycosaminoglycans

Suggested Use

▶ reduce the risk of a heart attack
▶ normalize blood lipids

Dosage: 1200 mg of glycosaminoglycans 3 times daily

Essential Fatty Acids

Whereas earlier studies examined the effects of polyunsaturated fatty acids as a group, recent research has focused on those polyunsaturates that are also essential, that is, fatty acids that we must have but are unable to make within our bodies. These belong to either the omega-6 or the omega-3 family and serve as precursors to the *prostaglandins,* which are hormone-like substances with important biologic effects.

Omega-6 Fatty Acids

Linoleic acid, the parent compound of the omega-6 fatty acids, is found in abundance in safflower and a number of other commonly used vegetable oils. In the body, it is transformed into the 1-series prostaglandins in a series of steps: first it becomes gamma-linolenic acid (GLA) and then dihomogamma-linolenic acid (DGLA), the immediate precursor of prostaglandin E_1 (PGE_1).

PGE_1 and its precursors can reduce elevated cholesterol levels and the tendency for arterial thrombosis. In a number of studies, the lower the amount of linoleic acid in the diet and the lower the levels of the omega-6 fatty acids in the body, the greater the risk of coronary heart disease.[80,81,82]

Though an inadequate intake of linoleic acid can result in a low level of PGE_1, other factors also affect PGE_1 stores. Eating a lot of refined carbohydrates, saturated fats or hydrogenated fats, or drinking a lot of alcohol reduces PGE_1 levels. Vitamin B_6 and zinc deficiencies—as well as aging, viral infections, chemical carcinogens, and radiation—have the same effect.

Thus, in certain people, PGE_1 may be deficient despite an adequate amount of linoleic acid in the diet. Reducing the intake of saturated and hydrogenated fats while ensuring adequate supplies of zinc and vitamin B_6 appears prudent. Sometimes, however, because of genetics or due to aging, the blocking factors of the conversion of linoleic acid to PGE_1 cannot be overcome. The solution may be to add GLA to the diet. (Adding GLA bypasses the transformation of linoleic acid into GLA, which is the major biochemical hurdle in the transformation of linoleic acid to PGE_1.) This can be done by taking supplements containing a plant oil that has a relatively high content of GLA, such as evening primrose oil.[83]

NUTRITIONAL HEALING PLAN: Omega-6 Fatty Acids

Suggested Use

▶ reduce the risk of atherosclerosis
▶ normalize blood lipids
▶ protect against coronary thrombosis

Preparations and Dosages

3 tbsp of cold pressed safflower oil daily, **or**
1 g of evening primrose oil 3 times daily

Omega-3 Fatty Acids

Just as linoleic acid is parent to the omega-6 family of fatty acids, alpha-linolenic acid is parent to the omega-3 family, and is transformed into the 3-series prostaglandins by a slightly longer series of steps. Earlier I noted that adequate dietary linoleic acid does not insure adequate supplies of the 1-series prostaglandins; neither does adequate dietary alpha-linolenic acid insure adequate supplies of the 3-series prostaglandins. In fact, in both families, the same factors influence the conversion of the parent fatty acid to its prostaglandin form. An additional problem in regard to the omega-3 family is that alpha-linolenic acid is found in greatest quantities in oils from northern plants such as flaxseed oil, whereas oils from southern plants are currently more widely available in most Western countries; thus alpha-linolenic acid, more than linoleic acid, is likely to be low in our diet.

Just as oils such as evening primrose oil can supply the important omega-6 fatty acid GLA, the oils of cold water fish can supply the equivalent omega-3 fatty acids: *eicosapentaenoic* (EPA) and *docosahexaenoic* (DHA). In both cases, these fatty acids are sometimes preferable to their parent compounds, linoleic and alpha-linolenic acids, because they are structurally closer to the prostaglandins and past the biggest biochemical hurdle for their conversion into prostaglandins.

The relationship between fish oils and atherosclerosis appears to be an intimate one. The higher the consumption of fish, the lower the risk of dying from coronary heart disease. In people with coronary heart disease, fish oils may reduce the risk of thrombosis, reduce the pain of angina, and improve cardiac function. There is even preliminary evidence that they may inhibit the development of atherosclerosis.[84,85,86,87,88]

Omega-3 fatty acids are the only polyunsaturates that lower serum triglyceride levels. Their effect on cholesterol is still uncertain.[89,90]

NUTRITIONAL HEALING PLAN: Omega-3 Fatty Acids

Suggested Use

▶ reduce the risk of atherosclerosis
▶ normalize blood lipids
▶ reduce the pain of angina and improve heart function
▶ protect against coronary artery thrombosis

Preparations and Dosages

3 tbsp of cold pressed linseed oil daily, **or**

fish oil (cholesterol-free): 1 g 3 times daily of omega-3 fatty acids

Example: MaxEPA™ 4 capsules four times daily

WARNING

Take under medical supervision.

Botanical Factors

Bromelain

Bromelain is the enzyme derived from the pineapple plant which is protocolytic (breaks down protein). When scientist Hans Nieper gave bromelain to 14 people with angina pectoris, their chest pains disappeared within four to ninety days, with the length of time related to the severity of their disease. This exciting finding has had some confirmation in other studies that suggest that bromelain may be able to dissolve coronary thromboses.[91,92]

It is hoped that large controlled clinical trials will be conducted to determine if bromelain is as effective as it appears to be.

NUTRITIONAL HEALING PLAN: Bromelain

Suggested Use

relieve angina pectoris by dissolving coronary thromboses

Dosage: uncertain, but 500 mg three times daily would be reasonable

---

Combined Nutritional Supplementation

While everyone with coronary heart disease should be on the Healing Diet, Nutritional Healing plans need to be selected according to the needs of the individual. The following example of a specific treatment program is taken from my own practice:

A 75-year-old woman developed increasing chest pain that was found to be the result of advanced coronary atherosclerosis. Coronary bypass surgery and her cardiologist's many attempts to regulate her medications over a period of a year or two failed to prevent frequent episodes of anginal pain. She gradually developed leg pain while walking (intermittent claudication) which, like the angina, increasingly limited her activities. She then suffered a stroke, after which she became sullen and withdrawn and complained of confusion and restlessness.

At the time of nutritional evaluation, three years after her chest pains began, she was taking eight medications. She ate a high-saturated-fat, high-cholesterol, high-sugar diet, used a water softener in her home (which exchanged calcium and magnesium for sodium), and took no nutritional supplements. Her total cholesterol level was 391 (normal is below 200), her red blood cell magnesium level was 4.5 (normal range: 5.3–7.3), and her red blood cell potassium level was 49 (normal range: 89–101).

She was placed on a diet that was low in fat, cholesterol, and sugar, told to shut off the water softener and started on vitamin E, calcium, magnesium, fish oils, L-carnitine and ginkgo biloba.

One month later, her red cell magnesium level had risen to 5.4 and her red cell potassium had risen to 82, and her total cholesterol level had dropped to 294. She was given niacin supplements, and her cholesterol dropped further to 174.

Whereas previously the atherosclerotic changes had been rapidly progressing, her condition stabilized. Both her angina and leg pains rapidly and dramatically improved. Although she remained in need of some personal assistance, her levels of awareness improved substantially and her mental complaints were much reduced.

Five years after the initial visit, she was almost symptom-free except for the residual effects of her stroke. There was no evidence of further progression of her disease; in fact her cardiologist stopped almost all of her medications after they caused her blood pressure to drop too far.

CHOOSING A PERSONAL PLAN

If you suffer from coronary heart disease, or if you simply wish to reduce your risk of developing it, following the principles of the Basic Healing diet is the single most important recommendation I can make. Whether or not you wish to try any of the Nutritional Healing plans, first make a commitment to follow this diet.

Choosing from the many Nutritional Healing plans is difficult, especially since few studies have been done comparing their efficacy. Certain plans are indicated only in specific situations. For example, the major benefit of bromelain, carnitine, and coenzyme Q_{10} is to reduce the pain of angina pectoris, whereas folic acid appears to be worth trying only if your doctor finds elevated homocysteine levels.

As for the Nutritional Healing plans that seek to normalize blood lipid levels, expect them to take at least a month before you and your doctor can see results on laboratory testing; maximal results may even take up to six months. There is no way of knowing in advance how effective each one will be. Niacin is by far the best proven supplement, but it also is the only plan that has more than a very minimal chance of causing side effects.

ADDITIONAL SUGGESTIONS

An aerobic exercise program may increase HDL cholesterol levels and reduce your risk of coronary heart disease. However, if the program is too vigorous, it can be dangerous. Get your doctor's approval for your program and follow established guidelines for warming up, cooling down, and keeping within your proper heart rate range during exercise.

Stress can cause a coronary artery spasm that can trigger a heart attack. Seek to minimize stressful situations, especially after a heavy meal when you are more vulnerable to an inadequate blood supply to the heart.

Herpes Simplex

◈◈◈◈◈◈◈◈◈◈◈◈◈◈◈◈◈◈◈◈

The *herpes simplex* virus causes what are commonly called cold sores or fever blisters as well as genital infections. It affects possibly half of the world's population. The blisters often appear in the area of the lips following the start of a cold and are quite painful. Whereas canker sores are ulcerations, herpes lesions consist of clusters of small fluid-filled blisters immediately surrounded by a small area of inflammation. Though herpes of the lips is not dangerous, genital herpes in women can spread to the baby during vaginal delivery and cause serious illness.

DIETARY FACTORS

Arginine and lysine are amino acids that have an antagonistic effect on one another. Arginine promotes the growth of the herpes simplex virus, whereas lysine suppresses it, so a diet designed to minimize herpes outbreaks avoids foods that are rich in arginine, particularly those that have a high ratio of arginine to lysine.[1]

THE HEALING DIET

Increase your dietary lysine to arginine ratio.

LYSINE/ARGININE RATIOS OF FOODS

good	bad
meat	peanuts (1:3)
potatoes	chocolate (1:2)
milk	other nuts
brewer's yeast	various seeds
fish	cereal grains
chicken	gelatin
beans	carob
eggs	raisins

NUTRITIONAL HEALING PLANS

Vitamins

Vitamin C

Many studies have shown that vitamin C is important in fighting viral infections, and that supplementation with the vitamin may give the immune system an extra boost. When 38 people with recurrent cold sores started vitamin C supplementation, 30 of them reported no recurrences 4 years later, and the other 8 were able to reduce the severity of a recurrence by taking several grams of vitamin C at the first appearance of symptoms.[2]

NUTRITIONAL HEALING PLAN: Vitamin C

Dosage: 500 mg of vitamin C twice daily

Increase to 5 g daily during an outbreak

Vitamin E

Animal studies suggest that vitamin E supplementation may speed the healing of wounds in the moist mucus membranes of the mouth. There is a report of one person with herpes in the mouth whose blisters were treated by applying vitamin E directly to them. Symptoms stopped almost immediately, and the lesions healed promptly. Scientific studies need to be conducted to prove that vitamin E is effective.[3,4]

NUTRITIONAL HEALING PLAN: Vitamin E

Preparation

vitamin E capsules

> *Instructions:* Squeeze the contents of a capsule into a cotton ball and dab the blisters frequently with it.

Minerals

Zinc

Like vitamin C, zinc is believed to play a role in protecting the body against infection. In the test tube, it inhibits the herpes virus from multiplying.[5]

Oral zinc has not been tested except when combined with vitamin C. In a pilot study of recurrent genital herpes, so long as zinc and vitamin C supplementation was continued, some people stopped having eruptions. In others, a violent outbreak occurred after which the eruptions stopped; in the rest, eruptions were extremely mild and started to heal within 24 hours.[6]

In preliminary studies, zinc has also been used successfully when applied to herpetic lesions as an ointment or solution. Applications of the solution usually stopped the itching, burning, stinging, and pain within two to three hours. With regular application, recurrences were greatly reduced or eliminated.[7,8,9]

NUTRITIONAL HEALING PLAN: Zinc

Preparation to Take by Mouth

zinc sulfate

> *Dosage:* 100 mg twice daily
>
> *Instructions:* Take with copper 2 mg daily.

WARNING

Take under medical supervision.

Preparations to Apply Directly to the Blisters

0.01–0.25 percent zinc sulfate as an ointment or solution

> *Instructions:* Apply locally every 30 to 60 minutes when blisters first appear; then apply several times daily.

Lithium

Lithium is an element that has been found to inhibit the herpes virus. When taken orally, early reports suggest that it may prevent recurrent herpes infections. Although controlled studies have yet to be done, further evidence of the efficacy of lithium is the finding that people receiving it for the treatment of psychiatric illness are less likely to develop recurrent genital herpes infections. Oral lithium has many potential adverse effects, however, so it is not generally recommended for the treatment of herpes.[10,11,12]

What about applying lithium directly to the blisters? Though lithium ointment has not been tested alone, it was effective in a double-blind study of an ointment that combined lithium with small amounts of zinc and vitamin E to treat people with recurrent genital herpes. With regular applications, the ointment reduced the length of pain and discomfort from a herpes outbreak from seven days to only four days, and reduced the quantity of herpes virus that was shed from the blisters.[13]

NUTRITIONAL HEALING PLAN: Lithium

Preparation

lithium succinate 8% ointment combined with: zinc sulfate (0.05%) and d,l alpha tocopherol (0.1%)

Instructions: Apply to the blisters four times daily.

Other Nutritional Factors

Bioflavonoids

Bioflavonoids are a large group of naturally occurring plant compounds that are widely distributed in fruits, vegetables, grains, nuts, stems, leaves, and flowers. Though bioflavonoid supplementation has not been tested alone, in a double-blind study, people with recurrent herpes outbreaks received a combination of vitamin C and bioflavonoids or placebos for 3 days starting 48 hours after symptoms began. Whereas everyone taking placebos developed blisters, only about a third of those taking the vitamin C-bioflavonoid combination developed them. Moreover, those on the combination healed significantly faster.[14]

Since vitamin C supplementation may be effective by itself, these results fail to prove whether bioflavonoids have an additional benefit in treating herpes. In nature, vitamin C is usually found in sources that are also rich in bioflavonoids, and other studies have suggested that bioflavonoids often complement the effects of vitamin C. Thus, though their benefits are unproven, it would be reasonable to add bioflavonoids to vitamin C.

NUTRITIONAL HEALING PLAN: Bioflavonoids

Preparation

citrus bioflavonoids

Dosage: 500 mg twice daily

Instructions: Use in combination with vitamin C.

Lysine

Earlier, I discussed the value of eating foods high in lysine and low in arginine. Lysine supplementation has been shown to reduce both the severity of symptoms and the frequency of outbreaks in several scientific studies,[15,16] as shown by the following case:

A patient usually had three to four weeks of pain following the start of a herpes outbreak on the upper lip. However, when 1300 mg of lysine were taken daily as soon as the lesions appeared, the blisters stopped spreading by the second day and began to "dry up." After the fourth day, they were completely "dried up" and the pain was gone.[17]

NUTRITIONAL HEALING PLAN: Lysine

Instructions

For an acute outbreak, take 1000 mg of L-lysine 3 times daily between meals until the blisters are healed; then take 500 mg daily to prevent recurrences.

WARNING

If you take lysine regularly, make sure your physician monitors your cholesterol levels, as an animal study found evidence that lysine may stimulate the liver to increase the manufacture of cholesterol.[18]

Other Factors: Lactobacillus Acidophilus

Lactobacillus acidophilus is a healthy form of bacteria that lives in the bowels. Thirty-eight of a group of 40 people with herpes ulcerations in their mouths reported relief of their symptoms within 48 hours after starting acidophilus tablets. Controlled studies are needed to confirm these results.[19]

NUTRITIONAL HEALING PLAN: Lactobacillus Acidophilus

Preparation

Available in many forms. Look for a guarantee of 10 billion organisms per g.

Dosage: Follow the manufacturer's instructions; the dosage depends upon the potency of the specific preparation.

CHOOSING A PERSONAL PLAN

For a herpes outbreak, the Basic Healing diet combined with lysine supplementation is the best proven plan. The addition of vitamin C, bioflavonoids, and zinc is probably worthwhile. If you wish to try everything, add acidophilus.

Also, treat the blisters directly with local applications. If they are on the skin, I suggest an ointment consisting of lithium, zinc, and vitamin E. If it is not available, try zinc ointment or apply vitamin E directly from the capsule. If the blisters are on moist mucus membranes, try frequent applications of either a zinc solution or the contents of vitamin E capsules.

For frequent herpes outbreaks, consider a preventative program. Continue the Healing diet and the supplement program that I suggested for a herpes outbreak, but lower the doses of lysine and vitamin C.

ADDITIONAL SUGGESTIONS

Ice is a simple remedy which, though never studied formally, has been found surprisingly effective by many people. As soon as blisters appear, apply an ice cube wrapped in linen for up to two hours a few times a day. (Sometimes 45 minutes or even less is adequate.) Remove the ice cube every few minutes for 15 seconds to avoid "burning" the skin.[20]

The possible benefits of ice application are shown by the following case:

A person with recurrent cold sores normally had lesions that lasted ten days and two weeks. After one outbreak, ice was applied six hours after the blisters developed. This treatment was maintained for about two hours. The next day, a scab formed and the blister fell off four days later.[21]

Though colds are notorious for starting a herpetic eruption in the mouth, stress can cause herpes to emerge from hiding anyplace in the body. When you are under stress, practice relaxation exercises; they calm your body and can reduce herpes outbreaks.[22]

High Blood Pressure

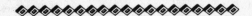

Blood pressure is the force exerted by the blood against the inner walls of the arteries due to the pumping action of the heart. High blood pressure, or *hypertension,* is undesirable because it places increased stress on the heart, kidneys, and blood vessels. Over time, this stress can lead to such serious problems as heart and kidney failure and strokes. In this chapter, we will limit our discussion to essential hypertension (hypertension of unknown cause), which accounts for nine out of ten cases of high blood pressure.

DIETARY FACTORS

Although we don't know exactly how excess weight induces the blood pressure to rise, it is well established that obesity is associated with an increased risk of high blood pressure. Moreover, overweight hypertensives who lose weight can achieve a substantial reduction in blood pressure. (See the chapter on obesity for help in losing weight.)[1]

Whether or not you are overweight, certain specific dietary changes can lower an elevated blood pressure. For example, reducing saturated fat in the diet is advisable. Don't stop drinking milk, however—just switch to nonfat milk. Probably because of its high calcium content, the regular intake of milk is associated with a **lower** risk of developing high blood pressure.[2,3]

Increasing dietary fiber tends to decrease blood pressure, and reducing sugar in the diet appears to be beneficial for the one in three people whose blood pressures are sugar-sensitive. Alcohol intake should be kept low.

Though caffeine may elevate the blood pressure of people who normally avoid it, people who regularly ingest caffeine appear to adapt to it so that it does not cause their blood pressure to rise.[4,5,6,7]

A vegetarian diet is clearly beneficial. Not only are vegetarians less likely to be hypertensive, but hypertensive meat eaters who switch to a vegetarian diet often find that their blood pressure goes down. Several features of this diet make it close to ideal for blood pressure regulation. These include its high content of fiber, potassium, and magnesium as well as its low content of fat and cholesterol.[8,9]

Sometimes (we don't know how often) elevated blood pressure may be due to food sensitivities. When that is the cause, elimination of those foods may lower the blood pressure to normal after the first five days:[10]

> *A 51-year-old hypertensive woman had lost 70 pounds over 18 months on a salt-free, low-protein diet and thyroid pills, but her blood pressure failed to improve. She noted that fruits made her skin itch. She was placed on a diet restricted to foods that were found on testing to be safe. Her blood pressure came down to the normal range, but it rose again after she began taking large, regular doses of cascara for constipation. Wheat products were also found to increase her blood pressure. Once these items were removed, her blood pressure again became normal.[11]*

THE HEALING DIET

1. Follow the Vegetarian Healing diet as described in Appendix A.
2. If the Vegetarian Healing diet is too restrictive for you, follow the Basic Healing diet also described in Appendix A.
3. Avoid foods found on testing to elevate blood pressure. *See Appendix B for information about diagnosing food sensitivities.*

NUTRITIONAL HEALING PLANS

Whether increasing vitamin intake prevents high blood pressure or lowers blood pressure in hypertensives remains to be proven. On the other hand, certain minerals have a definite effect on blood pressure.

Minerals

Sodium Chloride (Table Salt)

It is standard medical practice to recommend salt restriction to both prevent and treat high blood pressure. For the one-third to one-half of the population that is salt-sensitive, moderate salt restriction (avoiding table salt and minimizing the intake of foods high in sodium) can be expected to result in a slight decline in the average blood pressure *(see Appendix D for a list of high-sodium foods)*.[12,13]

Potassium

Though sodium restriction may be beneficial, dietary potassium may need to be increased. In fact, much of the supposed benefit of reduced sodium intake may actually be due to increased dietary potassium, since potassium intake usually increases when sodium intake is reduced (as when natural foods are substituted for processed foods). A reasonable approach would be to replace high-sodium, low-potassium processed foods with low-sodium, high-potassium natural foods *(see Appendix D for a list of high-potassium foods)*.[14,15]

Calcium

Calcium is a mineral whose influence on high blood pressure, although less well known than that of sodium and potassium, is of at least equal importance. Some experts even believe that alterations in calcium metabolism may cause salt sensitivity and hypertension. Reduced dietary calcium is more closely associated with elevated blood pressure than a high salt diet.[16,17]

As is the case with sodium, about one-third to one-half of hypertensives are believed to be calcium-sensitive. Your doctor can check the level of ionized calcium in your blood. A low level suggests that high blood pressure will respond to calcium supplementation, and that sodium restriction will probably also be helpful.[18]

NUTRITIONAL HEALING PLAN: Calcium

Preparation

calcium citrate

Dosage: 1 g daily

Trial Period

two months

Magnesium Deficiency

Magnesium is a potent blood vessel dilator. In one study of 61 dietary factors, the best predictor of high blood pressure was very low magnesium in the diet. Half of all people who are deficient in magnesium also have high blood pressure; once the deficiency is corrected, their blood pressure may return to normal.[19,20,21]

Since inadequate dietary magnesium is so common in industrialized societies, and magnesium supplementation is unlikely to be helpful unless you are magnesium-deficient, consider having your doctor test you for magnesium deficiency. (A magnesium-loading test is best; serum magnesium is least likely to be helpful.)[22,23]

To help protect yourself against a magnesium deficiency, make sure to regularly include in your diet foods that are high in magnesium *(see Appendix D for a list of high-magnesium foods)*.

NUTRITIONAL HEALING PLAN: Magnesium Deficiency

Dosage: 400 mg of magnesium daily

Trial Period

two months

Amino Acids

Taurine

Among the amino acids, *taurine* appears particularly promising for hypertension. The higher the levels of taurine in the diet, the lower the blood pressure. Moreover, in a placebo-controlled study, supplementation with taurine was shown to reduce high blood pressure.[24,25]

NUTRITIONAL HEALING PLAN: Taurine

Dosage: 2 g of taurine three times daily

Trial Period

one week

Tryptophan

Though low dietary levels of tryptophan have not been shown to be associated with high blood pressure, tryptophan is another amino acid that has been shown under double-blind conditions to reduce high blood pressure when added to the diet.[26]

NUTRITIONAL HEALING PLAN: Tryptophan

Dosage: 1 g of L-tryptophan 3 times daily

Trial Period

three weeks

Additional Instructions

1. Avoid protein for 90 minutes before and after ingestion.
2. Take with a carbohydrate (such as fruit juice).

Note: Since tryptophan supplements may not be currently available (see Introduction), you may wish to try foods with a high tryptophan to protein ratio (see Appendix A).

Fatty Acids

Though the intake of saturated fats should be minimized, certain fatty acids (which are found in fats) may be beneficial as long as total fat in the diet is kept low. A diet low in *alpha-linolenic acid,* an omega-3 fatty acid, is associated with high blood pressure. The body makes eicosapentaenoic acid (EPA) from alpha-linolenic acid, and supplementation with EPA, either by eating EPA-rich fish or by taking it in a concentrated form, has been shown in double-blind studies to lower high blood pressure.[27,28]

Pilot studies have also found that supplementation with linoleic acid (an omega-6 fatty acid) or with oleic acid (a fatty acid found in olive oil) may possibly prevent or treat high blood pressure. Controlled studies are needed before the efficacy of these fatty acids can be considered to be proven. In the meantime, I would suggest you eat fish at least twice a week as a source of fatty acids; taking a fish oil supplement would be the next best alternative *(see Appendix D for a list of fish that are rich in omega-3 fatty acids).*[29,30]

> ## NUTRITIONAL HEALING PLAN: Fatty Acids
>
> ### Preparation and Dosage
> cholesterol-free fish oil extract 3 g 3 times daily
> Example: MaxEPA™ 3 capsules 3 times daily
>
> ---
> ### WARNING
> Take under medical supervision.
>
> ---

Botanical Factors

Garlic

In animal studies, garlic has been shown to have a blood pressure-lowering effect in animals with high blood pressure. When, in a double-blind crossover clinical trial, normal volunteers were given garlic oil extracted from fresh garlic, their blood pressures significantly decreased, suggesting that humans also respond to the blood pressure-lowering effect of garlic. Whether the commercial extracts are as effective as fresh garlic or garlic oil remains to be proven.[31,32]

> ## NUTRITIONAL HEALING PLAN: Garlic
>
> *Dosage:* **3 fresh garlic cloves (9 g) daily or a garlic extract
> (dosage varies with each preparation)**
>
> ### Trial Period
> four weeks

Heavy Metal Toxicity

Excessive blood levels of cadmium may be associated with elevated blood pressure. In one study, untreated hypertensives were found to have three to four times the level of blood cadmium of people with normal blood pressure. Elevated blood cadmium is associated with reduced plasma zinc levels, and the results of an animal study suggest that zinc supplementation may reverse cadmium-induced hypertension. Like cadmium, lead is a heavy metal that can produce high blood pressure if too much enters the body. (Your physician can order a hair mineral analysis to discover if your cadmium or lead levels are elevated.)[33,34,35]

In the following case, hypertension was caused by heavy metal toxicity:

A 46-year-old industrial painter had a 3-year history of high blood pressure ranging from 156/100 to 180/110 mm Hg. All laboratory tests, including kidney X-rays, were normal. His diet was free of sugar, refined flour, caffeine, and added salt. He used potassium chloride as a salt substitute. He rarely ate fish, chicken, and red meats, and took daily supplements of 1 g of vitamin C and 200 IU of vitamin E.

Pubic hair mineral analysis revealed elevations of lead, cobalt, and cadmium, with the cadmium level especially high, whereas copper levels were normal. He was treated with 50 mg of zinc gluconate 3 times daily, up to 5–6 g of vitamin C 3 times daily as tolerated, a vitamin B complex with 100 mg of B6 daily (to prevent kidney stones), 100 mcg of selenium daily, 1 tbsp of linseed oil (a source of omega-3 fatty acids) daily, and an increase in vitamin E to 400 IU daily.

Six months later his average blood pressure had dropped to 154/96. Twelve months later, his blood pressure was 142/90, and 18 months later 134/80. In addition, his hair cadmium had dropped to a much more acceptable level. His level of nutritional supplementation was decreased, although zinc and vitamin C were continued at relatively high levels to prevent recurrence.[36]

CHOOSING A PERSONAL PLAN

If you have high blood pressure, buy a blood pressure cuff made for home use so that you can measure your blood pressure as frequently as you wish. With your own measurement device, you may be able to discover for yourself some of the factors that affect your blood pressure.

Consider trying the Vegetarian Healing diet. If that is too difficult, follow the Basic Healing diet. If you are overweight, losing weight should be part of your plan.

Test whether you are food-sensitive, salt-sensitive, or sugar-sensitive by following the three elimination diets for a few weeks one at a time or, if you wish, all together to see whether your blood pressure comes down.

Make sure your diet is rich in foods that are good sources of calcium, magnesium, and potassium, and try to eat at least two servings each week of fish.

Ask your doctor about measuring your serum ionized calcium and testing you for magnesium deficiency. (Remember that people with low ionized calcium are more likely to be salt-sensitive.) Though heavy metal toxicity is uncommon, testing to rule it out may also be worthwhile, especially if you may have been exposed to cadmium or lead in the past.

If none of the above is effective, try adding the nutritional supplements I have suggested. Test them one at a time to discover which lower your blood pressure, and which are ineffective.

ADDITIONAL SUGGESTIONS

1. Regular aerobic exercise can reduce blood pressure in people with mildly elevated blood pressure. It can be dangerous, however, to suddenly stress your cardiovascular system. Therefore start an exercise program slowly and with guidance from your doctor.
2. If you are stressed, tense, and anxious, the state of your nervous system may be raising your blood pressure. Consider ways of reducing stress and relaxing more often. Prayer or meditation may be helpful.
3. If you have difficulty relaxing even when you give yourself the time to do it, perhaps you can benefit from a training program that uses electronic biofeedback instruments to teach you how to successfully relax your body.

Hyperactivity

❖❖❖❖❖❖❖❖❖❖❖❖❖❖❖❖❖❖❖❖❖

Attention-deficit hyperactivity disorder is a behavioral disturbance that begins before age seven and may continue into adulthood. Characteristics include restlessness, short attention span, and distractability. The disorder may cause impairment in functioning at home, at school, and with peers.

DIETARY FACTORS

A high-protein diet may have a calming effect and may improve the capacity to learn. Though the reasons why this diet can improve behavior are not entirely clear, hyperactive children may need to eat more protein than other children because their bodies flush out nitrogen (which comes from protein) more readily.[1,2] The following case is a typical example:

> *An eight-year-old boy had a history of temper tantrums and overly aggressive behavior. He was also irritable and difficult to reach, particularly in the morning and around meal times. An uncle and some cousins were diabetic. His blood sugar level was found to be low whereas his insulin level was high, which suggested a prediabetic condition. After being placed on a high-protein, low-carbohydrate diet, he became calmer, his tantrums stopped, and he began to perform well in school.[3]*

Even if it is effective, a high-protein diet has possible risks. The typical Western diet already contains almost twice as much protein as is needed for optimal health, and excessive amounts of protein could theoretically promote cancer, kidney, and heart disease. It is unknown whether a

THE FEINGOLD DIET

1. *Foods Containing Natural Salicylates*

almonds
apples (cider and cider vinegars)
apricots
blackberries
cherries
cloves
cucumbers and pickles
currants
gooseberries
grapes or raisins
mint flavors
nectarines
oranges
peaches
plums or prunes
raspberries

high-protein diet has long-term adverse effects on health for hyperactive people who respond to the diet.

Some studies, but not others, have found sugar to worsen behavior; the results suggest that the majority of hyperactive children are not affected by it. However, the combination of sugar with starch (as in sugared breakfast cereals) may have more of an effect than sugar alone. Also, as in the above case study, low blood sugar levels due to excessive insulin production may cause symptoms in certain hyperactive children. Since sugar stimulates the pancreas to produce insulin, these children may do better on a sugar-free diet.[4,5,6,7]

Stimulant drugs often reduce hyperactivity. Caffeine is a natural stimulant that, for some hyperactive children, may be as effective as these drugs, but with fewer side effects.[8]

Food sensitivities can provoke hyperkinesis in some people, but how frequently they do so remains an issue for debate. The Feingold diet, a regimen that eliminates salicylates and food additives, has been particularly popular. Though only a small percentage of hyperkinetic children have had proven benefits from this diet, it is known that these children react adversely to both salicylates and food additives fairly often.[9,10,11]

THE FEINGOLD DIET *(CONT.)*

strawberries
tea
tomatoes
oil of wintergreen
wine and wine vinegars

2. *All Foods That Contain Artificial Colors and Flavors*

3. *Miscellaneous Items*

aspirin-containing compounds
medications with artificial colors and flavors
toothpaste and toothpowder (substitute salt and soda)
perfumes

SOURCE: Feingold, B. F. Hyperkinesis and learning disabilities linked to the ingestion of artificial food colors and flavors. *J Learn Disabil* 9(9):551–59, 1976.

The following case is a typical example of food sensitivities provoking hyperkinesis:

A seven-year-old boy had a history of severe hyperkinesis for several years. When at home, he stomped around, slamming doors, kicking walls, and charging oncoming cars with his bicycle. At school he was disruptive and unable to learn. Numerous pediatricians, neurologists, psychiatrists, and psychologists were consulted, and he had a complete medical and neurological work-up at a teaching medical center. All attempts at treatment failed until he was placed on a salicylate-free diet. Within a few weeks, he became well adjusted both at home and at school. Infractions of the dietary program led almost immediately to a recurrence of the hyperkinetic behavior patterns. [12]

THE HEALING DIET

1. Follow the High-Protein and Sugar-free diets as described in Appendix A.
2. Caffeine: 100–200 mg tablets 3 times daily (equivalent to between one and three cups of coffee 3 times daily).

WARNING

Caffeine at such doses may produce nausea, abdominal pain, or insomnia in children and should be tried only under medical supervision.

---

3. Avoid foods found on testing to provoke symptoms. *See Appendix B for information about diagnosing food sensitivities.*

NUTRITIONAL HEALING PLANS

Vitamins

Supplementation with high doses of specific vitamins of the B complex family appears effective for some hyperactive children. A child may be better on one B vitamin and worse on another; the response of each child is different.[13]

Though the reason is not known, it is possible that children who respond to a particular vitamin have an unusually high requirement for it; thus, even though they eat a normal diet, they may lack an adequate amount of that vitamin for optimal health.

Niacin (Vitamin B₃)

Supplementation with niacin (a form of vitamin B_3) in the form of niacinamide has been found effective for very disturbed hyperactive children. In addition to their overactive behavior, these children also have serious social and academic problems and often suffer from abnormal perceptions of reality. Commonly, one or both of the parents also need megadoses of niacin, a finding that suggests the need for abnormally high levels of niacin results from a genetic defect.[14]

NUTRITIONAL HEALING PLAN: Niacin

Preparation

niacinamide

Dosage: 500 mg to 2 g 3 times daily as tolerated

Note: The smaller the child, the lower the dosage.

WARNING

Because niacinamide can have adverse side effects, especially at this high a dosage, it should be taken only under a doctor's supervision.

Thiamine (Vitamin B₁)

Dr. Arnold Brenner, a member of the Department of Medicine at Baltimore County General Hospital in Baltimore, Maryland, gave thiamine (vitamin B$_1$) supplements to 100 hyperactive children. Eleven of them had a dramatic response but relapsed when they were given a placebo. After three months of thiamine therapy, four of these children were able to discontinue thiamine without relapsing, one required a second course, and four needed to continue thiamine for years afterward to avoid relapsing. The remaining four stopped responding to thiamine, but then responded to niacinamide.[15]

The benefits of thiamine supplementation are shown by the following case:

At age ten, a boy became hyperactive and was unable to concentrate. He was overly aggressive, easily frustrated and agitated, intolerant of noises, fearful of crossing the street, and confused while playing basketball. He suffered from nightmares and complained that his blankets felt like stones and that familiar objects in his bedroom appeared far away.

The Feingold diet was ineffective, and he was tried on nutritional supplements one at a time. Although a placebo had no effect, pyridoxine caused hallucinations, and both calcium pantothenate (vitamin B$_5$) and riboflavin also made him worse.

After starting daily supplementation with thiamine, his behavioral symptoms and nightmares disappeared. School performance, memory, and frequent emotional shifts improved dramatically, and letter reversals that he had experienced disappeared.

He did well until two months after thiamine was stopped; the hyperactivity, poor memory, letter reversals, and behavioral disturbances returned. Another three-month course of thiamine was as-

sociated again with dramatic improvement. In all, each of three trials of thiamine withdrawal and one placebo substitution were associated with relapse. On maintenance thiamine, he has continued to do well during three years of follow-up.[16]

NUTRITIONAL HEALING PLAN: Thiamine

Dosage: 100 mg of thiamine four times daily

WARNING
Only take under medical supervision.

Vitamin B₆

Serotonin is an important neurotransmitter that may affect hyperactivity. It is derived from the amino acid tryptophan, which comes entirely from the diet. Vitamin B_6 is required to transform tryptophan to serotonin. Double-blind studies have shown that hyperactive children whose blood serotonin levels are low may respond to supplementation with pyridoxine, a form of vitamin B_6; thus a simple blood test for serotonin can show whether a trial of the vitamin may be worthwhile.[17,18]

NUTRITIONAL HEALING PLAN: Vitamin B₆

Preparation

pyridoxine

Dosage: 500 mg 2 or 3 times daily for a 110 lb (50 kg) child, proportionately less for smaller children

---

WARNING
Close medical supervision is required for B_6 supplementation. This extremely high dosage of pyridoxine (the dosage used in the study) can cause a neuropathy (disorder of the nerves). It is possible, but unproven, that a much lower dosage (40 mg daily) is effective without the danger of this side effect. In addition, although unproven, pyridoxal-5-phosphate (the activated form of vitamin B_6) at a dosage of 50 mg daily may be considerably more powerful than the same dosage of pyridoxine and yet not risk this side effect.

Minerals

Calcium Deficiency

A deficiency of calcium is a relatively rare cause of hyperactivity but should be ruled out by the doctor with simple laboratory testing:

> *A nine-year-old boy diagnosed as hyperactive at age four had been treated with medication for two and a half years. On laboratory testing, he had a very low blood calcium level with a normal amount of calcium excreted in the urine. Within two months after increasing his intake of milk (as a source of calcium), he had a marked behavioral improvement and was able to stop medication. On retesting, his blood calcium level had returned to normal.[19]*

Copper Toxicity

Excessive levels of copper can occasionally cause hyperactivity along with other mental problems such as depression and psychosis. A doctor can eliminate this possibility by drawing blood for a serum copper level.[20]

Magnesium Deficiency

Children with inadequate magnesium may develop hyperactivity along with many of the same symptoms as other hyperactive children. The doctor can eliminate this possible cause of hyperactivity through a simple laboratory test.[21]

Zinc Deficiency

Hyperactivity is a common symptom of zinc deficiency, and hyperactive children may have lower zinc levels than normal children. At least one food additive (the yellow dye tartrazine) both increases their abnormal behavior and the loss of zinc through the urine, which suggests that reactions to food additives may be due to further lowering of already low zinc levels.[22]

If these are not enough reasons to consider zinc supplementation (which, unfortunately, has not been scientifically studied), zinc and copper decrease each other's absorption through the intestinal lining; thus zinc supplementation protects against hyperactivity due to excess copper.

NUTRITIONAL HEALING PLAN: Zinc

Dosage: not well established, but 25 to 100 mg daily, depending upon the child's weight, would be reasonable

---

Other Nutritional Factors

Essential Fatty Acid (EFA) Deficiency

Some hyperactive children are thought to be deficient in essential fatty acids (EFAs). Though the only scientific study of EFA supplementation found them to be generally ineffective, it is possible that they may be effective for a minority of children, especially allergic boys complaining of excessive thirst who have dry hair and skin:[23,24]

> A six-year-old boy with attention deficit disorder had episodes of irritability and crying that his mother attributed to eating sweets. He had been excessively thirsty since infancy, his nose was always congested, he had occasional coughing and wheezing, and he developed hives if licked by a dog.
>
> He had dry skin, lackluster hair, and puffy eyes. Blood tests suggested allergies, iron deficiency, and EFA deficiencies.
>
> After starting evening primrose oil, a source of omega-6 EFAs, he quickly became less thirsty. One week later, his teacher noted increased irritability while his mother noted a loss of appetite, so the dosage of primrose oil was reduced. After one month, his mother reported that he no longer developed hives when licked by a dog, he was less congested at night, his skin and hair were less dry, and he was calmer. An iron supplement and MaxEPA™ (a fish oil source of omega-3 EPAs) were added, and he was started on allergy shots.
>
> After nine months of treatment, primrose oil was stopped. Two weeks later, his parents noted increased thirst, along with sniffles, coughing and wheezing, irritability, and hives following contact with dogs. Primrose oil was restarted, and all symptoms improved within 14 days. He was followed for the next year and a half, and continued to do well.[25]

```
┌─────────────────────────────────────────────────────────────┐
│                                                               │
│        NUTRITIONAL HEALING PLAN: Essential Fatty Acids        │
│                                                               │
│                  Preparations and Dosages                     │
│     1. evening primrose oil 1 g 3 times daily                 │
│     2. cholesterol-free fish oil extract 1 g 3 times daily    │
│                                                               │
│     Example: MaxEPA™ 1 capsule 3 times daily                  │
│     ─────────────────────────────────────────────            │
│                         WARNING                               │
│     Take under medical supervision.                           │
│     ─────────────────────────────────────────────            │
│                                                               │
└─────────────────────────────────────────────────────────────┘
```

Heavy Metal Toxicity

Aluminum Toxicity

Hyperactive children may suffer from aluminum toxicity. In a study of 28 children with hyperactivity or learning disorders, their average aluminum levels in the blood were well above the normal range. Your doctor can evaluate aluminum levels with a simple blood test.[26]

Lead Toxicity

Lead is well known to interfere with normal brain function. For hyperactive children, the levels of lead in both the hair and the urine tend to be higher than in normal children. Usually these levels are not so high that they are above the normal range; sometimes, however, they do reach toxic levels. These tests can be ordered by your doctor. It is not known if treating high-normal lead levels is helpful for hyperactivity.[27,28]

CHOOSING A PERSONAL PLAN

Try the High-Protein and Sugar-free diets for at least two weeks. If you see improvement yet your child is reluctant to avoid sugar, return sugar to the diet to discover if it makes a difference. If you do not see improvement, try a food-elimination diet. (Both types of diets at the same time are too restrictive.) The Feingold diet can be tried alone, or it can be combined with a common food-elimination diet.

The B vitamins I discussed should be tried individually, since one may improve symptoms while another may worsen them. The better your child fits the classic picture (given in the case study above) of a positive response to evening primrose oil, the more likely a trial of primrose oil will be successful.

Several mineral abnormalities can be evaluated by a physician with simple laboratory tests. These include abnormalities of the nutrient minerals calcium, copper, magnesium, and zinc, and of the toxic metals aluminum and lead. Multimineral supplements containing copper should be avoided, as should sources of aluminum and lead *(see the chapter on dementia for a list of sources of aluminum)*.

My inclination would be against trying caffeine unless every other nutritional intervention had failed and your healthcare professional recommends medication. As a natural substitute for medication, caffeine has fewer adverse effects and thus may be worth a trial. If it does help, however, periodically try to wean your child off of it, and coordinate your efforts with your doctor and other healthcare professionals.

Infections

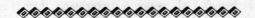

See also: COLDS.

Infections occur when infectious agents (bacteria, viruses, protozoa, parasites, and fungi) overwhelm the body's immune defenses. You can combat infections either by keeping these agents away from your body or by strengthening your immune defenses so that any infectious agent that may be present is destroyed.

DIETARY FACTORS

Malnutrition, which is especially common in the elderly, is associated with a decreased resistance to infections. There is also evidence that obesity and diets high in fat or cholesterol may do the same.[1,2]

Likewise, sugar ingestion weakens immune defenses against infection. In order to destroy bacteria, the *neutrophil,* one of the types of white blood cells, first engulfs them. Sugar is so potent in inhibiting neutrophils from protecting us that five hours after volunteers ingested sugar (in the form of glucose, fructose, sucrose, honey, or orange juice) their neutrophils had not yet regained their usual capacity to engulf bacteria.[3]

THE HEALING DIET

Follow The Basic Healing diet as described in Appendix A.

NUTRITIONAL HEALING PLANS

Vitamins

Vitamin A

Even a mild deficiency in vitamin A makes people more vulnerable to infections. People who are vitamin A-deficient, however, are not the only ones who can benefit from vitamin A supplements; there is considerable evidence that people with normal vitamin A levels can enhance their defenses against infections by increasing their daily intake of the vitamin. For example, when children with a history of frequent respiratory infections received either vitamin A or a worthless placebo, the children who received the vitamin subsequently had less frequent respiratory infections than those who received the placebo.[4,5,6]

NUTRITIONAL HEALING PLAN: Vitamin A

To Protect Against Infections

Dosage: 20,000 IU of vitamin A daily (8,000 IU daily during pregnancy)

To Treat Acute Infections

Dosage: 200,000 IU of vitamin A daily for no more than a few days

---

WARNINGS

1. Take under medical supervision.
2. Do not take this high a dosage of vitamin A if you are pregnant.

Vitamin C

When mammals develop a localized infection, the blood, urine, and tissue levels of vitamin C fall suddenly because the vitamin quickly travels to the site of the infection. Supplementation with this vitamin has been found to be effective in treating various infections due to bacteria, viruses, and *toxoplasma,* a protozoal parasite. Most of the double-blind studies of vitamin C have used daily doses of 2 g or less.[7,8,9,10]

Clinicians such as Dr.s Frederick Klenner and Robert Cathcart believe that these doses are far too low for optimal benefits. Dr. Cathcart recommends that vitamin C be taken up to a dose that is just below "bowel tolerance"; that is, the dosage at which diarrhea or abdominal cramps develop. Though both physicians have had extensive experience using megadosages of vitamin C for a wide variety of infections, their observations have not been put to the test of scientific investigation.[11,12]

NUTRITIONAL HEALING PLAN: Vitamin C

Dosage: 1 g of vitamin C twice daily

Note: Much higher doses and intravenous administration may be more effective. Consult a physician who is knowledgeable about nutritional medicine for assistance.

Vitamin E

Vitamin E is the third vitamin that plays an important role in infections. A deficiency makes people more vulnerable to infection, whereas supplementation increases resistance to infection. In a study of healthy people over age 60, the higher the blood level of vitamin E, the fewer the number of infections they had experienced over the previous three years.[13,14,15]

NUTRITIONAL HEALING PLAN: Vitamin E

Dosage: 400 IU of vitamin E daily

Minerals

Copper

While copper deficiency will make you more vulnerable to infections, copper excess will do the same; thus copper supplementation usually does not make sense unless your doctor finds that you are low in copper.[16,17]

Note: Zinc reduces copper absorption. If you are taking at least 50 mg daily of a zinc supplement, adding 1–2 mg of copper daily will protect you from the dangers of copper depletion.

Iron

A deficiency of iron increases the risk of infections; however, since iron excess fosters bacterial growth, I would not recommend iron supplements unless your doctor finds evidence of an iron deficiency. (A low level of iron in the blood during a bacterial infection does not prove that you are deficient, because the body removes iron from the blood to inhibit bacterial growth.)[18,19]

Zinc

A zinc deficiency is yet another nutritional factor that increases the risk of infections. Even when zinc levels are normal, supplementation with zinc may increase your resistance. Too much supplemental zinc, on the other hand, may actually **reduce** your resistance. Like iron, blood zinc decreases sharply in many infections, perhaps again to inhibit growth of the infectious agent, so low blood zinc levels during infections do not prove that the body is low in zinc.[20,21,22,23]

NUTRITIONAL HEALING PLAN: Zinc

Dosage: 50 mg of zinc daily

Botanical Preparations

Bromelain

Bromelain, an enzyme derived from the stem of the pineapple plant, has been found in several double-blind studies to be effective for a wide variety of infections. Moreover, it makes antibiotics more effective by increasing their blood and tissue levels.[24,25]

NUTRITIONAL HEALING PLAN: Bromelain

Suggested Use

▶ antibacterial agent
▶ increase the efficacy of antibiotics
   Dosage: varies, depending upon the individual preparation

Cranberry Juice

Cranberry juice has a long history of being used to treat acute urinary tract infections, and there is preliminary evidence that it may be of some value, although controlled studies remain to be done. The way it works is not well established. One theory is that it acidifies the urine; another is that it prevents bacteria from adhering to the urinary tract lining.[26,27,28]

NUTRITIONAL HEALING PLAN: Cranberry Juice

Suggested Use

acute urinary tract infections

Dosage: 500 ml (17 oz) of cranberry juice daily

Echinacea

Echinacea is a flower in the daisy family. Widely used in this country by both Native Americans and early settlers to combat infections, it has both antibacterial and antiviral activity. It does not kill germs but stimulates the body to fight the infection.[29]

NUTRITIONAL HEALING PLAN: Echinacea

Dosage: varies, depending upon the individual preparation

Garlic and Onions

Garlic, an ancient folk medicine, has been shown to fight a broad spectrum of infectious agents, particularly viruses and fungi. Unfortunately, most scientific studies were done using animals or by adding garlic to infectious agents in a test tube, so that there is still little proof of its efficacy in people. Onions, a close relative of garlic, may well be as effective as garlic but has been even less well studied.[30,31,32]

NUTRITIONAL HEALING PLAN: Garlic

Dosage: a few fresh garlic cloves daily **or** a deodorized garlic preparation (dosage varies with the potency of the preparation)

CHOOSING A PERSONAL PLAN

If you are already fighting an infection, I suggest you go on the Basic Healing diet. Any of the Nutritional Healing plans can be tried separately, or they may be tried in combination. Do not try to treat a potentially serious infection without the help of your doctor. Also, do not avoid taking antibiotics if your doctor believes they are needed; but, if you are placed on antibiotics, consider taking bromelain to increase their efficacy.

If your resistance to infections is low and infections are recurring frequently, consider taking supplemental vitamin A, C, E, and zinc in addition to following the Basic Healing diet. Try them for a reasonable period of time, perhaps three months, to see if they decrease the frequency, severity, or duration of your infections.

Infertility

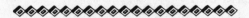

Men are infertile when their sperm are unable to fertilize the egg; women are infertile when they have failed to become pregnant after a year of regular intercourse. Infertility affects about 15 percent of couples and has multiple causes, some of which are affected by nutritional factors.

DIETARY FACTORS

Women who wish to become pregnant for the first time are more likely to succeed if they regulate their diet so that they are neither excessively under- or overweight. About 12 percent of infertility in women who have problems releasing eggs from the ovaries (ovulation) is due to weight; such cases are equally divided between women who are overweight and those who are underweight.[1]

In the male, alcohol is a reproductive tract toxin; the more alcohol ingested and the longer the period of alcohol abuse, the greater the impairment in fertility. Animal studies suggest that, following moderate periods of abstinence, male alcoholics with reproductive disorders due to alcohol could have at least a partial recovery.[2]

Alcohol may reduce a woman's fertility by increasing the level of the hormone *prolactin*. Excessive drinking elevates blood prolactin levels, and elevated levels are known to cause menstrual cycle dysfunction and infertility.[3]

The more caffeine a woman drinks, the more difficult she may find it to become pregnant. In one study, women who consumed more than the equivalent of one cup of coffee daily were half as likely to become pregnant, per cycle, as women who drank less. Though removing caffeine from the diet has not been proven to increase fertility, caffeine is known to reduce the blood prolactin level; a low level of prolactin, like a high level, is associated with infertility.[4,5]

THE HEALING DIET

1. Regulate food intake to achieve a normal weight.
2. Avoid alcohol.
3. Avoid caffeine.

NUTRITIONAL HEALING PLANS

Vitamins

Folic Acid (Folate) Deficiency

Women may become infertile because of a deficiency of folic acid (folate). Inadequate folate in the diet is only one of the causes of folate deficiency. Since folic acid is absorbed in the small intestines, any disease that affects the lining of the small intestines, such as celiac and tropical sprue, can be responsible for a deficiency. Also, a number of drugs may cause folate deficiency. These include drugs that reduce stomach acid (antacids and antihistamines), diphenylhydantoin (an antiseizure drug), and alcohol.[6]

A nutritionally knowledgeable doctor can easily evaluate you for folate deficiency. Infertility that results from a folic acid deficiency can be cured by folate supplementation.[7]

Vitamin B₆

Vitamin B_6 supplementation appears to be a successful treatment for some cases of female infertility, including infertility caused by amenorrhea (the lack of menstrual periods in younger women). Why it works is unclear, although in one study five out of seven infertile women had significant increases in the level of progesterone (a female hormone) following vitamin B_6 supplementation, and adequate progesterone is known to be necessary to maintain the uterine lining so that it can support the growth of the fertilized egg.[8,9]

NUTRITIONAL HEALING PLAN: Vitamin B₆

Preparation

pyridoxine

Dosage: 40 mg daily

Vitamin B₁₂ Deficiency

Vitamin B₁₂ deficiency may cause pernicious anemia. Although it is rare during the childbearing ages, pernicious anemia usually leads to infertility in both sexes. Vitamin B₁₂ supplementation restores fertility. As with folate deficiency, your doctor can easily perform blood tests to rule out pernicious anemia.[10]

Vitamin C

Infertile men may benefit from supplementation with vitamin C. Antibodies directed against sperm cause them to clump together (agglutinate); as sperm increasingly agglutinate, a man becomes less able to impregnate a woman.

When more than one-quarter of the sperm agglutinate, vitamin C is particularly effective for reducing this process. In one study of men with more than 20 percent of agglutinated sperm, the average blood level of vitamin C was on the low side of normal. After three weeks of C supplementation, only 11 percent of their sperm was agglutinated. In addition to reducing sperm agglutination, vitamin C has been shown to reduce sperm abnormalities and to increase sperm count, viability (ability to survive), motility (amount of movement), and maturity. All these factors influence fertility.[11,12]

Vitamin C supplementation for the treatment of male infertility has been compared with two drugs. When compared to treatment with mesterolone and clomiphene citrate, vitamin C supplementation was equally effective.[13,14]

NUTRITIONAL HEALING PLAN: Vitamin C

Dosage: 1 g of vitamin C daily

Minerals: Zinc

The liquid that is propelled out of the penis during orgasm is called the *semen* or *seminal fluid*. The level of seminal zinc varies with both the

number of sperm and their motility, whereas the level of blood zinc varies
with the level of the male hormones. When zinc is removed from the diet,
both the level of male hormones and the sperm count decrease, proving
that zinc deficiency affects both values.[15,16,17]

Conversely, zinc supplementation increases both sperm count and
sperm motility in men with low sperm counts. Among this group of men,
those with low blood testosterone may be the best candidates. Supplementation increases their plasma testosterone; this may be why they are
more likely to respond than infertile men with normal blood testosterone
levels.[18,19]

NUTRITIONAL HEALING PLAN: Zinc

Dosage: 60 mg of zinc daily

Amino Acids: Arginine

A deficiency of the amino acid *arginine* has an adverse effect on sperm.
Arginine supplementation is often an effective treatment for male infertility. In one study, arginine supplementation improved sperm counts in
three-quarters of a group of 178 men with low numbers of active sperm.
Men with severely low sperm counts, however, are less likely to respond.[20,21,22]

The benefits of arginine supplementation for sperm count are shown
by the following case:

> *A man who had been unable to impregnate his wife for 6 years had
> only 25 million sperm per ml in his ejaculate, less than 50 percent of
> which were motile. He was treated with L-arginine, 4 g daily. Six
> weeks later, his sperm count was "100 percent improved," and
> shortly afterward his wife became pregnant.*[23]

NUTRITIONAL HEALING PLAN: Arginine

Dosage: 4 g of L-arginine daily

CHOOSING A PERSONAL PLAN

If you are a woman with problems becoming pregnant, avoid alcohol and
caffeine. If your weight is well outside the normal range, make the neces-

sary dietary changes to normalize your weight. Supplementation with vitamin B_6 may also be helpful. Ask your doctor to evaluate you for folic acid and vitamin B_{12} deficiencies. If you have either, appropriate supplementation may have dramatic results.

If you are a man with a fertility problem, avoid alcohol. I suggest you try supplementation with vitamin C, zinc, and arginine, and have your doctor evaluate you for a vitamin B_{12} deficiency.

Inflammatory Bowel Disease

There are two major forms of chronic inflammatory disease of the intestines. *Ulcerative colitis* is a disease of the colon (large intestines) in which ulcers develop in the colonic lining. *Crohn's disease* (regional enteritis) is often found in the lower part of the small intestines (the ileum) but may also occur in the colon. It commonly progresses to involve all layers of the intestinal wall. Both diseases produce abdominal pain and diarrhea which, in ulcerative colitis, is usually bloody. (Irritable bowel syndrome, while it may also cause abdominal pain and diarrhea, is not an inflammatory disease.)

Depending on the activity of the disease, people with inflammatory bowel diseases may become seriously malnourished due to poor absorption of nutrients from the intestines into the bloodstream. It is therefore important to have your nutritional status monitored by your doctor, who can determine whether your basic needs for protein and energy are being met, and whether you have developed any of the many nutritional deficiencies that are possible in the course of the disease. In some cases, it will be necessary for your doctor to provide nutritional supplementation through injections in order to bypass the bowel altogether.

DIETARY FACTORS

People with active disease often eat poorly due to a lack of appetite. Moreover, nutrients are primarily absorbed in the small bowel, so if it is inflamed it is possible to become malnourished even with an adequate diet.

212

The evidence is mounting that a diet in which the carbohydrates are unrefined may have a beneficial effect on the course of inflammatory bowel disease. The process of refining grains and other high-carbohydrate foods to produce such products as sugar and white flour strips these foods of their natural fiber, and dietary fiber appears to reduce the activity of the disease. Also, a number of studies have found that people with Crohn's disease eat more sugar (a refined carbohydrate) than people without the disease—even compared to people with ulcerative colitis—although this difference only develops many months after the disease has been diagnosed.[1,2,3,4,5]

Evidence for the value of a high-fiber, low-refined-carbohydrate diet comes from many directions. For example, black populations in Africa rarely develop this disease so long as they consume their traditional diet, which is very high in fiber and free of refined sugar. When the diets of people with ulcerative colitis were studied and the course of their disease was followed over time, a fiber-poor diet was the only dietary factor found that predicted that ulcerative colitis in remission would relapse.[6,7]

In two studies, people with Crohn's disease were placed on a fiber-rich, unrefined carbohydrate diet to see how they would do over time as compared to their progress on other diets. In the first study, the other diet was high in refined sugar. Four out of 5 people on the therapeutic diet had symptom relief within eighteen months, whereas 4 out of 10 people on the high-refined sugar diet became too ill to be able to stay on the diet that long. In the second study, compared to people who were given no dietary instruction, people on a fiber-rich, unrefined carbohydrate diet had fewer and shorter hospital admissions and were less likely to need intestinal surgery over an average of more than four years.[8,9]

Food sensitivities have been implicated in provoking exacerbations of inflammatory bowel disease. Removal of specific foods or replacing the diet with a liquid artificial food (an elemental diet) has sometimes brought the disease into remission:

Bernard, a forty-nine-year-old traveling salesman, had a ten-year history of ulcerative colitis, with up to ten bowel movements a day, that was unresponsive to medication. Mild iron and zinc deficiencies were treated with supplementation, and he was placed on an exclusion diet; however, his diarrhea was only minimally improved. Since his symptoms were worsened by salicylate-containing medications, he was placed on a low-salicylate diet. Within three days his diarrhea was less, and within one week it had completely ceased. He gained more than fourteen pounds and went into a full remission, as confirmed by the gastroenterologist.[10]

There is no evidence, however, that food sensitivities are the underlying cause of inflammatory bowel disease.[11]

THE HEALING DIET

1. Follow the High-Fiber and Low-Refined-Carbohydrate diets as described in Appendix A.
2. Avoid foods found on testing to aggravate symptoms. *See Appendix B for information about diagnosing food sensitivities.*

NUTRITIONAL HEALING PLANS

Vitamins

Vitamin E

The levels of a number of vitamins may be reduced when inflammatory bowel disease is active. Though restoring normal levels of these nutrients is important for general health, in most cases there is no evidence that their normalization affects the course of the disease.

There is preliminary evidence, which has yet to be verified with scientific studies, that supplementation with vitamin E may reduce bowel inflammation. This finding is not surprising, since vitamin E supplementation is known to affect the functioning of the immune system; perhaps it affects the immune system in such a way that it helps the gut to combat the inflammatory process.[12,13]

The following case illustrates the possible benefits of vitamin E supplementation for Crohn's disease:

A woman who for several years suffered from Crohn's disease that had been treated surgically, was having up to ten diarrheal bowel movements daily and violent abdominal cramps. Examination of the involved areas of the bowel showed bleeding, abscesses, and four fistulas (abnormal passageways between sections of the bowel). Although oral steroids helped for two months, medication was unsuccessful in inducing a remission.

She was started on forty 400-IU capsules of vitamin E (alpha-tocopherol) daily. By the end of four weeks, the diarrhea had stopped and the fistulas were reduced to half their previous size. Subsequently the cramps became increasingly rare and she felt good for the first time since the disease began. By five and one-half months after starting supplementation, two of the fistulas had reduced to very small openings and two had closed completely. X-rays of the lower bowel failed to reveal signs of acute colitis or ulceration, either in the section of the small bowel left after surgery or in the colon or rectum. She reported one solid bowel movement daily and no cramps.[14]

NUTRITIONAL HEALING PLAN: Vitamin E

Dosage: uncertain, but 800 IU of vitamin E daily would be reasonable

Trial Period

four weeks for initial results

Minerals

Poor dietary habits and malabsorption from the gut are the primary reasons that several minerals may fall well below normal levels when bowel disease is active. These include calcium, iron (which may also be lowered by bleeding from the diseased area), magnesium, and zinc. Any of these minerals may become so deficient as to result in the development of a mineral-deficiency disease, and all should be carefully evaluated by your physician.[15]

Other Nutritional Factors

Omega-3 Fatty Acids

The omega-3 fatty acids, for which fish and linseed oils are excellent sources, have known anti-inflammatory effects. Recently, ten patients with mild to moderate cases of ulcerative colitis who had either failed to improve from conventional treatment or, in one case, had refused conventional treatment, were treated with fish oils that were rich in these fatty acids. Seven out of the ten had either moderate or marked improvement.[16]

These promising results were confirmed in a double-blind crossover study of thirty-nine people that found moderate improvement in the extent and severity of their bowel involvement after they started taking similar fish-oil supplements. Ulcerative colitis appeared to respond better than Crohn's disease, as only people with ulcerative colitis had symptom relief.[17]

NUTRITIONAL HEALING PLAN: Omega-3 Fatty Acids

Suggested Use

active ulcerative colitis

Preparation and Dosage

cholesterol-free fish oil extract in a quantity providing 2.7 g
of eicosapentaenoic acid (EPA) daily
   Example: MaxEPA™ 5 capsules 3 times daily

WARNING

Take under medical supervision

Trial Period

8 weeks minimum

CHOOSING A PERSONAL PLAN

Everyone with an inflammatory bowel disease should consider a trial of
combining the High-Fiber and Low-Refined-Carbohydrate diets. Consider
whether you may be food-sensitive; if you are suspicious, try a food-
elimination diet.

   Because there is so little scientific literature proving the value of nutritional supplementation for treating inflammatory bowel disease, the benefits from trials of vitamin E or omega-3 fatty acids are uncertain. The early
reports of a few people who have tried massive doses of vitamin E raise
the hope that it could be dramatically effective.

   If you have active ulcerative colitis, consider increasing your intake of
omega-3 fatty acids and combining it with vitamin E. The best way to do
this is by eating fish rich in these fatty acids at least twice a week *(see
Appendix D for a list of such fish)*. Taking a fish oil supplement is an
alternative.

   Remember, if your disease is active, you may be developing nutritional
deficiencies, so consider asking a nutritionally trained physician to evaluate you.

Inner Ear Dysfunction

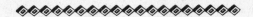

See also: HEART DISEASE.

Loss of hearing is one of the symptoms of inner ear dysfunction. When it results from a lesion in the ear canal or in the middle ear (the little bones just behind the eardrum), it is a *conductive* hearing loss; when it is caused by a lesion in the inner ear, either in the *cochlea* (where sounds are translated into nerve impulses) or in the nerve that carries these impulses to the brain, it is a *sensorineural* hearing loss. The other two symptoms are *tinnitus* (a ringing noise in the ear), which often accompanies hearing loss, and *vertigo* (the sensation of spinning in a direction), caused by a dysfunction in the inner ear's semicircular canals. People suffering from Ménière's disease, which is characterized by increased fluid pressure in the inner ear, may experience all three symptoms.

DIETARY FACTORS

Sensorineural hearing loss is frequently associated with elevated blood fats. When animals are fed a high-cholesterol diet to elevate their blood fats, their hearing deteriorates and they become more susceptible to noise-induced hearing loss. It is therefore likely that an elevated level of blood fats in humans is a cause of sensorineural hearing loss.[1,2]

Elevated blood fats appear to cause hearing loss by reducing the flow of oxygen and nutrients to the inner ear. They seem to accomplish this by restricting the movement of the red blood cells nourishing the inner ear, either by increasing the tendency of these cells to mass together or by making them less flexible so that they cannot flow freely through the small capillaries.[3,4]

A low-saturated-fat diet has been shown not only to protect against hearing loss (usually of the sensorineural type) but to partly restore hearing. Moreover, these relationships extend to children with elevated blood fats who have fluctuating sensorineural hearing loss in both ears. For a group of these children, the worse their hearing, the higher their blood fats. Moreover, when they were placed on a low-fat diet, their hearing improved.[5,6]

Sugar is suspected of causing inner ear dysfunction through its stimulation of the release of adrenalin, which causes constriction in the small blood vessels that feed the inner ear. Forms of sensorineural hearing loss, including Ménière's syndrome, fluctuant hearing loss, and sudden deafness, have all been shown to be associated with abnormal responses to sugar. In these disorders, replacement of sugar and other refined carbohydrates with either a high-protein or a high-unrefined-complex-carbohydrate diet is sometimes followed by a lessening of symptoms.[7,8,9,10,11]

Food sensitivities have been implicated in inner ear dysfunction, with symptoms sometimes remitting following food eliminations.[12,13]

A 49-year-old woman complained of a buzzing in the left ear associated with decreased hearing. She also had recurrent attacks of mild vertigo, recurrent headaches, and gastrointestinal complaints. Lobsters, and occasionally fish, caused diarrhea. She drank eight to nine cups of coffee daily. Though her physical exam was essentially negative, she had a mild low-tone sensorineural hearing loss in the left ear.

Food testing found that she was highly allergic to coffee. When she avoided coffee, her hearing became normal and the buzzing ceased.[14]

Though reports of improvement go back many years, scientific controlled studies on food eliminations to treat inner ear dysfunction still remain to be done.

THE HEALING DIET

For sensorineural hearing loss:

1. Follow the Basic Healing diet as described in Appendix A.
2. Avoid foods found on testing to provoke symptoms. *See Appendix B for information about diagnosing food sensitivities.*

NUTRITIONAL HEALING PLANS

Vitamin Deficiencies

Vitamin A Deficiency

The cochlea requires high concentrations of vitamin A; the special sensory receptor cells within it contain, or are functionally dependent upon, the vitamin. Low serum vitamin A levels are associated with decreased hearing, and feeding young rats a vitamin-A deficient diet causes changes in the cochlea that are visible under an electron microscope. When 300 people with documented hearing loss received injections of vitamin A, 83 percent reported improvement in hearing conversational tones.[15,16,17]

Since vitamin E protects vitamin A, it has been combined with vitamin A when treating sensorineural hearing loss. Particularly when the auditory symptoms are related to aging, the combination may cause a measurable improvement in hearing. Controlled studies have not yet been done to confirm these preliminary findings, and we do not know if vitamin A supplementation is beneficial when serum vitamin A levels are normal.[18,19]

NUTRITIONAL HEALING PLAN: Vitamin A Deficiency

Suggested Use

sensorineural hearing loss

Dosage: 20,000 IU of vitamin A daily

Instructions: Combine with 400 IU of vitamin E daily.

Vitamin D Deficiency

A deficiency of vitamin D appears to cause hearing loss by reducing the concentration of calcium in the fluid of the inner ear. *Otosclerosis,* a common cause of conductive hearing loss, is a condition in which a new formation of spongy bone interferes with sound transmission. Reduced serum vitamin D levels are fairly common among people with this condition. In a study of 47 people with inner ear symptoms due to otosclerosis, 21 percent were found to have abnormally low levels of vitamin D.[20,21]

People with both otosclerosis and low serum vitamin D levels may be candidates for vitamin D supplementation, since one study found that 19 percent of a group of 16 people in this category had significant improvements in their hearing following supplementation. Although the research is only preliminary, these same supplements may also be helpful to people with low vitamin D levels and hearing loss whose deafness has resulted from a disorder of the cochlea. Controlled studies are needed before the value of these supplements can be considered to be proven.[22,23]

NUTRITIONAL HEALING PLAN: Vitamin D Deficiency

Suggested Use

▶ otosclerosis
▶ sensorineural hearing loss

Dosage: 500–1000 IU of vitamin D daily

WARNING

Excess vitamin D can be unhealthy because of interference with calcium metabolism. Supplementation is suggested only if blood testing shows evidence of a vitamin D deficiency.

Minerals

Iron Deficiency

People with sensorineural hearing loss may have reduced serum iron levels. It has been shown that rats raised on an iron-deficient diet become hard of hearing; thus iron deficiency may be a cause of sensorineural hearing loss in humans. When a group of people with sensorineural hearing loss who also had low-serum iron levels were given iron supplementation, hearing improved in those whose serum iron increased.[24,25]

NUTRITIONAL HEALING PLAN: Iron Deficiency

Suggested Use

sensorineural hearing loss

Dosage: 30 to 60 mg of iron daily to 3 times daily

WARNING

Iron supplementation is recommended only for people with evidence of iron deficiency and therefore should be taken under medical supervision.

Zinc Deficiency

Zinc deficiency appears to be associated with sensorineural hearing loss, tinnitus, or both. The tinnitus associated with zinc deficiency tends to be continuous rather than intermittent. Pilot studies have reported improvement following zinc supplementation. In the absence of zinc deficiency, however, supplementation has been proven to be ineffective. Controlled studies are needed to prove the therapeutic benefits of zinc supplementation for people with zinc deficiency.[26,27,28]

NUTRITIONAL HEALING PLAN: Zinc Deficiency

Suggested Use

▶ sensorineural hearing loss
▶ tinnitus

Dosage: 60 to 120 mg of zinc daily

Other Nutritional Factors

Hydroxyethylrutoside

This bioflavonoid (which is related to rutin) has been proven effective in Ménière's syndrome in a double-blind, crossover study. There was no evidence of side effects. Sudden deafness caused by an insufficient supply of blood to the inner ear may also be responsive. In a pilot study, four people with this problem found that their hearing improved and their tinnitus disappeared after they started to take the bioflavonoid regularly.[29,30]

NUTRITIONAL HEALING PLAN: Hydroxyethylrutoside

Suggested Use

▶ Ménière's syndrome
▶ Sudden deafness of vascular origin

Dosage: 2 g of hydroxyethylrutoside daily

Botanical Factors

Ginger

Many people suffer from seasickness because of the effects of the rocking motion of the water upon the semicircular canals of the inner ear. In a double-blind study, administration of ginger root has been shown to reduce seasickness on the open sea. Specifically, people given ginger root vomited less often and were less likely to complain of cold sweats. Another double-blind, crossover study has shown that ginger root also reduces vertigo that has been intentionally induced in normal volunteers.[31,32]

The following case illustrates the benefits of ginger for vertigo:

> *After suffering six strokes in six months, a woman suffered from intense vertigo, nausea, and vomiting. Her blood pressure was very low (80/30 mm Hg), and she could take only 10 to 15 steps at a time. She began taking 1 tsp of ground ginger in hot water once daily. Soon she experienced a "remarkable improvement" in her symptoms.*[33]

NUTRITIONAL HEALING PLAN: Ginger

Suggested Use

▶ seasickness
▶ vertigo

Preparation

ginger root

Dosage: 1 g daily

Ginkgo Biloba

The extract from the leaf of the *Ginkgo biloba* tree has been proven effective in double-blind studies for reducing the symptoms of tinnitus, vertigo, and acute cochlear deafness. The ability of ginkgo to reduce vertigo has been further confirmed by using a special instrument that records changes in the subtle physical signs of vertigo.[34,35,36,37]

NUTRITIONAL HEALING PLAN: Ginkgo Biloba

Suggested Use

▶ sensorineural hearing loss
▶ tinnitus
▶ vertigo

Preparation

solid extract

Dosage: 40 mg 3 times daily

CHOOSING A PERSONAL PLAN

A number of nutritional treatments may be effective for sensorineural symptoms. The Basic Healing diet is generally recommended. If your doctor cannot find a physical explanation for your symptoms, especially if you have other unexplained symptoms, consider trying a food-elimination diet.

I especially recommend a trial of *Ginkgo biloba* extract, because of its proven efficacy in treating tinnitus, vertigo, and at least one form of sensorineural deafness, as well as its excellent safety record. Less has been published on the efficacy of hydroxyethylrutoside for inner ear dysfunction; however it has proven itself to be safe and effective in Ménière's disease as well as in a number of other disorders. Ginger root appears to specifically improve the functioning of the balance system within the inner ear, but there is no evidence that it is effective for other inner ear symptoms.

Since a deficiency of vitamin A, vitamin D, iron, or zinc can be the cause of sensorineural symptoms, consider having a nutritionally trained physician evaluate you for these deficiencies to determine whether a trial of supplementation is indicated. **Please note that a chronic excess of any of these four nutrients can be unhealthy.**

Finally, if your inner ear dysfunction is due to otosclerosis, the only Nutritional Healing plan that may be helpful is the plan for treating vitamin D deficiency. Even though only a minority of people with otosclerosis appear to respond to vitamin D supplements, I suggest you ask your physician to check your serum 25-hydroxyvitamin D level and, if it is low, to place you on supplementation.

ADDITIONAL SUGGESTIONS

If you suffer from tinnitus, relaxation training procedures may be helpful. Several years ago, I did a study on biofeedback-assisted relaxation training for the treatment of tinnitus. The results were most interesting. About two-thirds of my patients said that they had improved. Half of the group that improved noted that their tinnitus had clearly decreased or, occasionally, had disappeared; the other half noted that, though their tinnitus was unchanged, it no longer bothered them as much as it did before. These results suggest that relaxation may help either physiologically (by normalizing the way the body functions) or psychologically (by reducing the distress that the symptom causes).

Insomnia

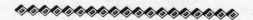

See also: ANXIETY, DEPRESSION, FATIGUE.

Since individual requirements for sleep vary greatly, insomnia exists only if you feel tired or sleepy, or find it hard to concentrate during the daytime. Insomnia is a common complaint with as many as 40 percent of adults dissatisfied with the quality of their sleep. Symptoms can include difficulty in falling asleep, frequent reawakenings with difficulty returning to sleep, or poor-quality sleep.

DIETARY FACTORS

Since alcohol has an initial sedative effect, many people mistakenly believe that drinking alcohol before going to bed will improve their night's sleep. In fact, alcohol interferes with deep sleep and therefore should be avoided by anyone with a sleeping problem.[1]

Caffeine is another substance that has been repeatedly shown to adversely affect sleep. The more caffeine people consume, the more likely it is that they will complain of insomnia. Among people who have no problem sleeping, the equivalent of 1 cup of coffee a half an hour before retiring has no effect, 2 cups primarily increases the amount of time it takes to fall asleep and the quality of sleep during the early part of the night, and 4 cups adversely affects all sleep measures.[2,3]

Insomnia has been attributed at times to food sensitivities. When extensive medical and psychological testing failed to find a cause for sleeplessness in eight infants, all eight were found to be allergic to cow's milk.

When cow's milk protein was removed from the diet, their insomnia was eliminated; when it was put back in the diet, their insomnia returned. How frequently food sensitivities are a cause of insomnia is unknown.[4]

THE HEALING DIET

1. Avoid alcohol and caffeine, especially in the afternoon and evening.
2. Rule out food sensitivities *(see Appendix B for information about diagnosing food sensitivities).*

NUTRITIONAL HEALING PLANS

Vitamins

Niacinamide (Vitamin B₃)

The most popular prescription sleeping medications are members of the *benzodiazepine family.* The ability of these drugs to induce sleep was initially discovered by testing them in animals. Similar animal studies suggest that niacinamide (a form of vitamin B_3) has hypnotic effects like those of the benzodiazepines. Though niacinamide has not yet been formally studied in humans for this purpose, it is likely that it will be found to have the same effect, although its potency, as compared to prescription drugs, is unknown.[5]

NUTRITIONAL HEALING PLAN: Niacinamide

Dosage: 1 g of niacinamide 30 minutes before bedtime

Amino Acids: Tryptophan

Serotonin is a neurotransmitter (a carrier of messages between nerve cells) that plays an important role in the regulation of sleep. In the body, serotonin is derived from *tryptophan,* an essential amino acid found in protein. Tryptophan supplementation has been studied extensively, and has been proven to be effective for improving sleep.

For younger insomniacs suffering purely from difficulty in falling asleep, it is effective starting the first night of supplementation. For more chronic and severe insomniacs with difficulties in both falling asleep and staying asleep, it may take several days or longer before improvement occurs; in fact, sometimes improvement occurs only after tryptophan is discontinued. For people fitting into this group, intermittent supplementation may be most effective.[6]

Sleep following tryptophan supplementation has a natural quality. Tryptophan does not impair coordination, thinking, or memory; does not interfere with the ability to awaken; and does not distort the natural progression of sleep stages during the night. Doses do not have to be raised over time, and significant side effects are very rare.[7,8]

The benefits of tryptophan for insomnia are shown by the following case:

> A two-year-old girl had always slept poorly, and it was difficult to keep her quiet and in bed at night. She was started on 500 mg of tryptophan crushed and added to a glass of milk, which she drank just before dinner. By bedtime she became sleepy and slept throughout the night. One night when the tryptophan-fortified milk was forgotten, she got up several times.

NUTRITIONAL HEALING PLAN: Tryptophan

Dosage: 1 g of tryptophan 30–45 minutes before bedtime (2–3 grams may be needed for people over age 40)

Additional Instructions

1. Avoid protein for 90 minutes before and after ingestion.
2. Take with a carbohydrate (such as fruit juice).

Note: Since tryptophan supplements may not be currently available (see Introduction), you may wish to try foods with a high tryptophan to protein ratio (see Appendix A).

Botanical Factors

Valerian

A perennial plant native to North America and Europe, *valerian* has been used as a sedative for more than 200 years. Its efficacy in treating insomnia has been confirmed recently in scientific studies that have reported improved sleep with a reduction in the time needed to fall asleep. Night awakenings and sleepiness the next morning, however, are relatively unaffected.[10,11]

Though research has shown that it is entirely safe to take on occasion, valerian has not yet been proven to be safe taken daily over a long period of time. For this reason, chronic daily use is not recommended.[12]

NUTRITIONAL HEALING PLAN: Valerian

Preparation

standardized aqueous extract (0.8 percent valeric acid)

Dosage: 150–300 mg 30–45 minutes before bedtime

CHOOSING A PERSONAL PLAN

Avoid drinking alcoholic and caffeinated beverages, especially after noon-time. Even if stopping them does not solve your sleeping problem, they may well contribute to it. You may wish to test yourself for food sensitivities, although these are unlikely to be a cause of insomnia unless the insomnia is just one of several suspicious symptoms of sensitivity.

Since tryptophan is the best proven of the Nutritional Healing plans, and its mechanism of action is well understood, I would try it first if the Healing diet is not of value. Valerian would be my second choice, and niacinamide my final choice. Should valerian be effective, avoid taking it nightly for a prolonged period of time.

ADDITIONAL SUGGESTIONS

Insomnia is often a manifestation of a high level of anxiety. If that is the case, the anxiety itself should be treated. Psychotherapy, biofeedback-assisted-relaxation training, acupuncture, and aerobic exercise are a few methods that may be helpful, in addition to nutritional treatment programs.

Depression, including the anxious (agitated) form of depression, may also cause insomnia, in which case treatment for the depression should be the primary goal. Sleep will improve once the depression is resolved. Conversely, sometimes depression resolves once adequate sleep is restored.

Irritable Bowel Syndrome

◇◆◇◆◇◆◇◆◇◆◇◆◇◆◇◆◇◆◇◆◇

See also: CONSTIPATION.

The key features of irritable bowel syndrome are abdominal discomfort accompanied by constipation or diarrhea (or both) without a known physical cause. While symptoms often resemble those of inflammatory bowel disease, the bowel is not inflamed. The most common disorder of the gastrointestinal tract in industrialized societies, irritable bowel syndrome is the cause of up to half of all consultations with a gastroenterologist. The disorder usually occurs in the middle years of life, and develops more frequently in women.

DIETARY FACTORS

Symptoms from this disorder are associated with spasms in the muscle lining the gut wall. Since fiber substantially increases fecal bulk, it is believed to reduce symptoms by providing more of a cushion to the contracting gut muscle.[1]

Though a high-fiber diet has been proven to be effective for constipation, a common complaint with this disorder, people have been shown to improve as much when they eat cookies every day to which no fiber is added, as when they eat cookies enriched with corn fiber or wheat bran. Such findings add evidence to the belief that there is frequently a substantial psychological component to the illness.[2,3]

Another possible explanation is that increased dietary fiber is beneficial only for people whose diets are too low in fiber. Bran was found to be effective, for example, when people suffering from irritable bowel syndrome were divided into two groups: one given a diet made low in fiber by removing whole-grain cereal products and the other given a diet made high in fiber by adding bran to their normal diet. Compared to the low-fiber group, the high-fiber group soon had less symptoms.[4]

The preferable way to add fiber is by switching from refined grains (which have had their natural fiber coverings removed) to whole grains, and by switching from refined sugars to whole fruits and vegetables. Alternatively, you can simply supplement your usual diet with fiber. For example, if you add 8 to 10 tsp of unprocessed wheat bran daily or 1 tsp of psyllium twice daily, along with plenty of fluid, your fiber intake will be adequate to minimize symptoms:

For several years a 14-year-old girl experienced increasingly severe abdominal cramps in varying locations throughout her abdomen; the cramps were largely relieved by antispasmotics. Her stools were normal, and defecation occurred once every two to three days. Dietary analysis revealed a lack of dietary bulk and fiber.

She was told to add raw, bulky, fibrous vegetables to her diet; to eat honey-sweetened granola for breakfast; and to take 2 tbsp of unprocessed bran daily. On follow-up one month later, she reported no further spasms.[5]

Not only are refined sugars devoid of fiber, but they may contribute directly to the symptoms of irritable bowel syndrome. Following the ingestion of fructose (fruit sugar) or sorbitol (a sugar alcohol used in candies and chewing gums), people with an irritable bowel may develop pronounced stomach distress as well as difficulty absorbing nutrients from the intestines. The ingestion of sucrose (table sugar) may also cause stomach distress, but not as much, and it does not cause malabsorption. It does, however, cause alterations in the gut that increase the risk of developing symptoms.[6,7]

Fat in the stomach stimulates colonic contractions. If you have an irritable bowel, a fatty meal can cause abnormal intestinal contractions that are often accompanied by stomach symptoms.[8]

Food sensitivities provoke symptoms in perhaps one out of two people suffering from an irritable bowel syndrome, especially those who suffer from classic (atopic) allergies. Both foods and food additives have been implicated. Of the foods, dairy products and grains are the most common offenders.[9,10,11]

Many people develop bowel symptoms because they are unable to tolerate milk sugar (lactose) due to a lack of the enzyme (lactase) needed to split it into its component sugars, glucose and galactose. These people do well by avoiding milk and most milk products or by taking lactose supplements. They may, however, be able to tolerate butter and some aged cheeses (because they are low in lactose) and yogurt (due to the lactase activity of the bacterial culture). (See the chapter on cataracts for a list of dairy products that are high in lactose.)

In the following case, stomach distress was caused by a lactose intolerance:

A 42-year-old woman with a diagnosis of irritable bowel syndrome had an 8-year history of almost daily bloating, loose stools, abdominal pain, and gas. Fourteen days after stopping all dairy products, she was symptom-free. The following day she drank three glasses of milk and ate a bowl of ice cream, and discovered that her symptoms returned worse than before. She tried avoidance and provocation twice more, each time with the same result.[12]

THE HEALING DIET

1. Follow the Basic Healing diet with an emphasis on high-fiber foods as described in Appendix A.
2. Avoid foods found on testing to provoke symptoms. *See Appendix B for information about diagnosing food sensitivities.*

NUTRITIONAL HEALING PLANS: PEPPERMINT OIL

Peppermint oil relieves the symptoms of stomach distress by reducing the contractions of the gut muscle. When given in the form of enteric-coated capsules to prevent premature release, it significantly reduces abdominal symptoms as compared to placebos.[13]

NUTRITIONAL HEALING PLAN: Peppermint Oil

Preparation

enteric-coated capsules containing 0.2 ml peppermint oil per capsule

Dosage: 1–2 capsules 3 times daily between meals

CHOOSING A PERSONAL PLAN

The Healing diet should be tried by everyone suffering from irritable bowel syndrome. Consider a trial of a food-elimination diet to see whether food sensitivities contribute to your symptoms.

If the Healing diet fails to relieve all symptoms, peppermint oil, a natural alternative to medication, is well worth trying.

ADDITIONAL SUGGESTIONS

The mind has a powerful influence on the tendency of the gut to spasm. Whatever the cause of your bowel becoming irritable, your mind may be capable of reducing your symptoms. There are a number of mentally based treatments, all of which have been shown to have some value:

1. Psychotherapy, when added to medical treatment (such as nutritional medicine), tends to result in greater improvement than medical treatment alone.[14]
2. Various forms of biofeedback training, such as bowel sound biofeedback, have been effective; they are often combined with other behavioral or psychological procedures in the belief that this adds to their efficacy.[15,16,17]
3. Hypnotherapy is frequently successful, even when all forms of medical treatment have failed.[18]

Kidney Stones

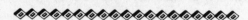

Since the beginning of this century, kidney stones have become increasingly common in the industrialized countries. Four out of 5 stone formers are men, and symptoms most frequently start between the ages of 20 and 30. The pain of passing a stone (renal colic) is in the flank; it starts suddenly and radiates down the abdomen toward the groin. There may be an urge to urinate, pain on urination, and blood in the urine.

In up to 80 percent of cases, a predisposing cause cannot be found. The stone is likely to be composed of calcium oxalate. The more calcium and oxalate in the urine, the more likely it is that stone will form. Urinary calcium and oxalate levels, however, are only two of the many other factors that influence the tendency for stone formation. Urinary uric acid, for example, interferes with the action of naturally occurring inhibitors of calcium oxalate stone formation; it also forms seeds around which calcium oxalate stones can develop. These factors and others that affect the development of kidney stones are strongly influenced by nutrition.

DIETARY FACTORS

There are several items that kidney stone formers should minimize or even avoid altogether. Animal protein is one of them. In addition to increasing the urinary excretion of both calcium and oxalate, animal protein increases the urinary excretion of uric acid. This increased uric acid excretion promotes calcium oxalate stone formation by interfering with the action of naturally occurring inhibitors in the urine, and by serving as seeds for stone formation and growth.[1,2,3]

Fats in your diet should also be minimized. Studies show that urinary stone formers tend to eat more fat than other people. When dietary fat is not fully absorbed from the gut, it may contribute to kidney stone formation by binding with calcium. Fat-bound calcium cannot bind with oxalate, so more oxalate is absorbed to later reappear in the urine where it can bind with calcium to encourage the development of stones.[4,5]

Sugar is another contributor to stone formation. The more sugar there is in your diet, the greater your risk of kidney stones. More than 70 percent of people who form kidney stones that have no known cause respond to sugar by increasing their urinary excretion of calcium, oxalate, and uric acid. Moreover, sugar increases the quantity of calcium oxalate dissolved in the urine and induces calcium-containing lesions within the kidney on which stones can start to form.[6,7]

Alcohol should also be avoided. The more alcohol you drink, the greater your risk of kidney stones. In fact, among stone formers, alcohol consumption is almost double that of people who don't form kidney stones.[8]

Finally, you probably should keep away from caffeine. While we don't yet know whether caffeine increases the risk of kidney stones, we do know that it substantially increases the amount of calcium in the urine, where it is available for stone formation. Caffeine also increases the amount of salt (sodium chloride) in the urine, and it appears that the level of urinary calcium increases as urinary sodium increases. (For that reason, a low-salt diet is also suggested.)[9]

Dietary oxalate makes a relatively small contribution to the level of urinary oxalate; however, if your level of urinary oxalate is high, limiting high-oxalate foods may reduce your risk of forming new stones.[10]

FOODS WITH THE HIGHEST OXALATE CONCENTRATION (25 MG/100 G)

beans
cocoa
coffee (instant)
parsley
rhubarb
spinach
tea

OTHER RELATIVELY HIGH-OXALATE FOODS

beet tops
carrots
celery
chocolate
cucumbers
grapefruit
kale
peanuts
pepper
sweet potatoes

Fiber is one item that you should eat more of. Stone formers eat less dietary fiber, and kidney stones are rare in Third World countries where the fiber intake is still high. When fiber is added to the diet, stone formers reduce their excretion of calcium in the urine by perhaps 40 percent.[11,12,13]

Consider a vegetarian diet. High in fiber, low in animal protein and, if reasonably planned, low in fat, a vegetarian diet can be an excellent means to reduce your risk of future kidney stones.

Your fluid intake also makes a difference. Inadequate body fluid due either to insufficient intake or fluid loss encourages stone formation by reducing the amount of urine and increasing its concentration of stone-forming minerals. Therefore, unless they have a tendency to retain fluid, stone formers should have a daily intake of 2 to 3 qt (2 to 2 ½ l) of fluid spread evenly throughout the day.[14]

Hard water is preferable for drinking water since the harder the local water, the lower the likelihood of people developing kidney stones. The higher calcium content of hard water may be one reason for its superiority; calcium and oxalate from the diet combine to form solid calcium oxalate in the intestines. Because this material is not absorbed into the bloodstream, the risk of solid calcium oxalate developing in the urine is reduced.[15]

THE HEALING DIET

1. Consider a vegetarian diet (high in fiber, low in animal protein, low in fat).

2. Avoid sugar, salt, alcohol, and caffeine.
3. Avoid high-oxalate foods.
4. Drink 2 to 3 qt (2 to 2 ½ l) of fluid daily.
5. Drink hard, rather than soft, water.

NUTRITIONAL HEALING PLANS

Vitamins

Vitamin B_6

Some stone formers are marginally deficient in vitamin B_6. Because vitamin B_6 is required for the breakdown of oxalic acid in the body, a deficiency causes oxalic acid to accumulate. This results in increased excretion of oxalic acid in the urine that, in turn, increases the risk that calcium oxalate stones will form.[16,17]

Stone formers with excess urinary oxalic acid often respond to supplementation with vitamin B_6. Although those with marginal vitamin B_6 deficiencies would be expected to be the best candidates, even people who fail to show evidence of a deficiency on testing have benefited from B_6 supplementation.[18,19]

NUTRITIONAL HEALING PLANS: VITAMIN B_6

Preparation

Dosage: 40 mg daily

Vitamin C

Since vitamin C can be broken down to oxalate, some physicians have been concerned that vitamin C supplementation may increase oxalate levels in the urine and thus increase the risk of stone formation. Generally, however, urinary oxalate excretion does not increase significantly unless the dosage of vitamin C exceeds 6 g a day. If, for some reason, you need more than 6 g of vitamin C daily, take it along with pyridoxine. As already noted, vitamin B_6 helps to break down oxalic acid; it may thus be able to reduce the tendency of vitamin C to increase oxalic acid in the urine.[20]

Minerals

Calcium

About one-third to one-half of stone formers have excess calcium in their urine for unexplained reasons. Calcium restriction is usually not indicated, however, for the following reasons:

1. Chronic high calcium intake (up to 2 g daily) in people with normal vitamin D levels does not significantly increase urinary calcium, presumably because of a feedback system that decreases the percentage of calcium absorbed. (If you are taking calcium supplementation to prevent osteoporosis, take it in the form of carbonate, citrate, gluconate, or lactate. These calcium salts make the urine more alkaline, which in turn decreases the amount of calcium that is excreted in the urine.)[21,22]

2. Restricting calcium may not reduce urine calcium levels. For some stone formers, high levels of urine calcium are due to the overproduction of vitamin D, which increases the absorption of calcium from the intestines.[23]

3. Urinary oxalate increases as dietary calcium is reduced—perhaps because dietary calcium precipitates oxalate in the intestines to form calcium oxalate, which is not absorbed.[24]

4. For women of menopausal age who have kidney stones and early osteoporosis, excess urine calcium may be due to excessive resorption of calcium from the bones because of an estrogen deficiency.[25]

Occasionally, calcium restriction reduces urine calcium and may thus be worthwhile. Since calcium is an important nutrient mineral, only your doctor should decide whether to restrict calcium, and only after performing the necessary laboratory tests.

Magnesium

Magnesium deficiency appears to be a cause of kidney stones. When placed on a magnesium-deficient diet, animals can develop stones. Magnesium appears to reduce the occurrence of kidney stones by inhibiting the formation of calcium oxalate in the urine. By combining with oxalate to form magnesium oxalate, magnesium reduces the amount of oxalate that is available to combine with calcium. Since, in contrast to calcium oxalate, magnesium oxalate has no tendency to become solid, stones will not form.[26,27]

Perhaps 5 percent of stone formers have low levels of magnesium in their urine, most likely due to inadequate magnesium in their diets, and the urine of more than one-quarter of stone formers has a relatively low level of magnesium for the amount of calcium it contains.[28,29]

In several clinical trials, supplementation with magnesium salts at meal times was found to successfully inhibit stone formation. For example, in one study 55 stone formers decreased their average rate of stone development by 90 percent after being given magnesium supplements.[30]

NUTRITIONAL HEALING PLAN: Magnesium

Dosage: 300 mg of magnesium daily with meals

Potassium

Potassium has a beneficial effect in kidney stone disease. When it is low in the blood, urine citrate (which inhibits stone formation) also tends to be low, whereas eating potassium-rich foods counteracts the tendency of meat in the diet to increase urine calcium levels (*see Appendix D for a list of high-potassium foods*).[31]

Other Nutritional Factors

Citrate

The lower the level of citrate in the urine of stone formers, the higher the level of calcium. When their urinary citrate level is low, citrate supplementation helps to prevent calcium oxalate from becoming solid and has been shown to successfully reduce stone formation. Calcium oxalate stone formers with elevated levels of uric acid in the urine may also benefit, even though their urinary uric acid level remains high.[32,33,34,35]

For supplementation, citrate is usually combined with magnesium or potassium to form a stable salt.

NUTRITIONAL HEALING PLAN: Citrate

Preparation

potassium citrate

Dosage: 2 g 3 times daily

Botanical Preparations: Cranberry Juice

Cranberry juice is one fluid that appears to be especially beneficial for kidney stone disease. Though cranberry juice has no effect on urinary calcium levels in people who don't form kidney stones, two pints of the juice have been shown to reduce urinary ionized calcium levels in stone formers by an average of 50 percent.[36]

Toxic Metals: Cadmium

People who are exposed to cadmium, a toxic metal, have an increased risk of developing kidney stones. Cadmium both damages the kidney, predisposing it to develop calcium deposits, and encourages oxalate in the urine to crystallize. Though you may think that cadmium toxicity is very rare, some cadmium is in the diet and, among stone formers, significantly elevated amounts of cadmium in the urine may be found.[37,38,39,40]

Cadmium competes with zinc and calcium for absorption from the gut. Therefore deficiencies of these minerals will increase cadmium absorption, while a diet high in zinc and calcium will reduce the danger of cadmium toxicity from foods. A diet high in protein, other minerals, and vitamins will increase your protection from cadmium toxicity even more.[41]

CHOOSING A PERSONAL PLAN

If you have recurrent kidney stones, consider following the principles of the Basic Healing diet. Simply improving your diet may be all you need to do to protect yourself from forming new stones.

As regards nutritional supplementation, since vitamin B_6 and magnesium are nutritional partners, it makes sense to try them at the same time. In fact, in some of the studies in which kidney stones were successfully reduced, vitamin B_6 and magnesium were given together. Potassium citrate is the other supplement you should consider. It has been demonstrated to be effective in several careful studies. (Magnesium citrate could be tried instead; however, if you choose to try it, don't take another form of magnesium supplementation at the same time.)

Though different people may form the same type of calcium oxalate stones, different metabolic abnormalities may be responsible. Finding out the specifics in your case may help to decide not only the best treatment, but also whether the treatment has corrected the abnormalities. A nutritionally knowledgeable physician can perform the appropriate laboratory testing. The following case is a typical example:

A man who passed 15 calcium oxalate stones over 9 years had an increased 24-hour urinary oxalate excretion, a low-normal calcium excretion, a high-normal phosphate excretion, a low magnesium ex-

cretion, and normal uric acid excretion. Serum calcium, phosphorus, and uric acid were normal, but magnesium was slightly low. Hair calcium and phosphorus were high-normal, whereas hair magnesium was quite elevated, suggesting a magnesium deficiency. (For reasons that remain unclear, the levels of magnesium and of certain other minerals sometimes rise in the hair rather than fall when the body becomes deficient in them.)

He was placed on 100 mg of chelated magnesium twice daily and 50 mg of pyridoxine twice daily. In addition, he was told to limit vitamin C to a maximum of 2 to 3 g daily, eliminate high-oxalate foods, and to limit calcium for a few weeks.

Three months later, his tests for magnesium and oxalate were normal; after six months, his elevated hair magnesium had reduced to nearly normal. On follow-up three years later, he had not passed any stones.[42]

Learning Disabilities

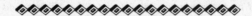

Learning requires adequate intelligence and motivation. Equally important, it requires the ability to concentrate, which can be compromised by undue restlessness or fatigue. Children are considered to be *learning disabled* when their academic achievements are at least two years behind the norms for their age; they are *dyslexic* if they have difficulty in mastering words and symbols.

DIETARY FACTORS

The diet must be nutritionally adequate, since malnutrition is a known cause of learning failure. Eating a healthy breakfast, while recommended for all children, has been shown to improve learning only in those children who were previously undernourished.

Though most research suggests that sugar in the diet is not a common cause of learning problems in children, eating foods and candies that are full of sugar can adversely affect the learning process. One of the ways in which sugar can interfere with learning may be by increasing adrenalin levels. In a Yale study, children, but not adults, had a dramatic rise in blood adrenalin after eating the equivalent of two frosted cupcakes for breakfast. Adrenalin may increase anxiety and irritability and reduce concentration, thus making learning more difficult.[1,2,3]

Caffeine is found in coffee, cola, and some teas. Since high levels of caffeine consumption may cause anxiety, depression, and various physical symptoms, too much caffeine is likely to interfere with learning. Evidence of this relationship comes from a survey of college students that found heavy caffeine consumers had poorer grades.[4]

Food sensitivities have not been proven to cause learning problems. This lack of evidence is striking when one considers that many studies have found a relationship between food sensitivities and attention-deficit hyperactivity disorder, which is common among people who are learning-disabled.

Despite the absence of an experimental literature, clinicians have encountered children for whom food sensitivities appeared to play an important role in causing their learning problems. The following case report is an example of learning disabilities and hyperactivity associated with food sensitivities:

> *Two days after delivery, a male infant broke out in a severe rash. The rash became chronic and was diagnosed as eczema. Later he developed difficulty pronouncing words, spoke in incomplete sentences, and appeared forgetful and confused. His symptoms were so severe that he was unable to sit quietly in his school classroom and failed to learn at a normal rate.*
>
> *When he was in the second grade, his mother tried a Feingold salicylate and food additive elimination-diet as well as nutritional supplements, with uncertain results. He was seen at the Learning Disabilities Unit of the Massachusetts General Hospital in Boston, where he was diagnosed as having a learning disorder with developmental dyslexia. Individualized teaching was unsuccessful because of "hyperactivity, distractability, moodiness, and unpredictable behavior."*
>
> *When examined at age nine and a half, his face was stark white, whereas his eyes were puffy and black. He had constant itchiness with scabs and scars from scratching, and he overreacted to loud noises. All dairy products were removed from his diet. Four days later, he had an episode of violent behavior; afterward he became relatively calm, and his school behavior markedly improved. The presence of multiple sensitivities was confirmed by placing solutions of various substances under his tongue. Numerous foods and chemicals provoked reactions, including changes in behavior and penmanship, fluid retention, nasal discharge, and sneezing.[5]*

THE HEALING DIET

1. Follow the Basic Healing diet as described in Appendix A.
2. Restrict caffeine consumption.

NUTRITIONAL HEALING PLANS

Vitamins

Vitamin C

It is well accepted that the classical vitamin deficiency diseases may interfere with learning. If, however, vitamins are not clearly deficient, there is very little evidence that they affect learning.

One bit of evidence that vitamins may affect learning is an intriguing study in which 72 pairs of students of kindergarten to college age were divided into 2 groups depending upon how high the ascorbic acid (vitamin C) level was in their blood. Not only was the average IQ of the higher ascorbic acid group higher but, after both groups received a glass of orange juice (an excellent source of vitamin C) daily for 6 months, the average IQ of the lower ascorbic acid group increased more than did that of the higher ascorbic acid group. The study was continued with 32 pairs of students for a second school year with similar results.[6]

This study suggests that children who are low in vitamin C are most likely to increase their IQ with supplementation. Hopefully, more studies will be done to further clarify the value of vitamin C supplementation in improving learning.

NUTRITIONAL HEALING PLAN: VITAMIN C

Dosage: 500 mg of vitamin C daily

Mineral Deficiencies

Iodine Deficiency

In studies from both Sicily and China, iodine deficiency in childhood has been shown to be associated with problems with thinking processes. If there is any reason to suspect that a child may not be receiving enough iodine in the diet, he or she should be medically evaluated; any deficiency should be treated by the doctor.[7,8]

Iron Deficiency

Many people wrongly believe that unless children are anemic they cannot be iron-deficient. Iron-deficient children have difficulties concentrating, and they do poorly in school. Although they often improve following iron supplementation, they may continue to have some problems in learning.[9]

Because of the possibility of adverse effects from iron supplementation, it should be given only under a doctor's supervision after an iron-deficiency has been diagnosed.

Magnesium Deficiency

Chronically magnesium-deficient children with normal IQ scores may experience learning problems. They are fidgety, anxious, and restless. A medical evaluation, including laboratory testing, can diagnose magnesium deficiency.[10]

Zinc Deficiency

Zinc-deficient children are irritable, tearful, and sullen, and are therefore prone to be poor students. Moreover, one study reported finding that the amount of zinc in the sweat of a group of dyslexic children was only two-thirds that of normal children, which suggests that a zinc deficiency may somehow contribute to the development of dyslexia.[11]

In the following case report, both zinc deficiency and sugar ingestion appeared to be important contributors to the behavior of a young girl with learning problems:

> *A 13-year-old girl had been diagnosed as having minimal brain dysfunction. In addition to learning problems, she was uncooperative, antagonistic, and displayed unprovoked raging temper tantrums. She was placed on a high-protein, sugar-free diet with vitamin C, niacinamide, and pyridoxine. Tantrums ceased after a few days but recurred after she ate candy.*
>
> *Because she was unusually alert and cooperative after eating oysters, which have a high zinc content, a trial of zinc supplementation was begun. Within 24 hours after zinc supplementation was started, her behavior improved dramatically. However, when the zinc supplements were stopped, her tantrums returned.[12]*

Combined Nutritional Treatments

Many scientific studies have explored the effects of dietary changes, sometimes along with nutritional supplementation, upon intelligence and school performance. Though, following these changes, significant improvements were sometimes found, other investigators have generally not been able to confirm these improvements. This may be because the studies did not select the children who were most likely to benefit. For example, dietary changes designed to improve nutrition would most likely benefit those children whose nutrition is poor, while elimination diets would most likely benefit those children who have been found to be sensitive to foods or food additives.

Perhaps the largest and most intriguing of these studies involved 803

New York City public schools. Over a period of four years, these schools introduced a policy that reduced the amount of sugar and synthetic food additives in school lunches. Before the dietary changes, from year to year students in these schools did almost exactly the same on an academic test as students at other American schools. Following the dietary changes, they achieved a 16 percent increase.

Moreover, before the diet changed, the smaller the percentage of children at a particular school who ate school food, the higher the school's performance on the test. After the dietary changes, the greater the percentage of children who ate school meals within each school, the greater that school's rate of gain in its ranking on the test.[13]

In the following case report, combined nutritional treatments were used to treat a dyslexic boy:

> *In the sixth grade, even though intelligence tests showed him to be in the high-average range, he had difficulty understanding the meaning of printed words. The neurologist had found only "slight clumsiness of gross motor activity" and he was diagnosed as dyslexic.*
>
> *On examination, he had very dry, patchy, dull skin, and both his skin and his hair failed to reflect light with a normal luster. His hair was easily tousled; when pulled between the fingers, it had a straw-like texture. He had dandruff, "chicken skin" (follicular hyperkeratosis) on the back of his arms, and his fingernails were soft and frayed at the ends.*
>
> *Because these findings were consistent with an essential fatty acid imbalance, blood was drawn to evaluate the essential fatty acids in addition to other nutritional factors. The results suggested that he needed larger amounts of polyunsaturated fats and less saturated fats in his diet. Also, his levels of vitamin B_6, iron, and zinc were low.*
>
> *His parents were told to reduce saturated fats in his diet, and he was given supplements of vitamins and minerals along with linseed and evening primrose oils to increase his levels of essential fatty acids. His symptoms markedly improved; at the same time his skin and hair regained their normal luster and texture.*
>
> *Because he had experienced milk intolerance in infancy, his parents were asked to remove all dairy products from his diet for five days and then to challenge him by feeding him a high quantity of them. His stuffy nose cleared noticeably by last day of the dairy elimination; when he returned to dairy products he became congested, cranky, and "spacey." He therefore agreed to avoid all dairy products.*
>
> *Less than a year after starting treatment, he was doing well in school and catching up in reading.[14]*

Note: Although there is no experimental literature suggesting a relationship between essential fatty acid deficiencies and learning problems, pilot studies suggest a possible relationship with schizophrenia and perhaps certain other psychiatric disorders.

Metal Toxicity

Aluminum

Findings of several studies suggest that aluminum toxicity may play a role in learning problems. For example, serum aluminum levels were higher in 28 children with learning disorders or hyperactivity than in a group of normal children. Similarly, hair aluminum has been found to be elevated in some of the studies of dyslexic or learning disabled children. Aluminum is also suspected of contributing to Alzheimer's dementia; however, more research is needed to establish whether aluminum toxicity is a common cause of impaired brain function.[15,16,17]

Cadmium and Lead

When 26 dyslexic children aged 6 to 14 were compared to normal children, they tended to have higher lead and cadmium concentrations in both their sweat and hair. Similarly, when 150 unselected school children were evaluated, the higher either their hair lead or hair cadmium levels, the lower their scores on measures of intelligence.[18]

One reason for the harmful effects of cadmium is its ability to masquerade as zinc and other essential minerals in biochemical reactions. When it successfully displaces an essential mineral, reactions which require that mineral fail to occur properly and brain functioning is impaired. (Adequate minerals in the diet may help to protect against the toxic effects of cadmium.)

The evidence against these metals is strongest for lead. The *Journal of the American Medical Association* published a statistical analysis of the results of 24 scientific studies investigating this relationship. The conclusion of the authors was that these studies presented strong evidence that low-level lead exposure impairs children's intelligence.[19]

Low dietary intakes of calcium, iron, zinc, or copper can increase the absorption of lead from the diet, causing higher tissue accumulation and exacerbated symptoms, while increased intake of these minerals reduces lead absorption and thus reduces symptoms due to lead exposure.[20] Among the vitamins, both thiamine and vitamin C help to combat the effects of lead poisoning.[21]

Manganese

Studies have shown that learning-disabled children have higher hair manganese levels than normal. When manganese is elevated in the hair, it may also be elevated in the central nervous system, where excessive manganese is known to have toxic effects. Moreover, since it inhibits the absorption of iron from the gut, elevated manganese can promote the development of iron deficiency, which we have already discussed as a cause of learning problems.[22]

Manganese toxicity has been reported to result from drinking water containing high manganese concentrations. Also, since infant formulas may contain 3 to 100 times the manganese content of breast milk, they could contribute to a manganese overload. Although more studies are needed to confirm a relationship between manganese toxicity and learning disabilities, laboratory studies can evaluate whether a child with learning problems has elevated manganese levels. When excess manganese is found, attempts can be made to reduce its sources in the diet.[23]

CHOOSING A PERSONAL PLAN

All students with learning problems should follow the principles of the Basic Healing diet; that is, a nutritionally sound diet that minimizes sugar and caffeine. In most cases, multivitamin supplements are helpful only if the student fails to eat a wholesome diet, although the occasional student, because of poor vitamin absorption or a biological need for an unusually high amount of a vitamin, could theoretically benefit from a supplement. (A nutritionally knowledgeable physician can determine whether a particular student could benefit.)

In most industrialized countries, the addition of iodine to salt has protected students from iodine deficiency, and iron, magnesium, and zinc deficiencies are rare if a student is eating a wholesome diet. As with vitamins, an occasional student may benefit from supplementation with one or more minerals; a medical evaluation, including laboratory studies, is the only way of determining who could benefit.

Laboratory studies can also identify students who have elevated levels of manganese, cadmium, lead, or mercury. If elevated levels are found, further exposure can be avoided. Moreover, it may be possible to reduce the body burden of that element. If that can be accomplished, then improvement in learning may be possible.

Menopausal Symptoms

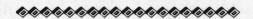

Menopause is the permanent cessation of the menstrual period because of ovarian failure, which occurs at an average age of 51 years. Before, during, and after menopause, there may be a wide range of symptoms due to estrogen deficiency, such as hot flashes, mood swings, depression, and vaginal irritation. As many as 75 percent of all postmenopausal women have hot flashes and excess perspiration that is bothersome enough for them to consult their physicians.

NUTRITIONAL HEALING PLANS

Vitamins

Vitamin E

With the reduction in stimulation of vaginal tissues that accompanies menopause, the vaginal lining becomes thinner and drier, sometimes making sexual intercourse painful. This condition is called *senile vaginitis.* In 1942, the *Journal of Obstetrics and Gynecology of the British Empire* reported that after supplementation with vitamin E, postmenopausal women suffering from senile vaginitis reported symptom relief. Following at least four weeks of supplementation, biopsy specimens showed what appeared to be a proliferation of new blood vessels in the vaginal wall.[1]

These results were later confirmed by a study reported in the *British Medical Journal.* In this study, 50 percent of all postmenopausal women with senile vaginitis responded to prolonged treatment with high doses of vitamin E.[2]

Between 1945 and 1952 several authors reported that hot flashes, sweats, depression, anxiety, and a number of physical complaints such as dizziness, palpitations, difficulty breathing, and fatigue all improved following supplementation with vitamin E. Three of these studies gave placebos to some of the women; in two of them, vitamin E was more effective than the placebo. Unfortunately, this exciting early work has not stimulated further studies in recent decades.[3,4,5]

The following case from my own practice is an example of the benefits of vitamin E supplementation for menopausal symptoms:

A 57-year-old postmenopausal woman who was not on estrogen replacement had a 12-year history of episodic hot flashes, palpitations, and shortness of breath. The hot flashes came in waves, lasted about 90 seconds, and were associated with a feeling of malaise. The palpitations were sometimes associated with the hot flashes but could also occur alone. Two years earlier her doctor had found that during an episode of palpitations, her pulse rate was 220 beats per minute, well above the normal range of 60 to 80 beats per minute. She described her breathing problem as a constant need to yawn, sigh, or try to take a deep breath, and noted that it seemed worse when she was nervous or in a rush.

She was given a trial of 200 IU of vitamin E daily. Three months later, she reported that she had also begun to take a "megavitamin." Her hot flashes were better, although not entirely gone. She was generally much calmer, her pulse rate was slower, and she stated that her shortness of breath was 75 percent improved. In addition, she felt more energetic and was able to do more physical work before tiring.

NUTRITIONAL HEALING PLAN: Vitamin E

Dosage: 400 IU of vitamin E daily

Trial Period

six weeks

Other Nutritional Factors

Hesperidin

In pilot studies, *hesperidin,* a bioflavonoid found in citrus fruits, seemed effective for reducing certain menopausal symptoms. Given alone, it has been reported to reduce flushing. Given along with vitamin C, nocturnal leg cramps, easy bruising, and spontaneous nosebleeds all appeared to respond.[6,7]

Other research suggests that the combination of bioflavonoids and vitamin C may be more effective than either nutrient alone, and vitamin C in nature is usually found in combination with bioflavonoids. Therefore, if you wish to try hesperidin, I suggest that you take vitamin C along with it.

NUTRITION HEALING PLAN: HESPERIDIN

Suggested Use

- ▶ bruising
- ▶ flushing
- ▶ leg cramps (at night)
- ▶ nosebleeds

Preparation

hesperidin methyl chalcone

Dosage: 250–500 mg 3 times daily; take with 1 g of vitamin C daily

---

L-Tryptophan

Depressed women who have recently gone through menopause tend to have low tryptophan levels. This suggests that tryptophan supplementation, which is often effective for treating depression, may be especially indicated for menopausal depression.[8]

NUTRITIONAL HEALING PLAN: Tryptophan

Dosage: 2 g of L-trytophan 3 times daily

Additional Instructions

1. Avoid protein for 90 minutes before and after ingestion.
2. Take with a carbohydrate (such as fruit juice).

Note: Since tryptophan supplements may not be currently available (see Introduction), you may wish to try foods with a high tryptophan to protein ratio (see Appendix A).

Suggested Use

depression

Botanical Extract

Gamma-Oryzanol

In several pilot studies, an extract of rice bran, *gamma-oryzanol,* has been reported to relieve a wide variety of menopausal symptoms in as many as 85 percent of women. Symptoms relieved included hot flashes, weakness, joint and muscle pains, headaches, insomnia, nervousness, and depression.[9]

NUTRITIONAL HEALING PLAN: Gamma-Oryzanol

Dosage: 100 mg of gamma-oryzanol 3 times daily

Trial Period

two to eight weeks

CHOOSING A PERSONAL PLAN

If you suffer from a depression that appears to be related to going through menopause, consider a trial of tryptophan first. For easy bruising or frequent nosebleeds, I would recommend the combination of hesperidin and vitamin C. No matter what the symptom, you may wish to include vitamin E. Gamma-oryzanol appears worth a trial if other Nutritional Healing plans are ineffective.

Menstrual Cramps

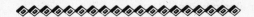

Assuming that the cramps are not due to a disease process, menstrual cramps are usually described as intermittent sharp, spasmodic pains localized just above the pubic bone and radiating to the thighs and back. In some women, they can be so severe as to be incapacitating. Menstrual cramps are commonly accompanied by other symptoms such as nausea, diarrhea, palpitations, flushing, dizziness, and headache.

NUTRITIONAL HEALING PLANS

Vitamins

Niacin (Vitamin B₃)

In the 1950's, Dr. Archibald Huggins reported that, in his experience, about 90 percent of 80 women whose menstrual cramps had been severe enough to require bed rest, heavy sedation, or loss of time from work, found relief from their cramps by taking niacin (a form of vitamin B_3). He believed that they did best if their dosage of niacin was adequate to produce flushing—although he thought that niacinamide (a derivative of niacin that does not produce flushing) worked just as well—and warned his patients in advance to expect flushing or itching, and occasionally slight dizziness. He also believed that niacin was more effective when given along with vitamin C and rutin (a bioflavonoid).[1]

Unfortunately, his observation has yet to be confirmed by controlled studies; nevertheless, his extremely high rate of success makes niacin supplementation a very promising treatment. In the meantime, we do not know if his patients responded merely because they believed in the treatment, or if niacin itself was largely responsible for their relief.

NUTRITIONAL HEALING PLAN: Niacin

Preparation

niacin or niacinamide

Dosage: 100 mg twice daily; increase to 100 mg every 2 to 3 hours during cramps

---

WARNING

Niacin may have side effects and should therefore be medically supervised.

Instructions: Take with 300 mg of vitamin C daily and 60 mg of rutin daily.

Vitamin E

In 1955, *Lancet* published a study in which 100 young women with menstrual cramps received either vitamin E or a placebo for 10 days before their menstrual periods and for the next 4 days. After 2 menstrual cycles, 68 percent of the women in the supplemented group improved, compared to only 18 percent of the women who received the placebo.[2]

Recent Russian studies have discovered one reason why vitamin E may relieve the pain of menstrual cramps. The body produces its own narcotics called *endorphins,* which are endogenous morphinelike compounds. Endorphins can be blocked from relieving pain by an injection of naloxone, a drug that prevents narcotics from working. When women who had just been relieved of cramps by a vitamin E injection were given naloxone, many reported the pain returning; this suggests that vitamin E had provided these women with pain relief by stimulating their bodies to release endorphins.[3]

Since there was evidence of endorphin release only 15 minutes after vitamin E was given, it is possible that vitamin E supplementation may be effective even when given after the start of menstrual cramping. However, an important cause of menstrual pain is the release of hormonelike substances called *prostaglandins.* In addition to activating the endorphin system, vitamin E may regulate prostaglandins in a beneficial way; to take full advantage of this latter effect, supplementation is likely to be more effective if started at least several days prior to the menstrual period.

NUTRITIONAL HEALING PLAN: Vitamin E

Dosage: 100 IU of vitamin E 3 times daily for 14 days starting 10 days prior to the menstrual period

---

Minerals

Iron Deficiency

In 1965 Dr. Nathaniel Shafer of the Department of Medicine, New York Medical College, learned from two patients receiving iron supplementation for iron-deficiency anemia, that their severe menstrual cramps had disappeared. Curious, he proceeded to question another four patients whom he had treated for iron-deficiency anemia, and to treat another six patients complaining of menstrual cramps (several of whom also had iron-deficiency anemia) with iron, without informing them that the treatment might relieve their menstrual pain. All reported that pain diminished or completely disappeared after they began iron supplementation.[4]

As intriguing as these findings are, Dr. Shafer's preliminary findings have yet to be confirmed by further studies. Moreover, iron supplementation is not recommended unless your doctor first finds evidence of an iron deficiency.

Magnesium

Recent studies have reported that magnesium supplementation appears to be effective for treating uncomplicated menstrual cramps. It relaxes the uterine muscle and its blood vessels, and appears to inhibit the synthesis of an inflammatory substance (prostaglandin PGF_2 alpha).[5,6]

Since vitamin B_6 increases the movement of magnesium into the cells of the uterine wall, it may increase magnesium's efficacy, although this hypothesis has yet to be tested.

NUTRITIONAL HEALING PLAN: Magnesium

Dosage: 100 mg of magnesium 4 times daily; increase to 100 mg every 3 hours while awake during menses

---

Botanical Extract

Bilberry Anthocyanosides

Extracts of *anthocyanosides,* flavonoid components of the fruit of the bilberry shrub, have smooth muscle relaxant effects. Since the uterine muscle is a smooth muscle, Italian investigators gave it or a placebo to women suffering from menstrual cramps. Their study found it to be an effective treatment.[7]

NUTRITIONAL HEALING PLAN: Bilberry Anthocyanosides

Preparation

bilberry extract (25% anthocyanidin content)

Dosage: 80—160 mg 3 times daily

CHOOSING A PERSONAL PLAN

Of the several nutritional treatments we have discussed, vitamin E is the best proven. Not only has it been shown to be effective for menstrual cramps, but it has also been shown to be effective for both premenstrual and menopausal symptoms. Moreover, we have some idea of how it works.

There is also a scientific basis for a trial of magnesium, which has been found to be an effective muscle relaxant for other smooth muscle tissues in the body. Like vitamin E, not only has it been shown to be effective, but we know a good deal about how it exerts its beneficial effects.

In contrast to vitamin E and magnesium, we know very little about the use of niacin or iron for treating menstrual cramps. Also, there are some concerns about possible side effects with both of them. The niacin flush can be uncomfortable, and occasionally niacin causes other adverse effects. Unless iron is deficient, supplementation can stress the liver; it should therefore be administered only under a doctor's supervision. Moreover, iron supplementation can cause gastrointestinal side effects.

In early studies, bilberry anthocyanosides have shown promise, and we do have some information about how they appear to work in reducing menstrual cramps. Though further studies are needed to evaluate them more fully, they appear worthy of a trial.

Migraine Headache

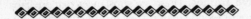

See also: PAIN.

Though their cause is quite complicated, migraine headaches are associated with the dilation of sensitive blood vessels in the head. If these blood vessels first constrict, the victim initially experiences a change in vision often referred to as an *aura* and the headache is called a classic migraine. (If there is no aura, it is called a common migraine.) Pain begins when the vessels dilate. Migraine pain is typically pulsating, often on one side of the head. It may be associated with nausea and vomiting as well as sensitivity to bright lights and loud noises. The pain can be so severe as to be incapacitating, forcing the victim to lie down in a quiet, darkened room until it subsides.

It is interesting that there are almost no studies showing that nutritional medicine is effective for treating common muscle contraction headaches; this suggests that this type of headache may be primarily related to stress and tension. By contrast, although migraine headaches may also be triggered by stress and tension, a growing literature suggests that nutritional factors often play a role in their genesis.

DIETARY FACTORS

Food Sensitivities

By far, the best-proven area of nutritional research concerns the role of foods as triggering agents of migraine headaches. Results of food-elimination diets have been so impressive that a conservative estimate is that one out of three migraine sufferers would benefit markedly from food avoidance. In fact, in one study 93 percent of 88 children with severe, frequent migraines did so well that the authors titled their study, "Is migraine food allergy?"[1,2]

Because of their specific ingredients, certain foods are more likely than others to provoke a migraine. Here are six incriminating ingredients:

1. **Vasoactive amines.** These are substances that are capable of changing the size of blood vessels. They include tyramine and phenylethylamine.[3,4] Tyramine can be found in

   - aged cheese
   - chicken liver
   - pickled herring
   - dry, fermented sausage
   - sour cream
   - red wine (especially Chianti)
   Phenylethylamine is found in
   - cheese
   - chocolate

2. **Nitrites.** These substances, which are added to meats as preservatives and turn them red, may provoke migraines in susceptible people.[5] Nitrites are found in:

   - bologna
   - hot dogs
   - salami
   - sausage

3. **Lactose (milk sugar).** Lactose can cause migraine headaches in people who are low in the enzyme *lactase* that normally digests it in the intestines.[6] Lactose is particularly high in:

   - buttermilk
   - cottage cheese
   - cream
   - ice cream
   - milk
   - yogurt

4. **Caffeine.** The greater your caffeine intake, the greater your chances of having headaches. For people consuming 240 mg daily (about 4 to 5 cups of coffee) as compared to non-coffee-drinkers, the relative risk of having headaches is 30 percent greater for men and 20 percent greater for women. When a habitual coffee drinker abstains, a caffeine-with-

drawal headache may start in about 18 hours and peak 3 to 6 hours later. This headache typically starts with a feeling of "fullness in the brain" and quickly develops into a diffuse, throbbing pain that is worsened by exercise.[7,8] Caffeine can be found in:

- ► coffee
- ► soft drinks
- ► tea (herbal teas may be caffeine-free)

5. **Copper.** This element is involved in the metabolism of the vasoactive amines (amines that affect tone and size of blood vessels), and its metabolism may be abnormal in migraine sufferers. Foods that have a high-copper content or that affect its absorption or transport in the body may provide a migraine stimulus.[9] Foods with a high copper content include:

- ► chocolate
- ► nuts
- ► shellfish
- ► wheat germ
  Citrus fruits also increase intestinal copper absorption. One food additive that binds and transports copper is monosodium glutamate (MSG).

6. **Aspartame (NutraSweet).** An artificial sweetener used in some low-calorie foods, aspartame has been shown in some studies to provoke migraine headache.[10]

In the following case, a food-elimination diet was used to reduce migraine headaches

A long-standing sufferer from common migraines learned how important food sensitivities could be when one day his high intake of aspirin caused gastrointestinal bleeding. In order to heal, he was forced to go on a bland diet that eliminated many of the foods he had been eating. Shortly thereafter, he became headache-free. When he challenged himself with single-food challenges, he learned that bananas, citrus fruits, and cheese (all of which contain vasoactive amines) caused headaches that would occur up to 72 hours following the ingestion of the provoking foods.

He happened to have kept detailed records of the frequency of his headaches and of the medication taken. They showed that during the year prior to his discovery he had headaches on 326 days and took 1,316 aspirin tablets. The year following it, in which he eliminated offending foods, he had headaches on only 8 days and took 16 aspirin.[11]

Serotonin and Migraines

Tryptophan is an amino acid in the diet that is transformed in the body to the neurotransmitter *serotonin.* In the brain, serotonin appears to reduce the experience of pain. One trick for increasing brain serotonin levels is to eat a high-carbohydrate diet. Carbohydrates increase brain tryptophan by provoking the pancreas to secrete insulin. Insulin, in turn, increases the relative concentration of tryptophan in the bloodstream by causing the body tissues to soak up competing amino acids from the blood; thus tryptophan has less competition transferring from the blood into the brain.[12]

Though increasing serotonin within the brain may seem to be a good idea, rising levels of serotonin in the bloodstream may actually set off a migraine in certain people. Such people may improve on a low-tryptophan diet. Fortunately, I can give you some clues to determining the odds of such a diet reducing your migraines: Good candidates often report symptoms of flushing and itchiness so severe that they can't help but scratch their skin, or hives. Also, people who have classic migraines may be more likely to benefit from the diet.[13,14,15]

In a pilot study, a high-carbohydrate diet was combined with a low-tryptophan diet. Three out of the four people with classic migraines, but none of the three other migraine sufferers in the study, noted a marked improvement within four weeks of starting the diet. Controlled studies are needed to confirm the value of this diet. Also, as it is low in protein, your doctor should agree that it is appropriate for you to try it.

Low Blood Sugar (Reactive Hypoglycemia) and Migraines

A high-carbohydrate diet may reduce migraines by another mechanism. Low blood sugar, or *hypoglycemia,* may be associated with a headache in some sufferers. People with diabetes and those whose headaches tend to occur when they fail to eat every few hours should be the most suspicious of such a relationship, which can be verified by your doctor with proper testing. When hypoglycemia touches off headaches, a high-complex-carbohydrate diet in which the carbohydrates are unrefined and sugars are strictly avoided is often effective in minimizing up and down swings in blood sugar and, according to a pilot study, appears to be strikingly effective in reducing migraines.[16,17,18]

THE HEALING DIETS

1. Avoid foods found on testing to provoke headaches. *See Appendix B for information about diagnosing food sensitivities.*
2. Try the High-Complex-Carbohydrate diet described in Appendix A to increase brain serotonin and/or to stabilize blood sugar levels.
3. Try the Low-Tryptophan diet described in Appendix A to decrease blood serotonin.

NUTRITIONAL HEALING PLANS

Minerals: Magnesium Deficiency

Low levels of magnesium in the blood are associated with increased irritability and spasms of the muscles, including the smooth muscle in the lining of blood vessels. Thus, when magnesium is marginally deficient (which is not uncommon in industrialized societies), migraine sufferers are more headache-prone.

Both men and women can have migraines as a result of low magnesium, but women are especially prone to low-magnesium headaches at the time of their menstrual periods and during the latter part of pregnancy. In a pilot study, 80 percent of a group of 3000 women appeared to have a good response to magnesium supplementation. (Combining a magnesium supplement with vitamin B_6 to help raise magnesium levels may make it more effective.)[19,20]

NUTRITIONAL HEALING PLAN: Magnesium Deficiency

Dosage: 200 mg of magnesium daily

Trial Period

two months

Other Nutritional Factors

Omega-3 Fatty Acids

Fish oils are an excellent source of omega-3 fatty acids, one of the two families of fatty acids that we must get from our diets. In double-blind studies, people suffering from severe, chronic migraines found that their headaches developed less often and were less painful after starting fish oil supplementation. (Cod liver oil is not recommended because of its excessive content of vitamin A.)[21,22]

NUTRITIONAL HEALING PLAN: Omega-3 Fatty Acids

Preparation

cholesterol-free fish oil extract
Example: MaxEPA™

Dosage: 3 g 3 times daily

WARNING

Take under medical supervision.

Trial Period

three to six weeks

Botanical Preparation: Feverfew

The results of two double-blind studies in leading medical journals have suggested that the herb feverfew is effective for at least some migraine sufferers. It is believed that this herb may work by inhibiting the release of serotonin from the platelets, the irregularly shaped disks found in blood that are involved in the process of clotting.[23,24,25]

NUTRITIONAL HEALING PLAN: Feverfew

Dosage: 20 to 60 mg daily of the feverfew extract **or** 1 to 3 leaves daily

Instructions: Take with meals.

WARNINGS

1. Sudden discontinuation after prolonged regular use may cause withdrawal symptoms such as increased headaches, joint and muscle pain, nervousness, tension, and insomnia.[26]
2. Though many people have taken this herb for years without problems, careful studies proving its long-term safety have yet to be done.

CHOOSING A PERSONAL PLAN

Every migraine sufferer should try a food-elimination diet in order to discover whether certain foods provoke headaches. If you find that your headaches begin when you have not eaten for at least a few hours or if your doctor has found that you have reactive hypoglycemia or noninsulin-dependent diabetes, you may benefit from the High-Complex-Carbohydrate diet. If you suffer from flushing, hives, or intense itchiness, you may wish to try the Low-Tryptophan diet.

Women who have migraines that are associated with pregnancies or menstrual periods are the most likely group to benefit from magnesium supplementation. (Your doctor can check the level of magnesium in your red blood cells to give you a better idea of whether magnesium supplementation will be effective.) Finally, as far as we know, everyone has an equally good chance of responding to feverfew or the fish oils.

Mitral Valve Prolapse

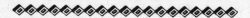

After the left ventricle of the heart contracts to pump blood into the major arteries, the mitral valves close to prevent blood from flowing back into the heart. A sinking downward, or *prolapse,* of these valves is the most common disorder of the heart valves in industrialized nations. Often the diagnosis is made by the physician on an asymptomatic patient. At other times the disorder is associated with chest pains, palpitations, and other symptoms.

NUTRITIONAL HEALING PLANS

Minerals: Magnesium Deficiency

Spasmophilia, or *latent tetany,* refers to a state of muscular hyperexcitability in which the muscles are irritable and readily spasm. *Chvostek's sign,* a popular test, consists of lightly tapping with a physician's hammer over the facial nerve (which runs forward from just beneath and in front of the ear) on one side of the face; when the test is positive, the muscles beneath the hammer go into spasm. If the facial muscles are hyperexcitable, others may be in a similar state.

Though latent tetany is not the only cause for mitral valve prolapse, it is probably the most common cause. For example, 85 percent of a group of people with mitral valve prolapse showed evidence of electrical changes in their muscles suggestive of latent tetany, and 73 percent of them had a positive Chvostek's sign. Similarly, one quarter of another group of people evaluated because of irritable muscles who were found to have latent tetany were also found to have prolapsed mitral valves, whereas mitral valve prolapse was not found in anyone in that group who did not have latent tetany.[1,2]

Latent tetany is believed to be due to a magnesium deficit, and mitral valve prolapse can develop when latent tetany goes untreated. Once prolapse has developed, magnesium supplementation, though essential, may take·months to be fully effective and is not always curative; therefore medications may still be required to control symptoms.[3,4]

NUTRITIONAL HEALING PLAN: Magnesium Deficiency

Dosage: 500 mg of magnesium daily

Other Nutritional Factors

Carnitine

Carnitine is a naturally occurring compound found in the diet that is involved in the transformation of food into energy for the body. Though unproven, decreased availability of carnitine to the heart muscle is suspected of promoting the development of mitral valve prolapse.

In the *Texas Heart Institute Journal,* a group of doctors described a patient with mitral valve prolapse and numerous associated symptoms who was resistant to drug therapy. Because both blood and urine carnitine levels were low, a trial of carnitine was begun as an experiment. Four months after starting treatment, the symptoms had successfully been resolved. Intrigued, they randomly sampled carnitine levels of four other patients with mitral valve prolapse; all were also found to have low levels of blood and urine carnitine.[5]

Since 1984, when their paper was published, no further studies on carnitine for mitral valve prolapse have been reported, although carnitine continues to be investigated for its promising benefits for other cardiac conditions. According to the Food and Drug Administration, gastrointestinal symptoms are a common side effect; they can be reduced or eliminated by a reduction in dosage.

NUTRITIONAL HEALING PLAN: Carnitine

Preparation

L-carnitine

Dosage: not well-established; 1 g 4 times daily was the dosage given to the patient described above, but a lower dosage may be effective

---

WARNING

For the treatment of symptoms of mitral valve prolapse, L-carnitine should be taken under close medical supervision.

Coenzyme Q_{10}

Like carnitine, *coenzyme Q_{10}* (CoQ_{10}), which is found primarily in the heart muscle, plays an important role in energy metabolism. In a Japanese study of 400 children between the ages of 8 and 16 with mitral valve prolapse, CoQ_{10} was highly effective. With adequate doses, heart function returned to normal within only one week, and there were no side effects. Although symptoms returned when CoQ_{10} was withdrawn, the dosage could be gradually reduced to a lower maintenance level.[6]

NUTRITIONAL HEALING PLAN: Coenzyme Q_{10}

Dosage: not well established; generally around 3 mg/kg (7 mg/lb) initially, which can be reduced to perhaps 0.6 mg/kg (1.3 mg/lb) once improvement has occurred

---

WARNING

Despite its excellent safety record, this high a dosage of CoQ_{10} should be taken only under close medical supervision, with the final dosage dependent on both symptoms and the results of medical testing.

CHOOSING A PERSONAL PLAN

Unless the prolapse is due to another disease, anyone suffering from mitral valve prolapse should probably take magnesium supplements. Moreover, consider having your doctor perform a thorough evaluation for latent tetany.

You may first wish to give magnesium supplementation some time to work, but it does not have to be taken alone. Under medical supervision, magnesium could be combined with either L-carnitine or CoQ_{10} for a reasonable trial period.

Muscle Cramps

See Also: CARPAL TUNNEL SYNDROME, PAIN.

Muscle cramps, painful involuntary contractions of the "voluntary" (skeletal) muscles, are fairly common and are caused by overexcitability of the nerves controlling the affected muscles. They are particularly common in growing children and during pregnancy. In most cases, they are unrelated to any disease process.

DIETARY FACTORS

Dr. H. J. Roberts has treated more than 350 patients with severe symptoms of either spontaneous leg cramps or restless legs. With few exceptions, they also experienced typical features of low blood sugar, or *hypoglycemia*. This diagnosis was confirmed by glucose tolerance testing. (Glucose tolerance testing is a procedure in which the level of blood sugar is measured over several hours after the ingestion of a standard amount of glucose.) Sometimes a muscle cramp occurred just as the blood sugar levels reached their lowest level during testing, providing further evidence for a relationship between the cramps and hypoglycemia.

Though scientific research has not been done, Dr. Roberts found that a sugar-free, high-protein diet with snacking was an effective treatment for the "vast majority" of his patients. Moreover, when cramps recurred, they were usually related to a dietary indiscretion within the preceding 24 hours.[1]

More recently, Dr. James W. Anderson, a leading researcher, has noted that he had better results in treating symptoms due to hypoglycemia by adding fiber to the diet rather than protein (in addition to removing sugar).[2] Since the Western diet is already too high in protein for optimal health, this latter diet is probably preferable.

THE HEALING DIET

Follow the Sugar-free and High-Fiber diets with in-between meal and late evening snacks as described in Appendix A.

NUTRITIONAL HEALING PLANS

Vitamins

Vitamin B$_6$

Carpal tunnel syndrome refers to pain, swelling, and numbness in the hand resulting from the compression of a tunnel in the wrist through which the nerves, tendons, and blood vessels have to pass. Dr. John Ellis has proposed that carpal tunnel syndrome can often be successfully treated with pyridoxine (a form of vitamin B$_6$), and his observation has been confirmed by a number of studies *(see the chapter on carpal tunnel syndrome for further information)*. In addition, he has noted that some people with carpal tunnel syndrome complain of muscle spasms in their extremities at night. As with the symptoms of carpal tunnel syndrome, he has found that these muscle spasms respond to pyridoxine supplementation,[3] as illustrated by the following case:

> *A 69-year-old tractor driver experienced stiffness in both hands. They were swollen, and flexion was very limited. He also complained of frequent cramps in his thighs during the day and nocturnal leg cramps about twice a week. Four weeks after starting on 50 mg of pyridoxine daily, his hand stiffness was dramatically relieved, and he reported that, after one week on pyridoxine, his leg cramps vanished.[4]*

Whether people with muscle cramps who do not have carpal tunnel syndrome respond to pyridoxine is not known.

NUTRITIONAL HEALING PLAN: Vitamin B₆

Special Use

carpal tunnel syndrome

Preparation

pyridoxine

Dosage: 100 mg daily

Trial Period

three months

Vitamin E

Vitamin E supplementation has been reported to be highly effective in providing relief for recurrent muscle cramps, although this remains a clinical observation unconfirmed by scientific studies.

The largest group studied consisted of 125 people with nocturnal leg and foot cramps, over half of whom had suffered for more than 5 years. Following supplementation, 82 percent reported complete or nearly complete relief usually within 1 week, whereas another 16 percent had a moderate to good response. Similar success was obtained with nighttime rectal cramps, stomach muscle cramps, and cramps following heavy exercise. Many people had to continue taking vitamin E to prevent cramps from recurring.[5]

The benefits of vitamin E supplementation for muscle cramps is illustrated by the following case:

> *A woman suffered from severe leg cramps every night after going to bed. By trial and error, she found that if she took vitamin E at precisely 5 P.M. each day, the cramps would not occur.*[6]

NUTRITIONAL HEALING PLAN: Vitamin E

Dosage: 300–600 IU of vitamin E daily

Trial Period

one month

Minerals

Calcium

A low blood calcium level (hypocalcemia) is sometimes associated with muscle cramps that respond to calcium supplementation. Calcium supplementation is a popular remedy for muscle cramps even in the absence of low blood calcium levels; experimental studies, however, have concentrated on its possible efficacy for relieving leg cramps related to pregnancy.

In a recent scientific study, calcium was no more effective than vitamin C in relieving pregnancy-related leg cramps; however, 41 out of 60 women (68 percent) who received one or the other supplement responded. The high response rate raises the possibility that vitamin C, rather than serving as a placebo, may also be an effective treatment. Hopefully, new studies will clarify the meaning of these findings.[7]

The benefits of calcium supplementation are shown by the following case:

> At age 75, a woman had been suffering for many years from cramps in the soles of the feet at night when turning or stretching. Within one or two days of starting supplementation with calcium lactate, the cramps disappeared. Previously, she wore arch supporters and stayed away from walking on the beach barefoot because she would experience pain after each walk. Now a daily beach walk of four to five miles never causes her cramps.[8]

NUTRITIONAL HEALING PLAN: Calcium

Special Use

pregnancy-associated leg cramps

Preparation

calcium citrate

Dosage: 1 g of calcium twice daily

Trial Period

four weeks

Magnesium

Low blood magnesium levels (hypomagnesemia) may be associated with muscle cramps that respond to magnesium supplementation. In a study of pregnant women with leg cramps, 19 out of 21 responded to magnesium compared to only 7 out of 21 women who had been given a placebo. It is uncertain whether magnesium supplementation is beneficial in the absence of a deficiency.[9]

NUTRITIONAL HEALING PLAN: Magnesium

Dosage: 400 mg of magnesium daily

Trial Period

four weeks

Potassium

Like calcium and magnesium, low blood potassium (hypokalemia) may be associated with muscle cramps that will respond to potassium supplementation:

> *A woman who had foot cramps for months realized that they always occurred ten days before her menstrual period. She began to increase her dietary potassium intake at that time in her monthly cycle, and her foot cramps ceased. When, however, she forgot to change her diet, the cramps would return.*[10]

It is not known whether potassium supplementation may be effective when the serum potassium level is normal. *See Appendix D for a list of foods that are high in potassium.*

CHOOSING A PERSONAL PLAN

If, in addition to muscle cramps, you have symptoms suggestive of low blood sugar (hypoglycemia)—such as episodes of weakness, dizziness, or anxiety—consider combining the Sugar-free and High-Fiber diets for a trial. (Evidence of low blood sugar on a glucose tolerance test would suggest that you are a particularly good candidate for this diet.)

Though not yet tested scientifically, vitamin E supplementation may well bring relief. Pyridoxine (vitamin B_6) supplementation may be more likely to be effective if you have symptoms of carpal tunnel syndrome. If you are considering a trial of either pyridoxine or magnesium, take them at the same time since they help one another to work.

For some people, calcium, magnesium, or potassium may be effective. Speak to your doctor about testing your blood to see if you have reduced levels of any of these three minerals, although supplementation may be effective even if your blood levels are normal.

ADDITIONAL SUGGESTION

Consider regular, gentle muscle-stretching exercises. They often reduce the tendency of muscles to spasm.

Obesity

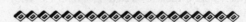

Obesity is a condition in which abnormal fat accumulation in body tissues causes people to weigh at least 20 percent more than their ideal weight. In industrialized societies, obesity is a common problem, with one out of four people classified as obese. It is also a potentially serious medical problem, since obesity is associated with an increased risk of death from heart disease, cancer, high blood pressure, stroke, and diabetes—the latter two being the leading causes of death from disease.

DIETARY FACTORS

In order for the average person to lose 1 lb per week, caloric intake must be reduced by 500 calories per day. Most people begin to lose weight when they reduce their daily calorie intake to less than 1,500 calories; some may require fewer than 1,000 calories to lose weight. (Detailed lists of the calories contained in individual foods are available at your local bookstore.)

Weight Reduction Diets

Calories come from the three macronutrients, namely carbohydrate, protein, and fat. While based on their weight, carbohydrate and protein each contain the same amount of energy (measured in calories), fat contains more than double that amount. That is why fatty foods promote weight gain and why, if you wish to lose weight, your fat intake should be minimized.

Weight reduction diets reduce the amount of one or more of the macronutrients in the diet, thereby increasing the percentage of calories which come from the remaining one(s). Thus, since weight reduction diets usually reduce both the total calorie count and the amount of fat, a high-carbohydrate diet is likely to be relatively low in protein, while a low-carbohydrate diet is likely to contain a high percentage of protein.

Balanced low-calorie diets are considered to be the safest for weight loss. They generally provide for 800 to 1500 calories daily using a wide variety of foods. High-carbohydrate diets provide more limited food choices, and some versions are nutritionally unbalanced.[1,2]

One reason that low-carbohydrate diets are popular is that they are generally associated with fewer hunger pangs than other weight-loss diets. Since carbohydrate is less available as a source of energy, body fat is converted into ketone bodies and free fatty acids to provide for energy needs. This metabolic state, called *ketosis,* quickly causes a loss of body fluid resulting in rapid initial weight loss. The ketone bodies, as well as the relatively high proportion of protein and fat, probably account for the ability of low-carbohydrate diets to satisfy hunger. Also, if you consume the same number of calories, you will lose more weight on low-carbohydrate diets than on high-carbohydrate diets.[3]

However, even if they are designed to be nutritionally adequate, low-carbohydrate diets have a number of health risks. Though in some people they produce a feeling of euphoria, others complain of fatigue and note feelings of dizziness upon standing due to low blood pressure. Either diarrhea or constipation may occur, and there may be medical problems resulting from the elevation of uric acid in the blood, sodium and potassium loss, blood sugar problems, or elevation of blood fats.[4]

Closely related to low-carbohydrate diets are high-protein diets. These tend to severely limit food choices and, if the protein comes mainly from animal sources, are high in cholesterol. Furthermore, they are commonly deficient in vitamins and minerals.[5]

Very-low-calorie diets generally contain 300 to 400 calories per day. Compared to balanced diets of equal calories, these diets may initially produce greater weight loss due to a larger amount of fluid loss. In order to reduce hunger and to improve bowel function, these diets are often improved by the addition of dietary fiber.[6,7]

Because of the possibility of medical complications, consider a very-low-calorie diet only if you are at least 30 percent and 40 lb (18 kg) overweight, and first see your physician for a physical examination and an electrocardiogram. The diet is not recommended for people with signifi-

CLASSIFICATION OF TYPICAL POPULAR DIET PLANS

Low-Calorie Balanced Diets
American Diabetes Association
Diet Center
La Costa Spa
Nutri/System
Prudent
Setpoint
TOPS (Take Off Pounds Sensibly)
Weight Watchers

High-Carbohydrate Diets

BALANCED
Pritikin

UNBALANCED
Beverly Hills
Macrobiotic (some earlier versions)
Rice

cant psychiatric illness, cancer, type I diabetes, or for those who have had strokes, or have heart, kidney, or liver disease and should be medically supervised.[8]

The "Fit for Life" diet, designed by Harvey and Marilyn Diamond, doesn't fit any of the usual categories. It is based on a number of generally unaccepted and unproven claims. For example, the authors state that eating two concentrated foods simultaneously will cause them to rot.[9]

Though fasting may seem to be the quickest way to lose weight, over the long term the results of temporary or intermittent fasting are sometimes disappointing. During a prolonged fast, such as one lasting 24 days, one-third of the weight lost is fluid and lean body mass. The longer a fast lasts, the greater its potential medical dangers, which include muscle wasting, liver and kidney impairment, and gout.[10,11,12]

CLASSIFICATION OF TYPICAL POPULAR DIET PLANS *(CONT.)*

Low-Carbohydrate Diets
>Dr. Atkins'
>Dr. Stillman's
>Endocrine Control
>Scarsdale

High-Protein Diets
>Berkowitz
>Richard Simmons' Never-Say-No
>Southampton

Very-Low-Calorie Diets
>Cambridge
>Liquid Protein
>Optifast
>Protein-Sparing Modified Fast

Dietary Constituents

Increasing dietary fiber adds noncaloric bulk; the result is that satiety (loss of hunger) develops after lower food intake, leading to weight loss. Several specific sources of dietary fiber appear to be effective in promoting weight loss, including bean husk, glucomannan, guar gum, and xanthan gum. Rather than supplementing your diet with a specific fiber, the best way of utilizing dietary fiber to lose weight is to emphasize high-fiber foods such as fruits, vegetables, and whole grain cereals.[13,14,15,16,17,18]

Sucrose (table sugar) consists of a molecule of glucose attached to a molecule of fructose; it appears to stimulate increased calorie consumption in obese people and should thus be restricted. As a source of sugar, fructose may be preferable. When volunteers were given drinks containing either glucose, fructose, or aspartame before a meal, those given the fructose drinks consumed fewer calories and less fat.[19,20]

Eating more than somebody of normal weight who is of the same sex and is similar in size and build is one cause of obesity. Another cause may be difficulty in converting food into energy in a process called *thermogenesis.* In such a case, food would be more readily stored as fat. Fructose, besides its advantage over other common forms of sugar in decreasing subsequent fat consumption, causes greater thermogenesis than glucose. This may be another reason for choosing it as the source of sugar.[21,22]

Caffeine is another promoter of thermogenesis; however, because of its many other effects, some of which appear to be unhealthy, I would not recommend a high consumption of caffeine on a regular basis.[23]

Food Sensitivities

On the basis of his experiences in medical practice over the years, Dr. Theron Randolph has suggested that obesity may result from cravings for frequently eaten foods to which people have become sensitized. The cravings develop, he believes, because avoidance of those foods causes a variety of mental and physical symptoms; people feel better when they eat those foods because eating them causes the symptoms to rapidly subside.[24]

For people who have become sensitized to certain foods, Randolph believes that a weight reduction diet is exceedingly difficult until the masked food allergens have first been avoided for several days in order to clear the person's body of withdrawal symptoms. He has found that corn, wheat, and milk are the most frequent offenders. Though others have reported similar observations, his hypothesis has yet to be explored scientifically.[25]

The following case is an example of food sensitivities affecting weight gain:

> *A 33-year-old chronically obese woman also had a history of depression, migraine headaches, irritability, perceptual and learning problems, periodic motor problems, and childhood hyperactivity. Upon repeated testing, several foods were found to produce consistent irregular behavioral and physiological states. By avoiding these substances, she was more effective in controlling her weight and greatly improved in other problem areas. Although calorie intake remained constant during her evaluative period, she gained weight during six-day phases when sensitive foods were eaten, and lost weight during phases when nonsensitive foods were eaten.*[26]

THE HEALING DIET

1. Eat a reduced calorie diet.
2. Increase consumption of dietary fiber.
3. Minimize fat consumption.
4. Minimize sugar and caffeine.
5. Substitute fructose for table sugar.

6. Avoid foods found on testing to be allergenic. *See Appendix B for information about diagnosing food sensitivities.*

NUTRITIONAL HEALING PLANS

Vitamins

Vitamin C

Only a few nutritional factors have been identified that, when added to the diet, may promote weight loss in people suffering from obesity. Vitamin C is the only vitamin for which there is some evidence of benefit. In a double-blind study, vitamin C supplementation was associated with significant weight loss in very obese women (women at least 50 percent above ideal body weight) who had previously failed to lose weight in various reducing programs. Further studies are needed to confirm this hopeful finding.[27]

NUTRITIONAL HEALING PLAN: Vitamin C

Dosage: 1 g of vitamin C 3 times daily

Other Nutritional Factors

Coenzyme Q_{10}

Some early work suggests that there may be a relationship between the blood level of coenzyme Q_{10} (CoQ_{10}), a vitaminlike substance, and obesity. About half of a group of 27 obese patients were found to have reduced levels of CoQ_{10}. Moreover, when nine obese patients were placed on a low-calorie diet and supplemented with CoQ_{10}, the mean weight loss of the five patients who had been found to have reduced CoQ_{10} levels was significantly greater than that of the rest of the group. If these findings are confirmed in larger studies, perhaps one out of every two obese patients may lose weight more easily with CoQ_{10} supplements.[28]

NUTRITIONAL HEALING PLAN: Coenzyme Q_{10}

Dosage: 50 mg of coenzyme Q_{10} twice daily

Omega-6 Fatty Acids

Most preliminary data suggests that *evening primrose oil,* which is rich in essential fatty acids of the omega-6 family, may promote weight loss in obese people who have failed to lose weight despite following an appropriate diet. Their difficulty in losing weight may be due to reduced brown fat activity, which is important to the process of converting food into energy. Evening primrose oil appears to help normalize reduced brown fat activity.

Though one double-blind study with an unselected group failed to find any benefit from evening primrose oil, a similar study that treated only people who had a family history of obesity found evening primrose oil to be effective in promoting weight loss. When combined, these findings suggest that the best candidates for a trial of evening primrose oil may be people with a family history of obesity. More clinical trials are needed, however, before the efficacy of primrose oil can be considered to be proven.[29,30]

NUTRITIONAL HEALING PLAN: Omega-6 Fatty Acids

Dosage: 1 g of evening primrose oil 3 times daily

CHOOSING A PERSONAL PLAN

Of the various types of weight reduction diets, balanced low-calorie diets that reduce fat intake to perhaps 20 percent of total calories are generally preferable. If you are in good health, medical supervision of this type of diet is unnecessary.

Other types of weight reduction diets sometimes have the advantage of resulting in faster weight loss and thereby provide the psychological boost you may need to enable you to stick to a diet. Also, low-carbohydrate diets may cause reduced feelings of hunger. However, because these types of diets are more stressful to the body, I suggest that you see your physician for medical supervision if you wish to try them.

Whether or not you place yourself on a weight reduction diet, adding fiber and restricting table sugar may assist you in losing weight. If you overeat due to intense cravings for particular foods, and especially if you have a number of vague symptoms relating to various body systems, consider trying a food-elimination diet.

The value of nutritional supplements in promoting weight loss has yet to be well proven. However, a trial of vitamin C, evening primrose oil, and/or coenzyme Q_{10} appears to be reasonably safe if you wish to experiment.

ADDITIONAL SUGGESTIONS

For optimal results, every weight reduction diet should be combined with an exercise program and a psychological and/or behavioral program. An exercise program speeds weight loss and helps to ensure that fat is lost from the right places. A psychological program is helpful to people who overeat because of emotional problems, whereas a behavioral program teaches you strategies to make dieting easier.

Osteoarthritis

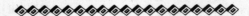

See also: PAIN.

Second only to diseases of the heart and blood vessels in producing
severe chronic disability, *osteoarthritis* is a common joint disease in
people over age 55. Pain, deformity, and limitation of motion are caused
by slow, progressive degeneration of the cartilage protecting the joint,
along with changes in the bone immediately beneath it.

DIETARY FACTORS

There is a rapidly growing scientific literature implicating food sensitivities
as a cause of exacerbations of rheumatoid arthritis. By contrast, very little
has appeared on food sensitivities causing pain in joints that have proven
to be osteoarthritic.

We do know that the popular nonsteroidal anti-inflammatory drugs
(NSAIDs)—such as ibuprofen, indomethacin, and naproxen—increase
the ability of food antigens to cross the gut lining into the bloodstream,
thus increasing the chances of developing food sensitivities. A few reports
have appeared that suggest that the elimination of certain foods may result
in dramatic improvement in symptoms. One group of foods that has been
placed under suspicion is the nightshades (white potato, tomato, eggplant, and pepper except for black pepper.[1,2,3])

The following case is a typical example:

*Two brothers with osteoarthritis began a nightshade-elimination
diet. Within the next several months, they both improved dramatically.*[4]

Proof that eating certain foods can provoke symptoms in osteoarthritic joints, however, will have to await the publication of double-blind trials.

THE HEALING DIET

Avoid foods found on testing to aggravate osteoarthritic symptoms. *See Appendix B for information about diagnosing food sensitivities.*

NUTRITIONAL HEALING PLANS

Vitamins

Niacinamide (Vitamin B₃)

William Kaufman is a medical doctor who has used large doses of niacinamide (a form of vitamin B₃) for half a century to reduce the symptoms caused by osteoarthritis. In an article published in 1955 in the *Journal of the American Geriatric Society,* he showed that hundreds of patients treated with large doses of niacinamide had a greater range of motion in their affected joints than similar patients who were untreated. He also found that treatment was associated with greater joint strength and reduced pain:[5]

> *A 77-year-old woman with osteoarthritis was severely crippled, with joint dysfunction that was almost in the extremely severe category. She was unable to get into or out of a chair or a bed and had difficulty standing, walking, and keeping her balance.*
>
> *She started taking 250 mg of niacinamide every 1½ hours for a total of 10 doses a day and began to show signs of improvement by the end of the first week. By the third month, she had regained her strength, was no longer excessively fatigued, and had a normal sense of balance. She was able to sit down and get up from a chair or bed without assistance and was able to walk on her own.*
>
> *Over the next three years, she continued to do well, although overuse of her fingers and wrists in crocheting or knitting would temporarily reduce her flexibility in those joints.[6]*

NUTRITIONAL HEALING PLAN: Niacinamide

Dosage

1. The greater the joint dysfunction, the higher the dosage needed for maximal benefits.
2. Dosage varies from 150–250 mg every 3 hours (6 doses daily) to 250 mg every hour (16 doses daily) depending upon the severity of the joint dysfunction.

Special Considerations

1. Niacinamide is believed to be particularly effective for osteoarthritis of the knee.
2. Side effects include nausea and liver dysfunction.
3. Medical supervision is strongly recommended.

Trial Period

Improvement may be seen within one week but can take months.

Vitamin C

Though the value of vitamin C in the treatment of osteoarthritis is not known, vitamin C supplementation has been proven to inhibit the progression of experimental osteoarthritis in guinea pigs. Also, we know that an excess of the vitamin is necessary to stimulate the growth of human cartilage cells.[7,8]

NUTRITIONAL HEALING PLAN: Vitamin C

Dosage: not well established, but 1 g of vitamin C twice daily would be reasonable

---

Vitamin E

Two double-blind studies have proven that vitamin E supplementation can provide effective pain relief. It appears that, like vitamin C, vitamin E may also retard the development of osteoarthritis, but this possibility has not yet been proven.[9,10]

Though we still have a lot to learn about how vitamin E works, one reason that it helps people with osteoarthritis is that it appears to function much like the NSAIDs in inhibiting substances (prostaglandins) that promote inflammation.[11]

NUTRITIONAL HEALING PLAN: Vitamin E

Dosage: 400 IU of vitamin E once or twice daily

Trial Period

1. for pain relief: ten days
2. to retard disease progression: indefinite

Minerals

Boron

Studies from a number of different countries have found that the lower the level of boron in the soil, the more often people develop osteoarthritis. One physician reported that, in his experience, 90 percent of his osteoarthritis patients improved with boron supplementation, and that most had complete remission of their symptoms. Moreover, under double-blind conditions, five of ten osteoarthritis patients given boron supplements improved, compared to only one of ten given a placebo. There were no side effects.[12,13,14]

The human requirement for boron is not yet established, and long-term toxicity studies have yet to be reported. Therefore, I suggest that instead of taking a boron supplement, you increase your boron intake by increasing the amount of boron in your diet *(see Appendix D for a list of foods that are rich sources of boron)*.

Sulfur

Sulfur, an essential mineral, is known to be an important mineral in cartilage, and sulfur baths have a long history as a popular treatment for arthritis. Although modern investigators seem to have forgotten sulfur, studies from the 1920s and 1930s have provided limited support for its use. There is some evidence, for example, that people with arthritis have low levels of sulfur in their tissues. Not only have sulfur baths been shown to increase blood sulfur levels, but arthritic pain and swelling have disappeared after sulfur injections. Scientific studies are badly needed to assess the value of sulfur treatments.[15,16,17]

NUTRITIONAL HEALING PLAN: Sulfur

1. It is not well established whether increasing sulfur through diet or supplementation is of any value.
2. Injections of sulfur, or the use of sulfur baths, may be beneficial.

Other Nutritional Factors

Glucosamine Sulfate

Glucosamine is the building block of the proteoglycans from which cartilage is made. It appears to be most effective against osteoarthritis when combined with sulfur to form glucosamine sulfate. Studies have shown that, while the NSAIDs inhibit the synthesis of proteoglycans, glucosamine prevents proteoglycans from breaking down.[18,19]

Glucosamine sulfate has been proven to be effective in several double-blind studies. When given orally, it has been shown to relieve pain, joint tenderness, and swelling so that joint movement can increase. Furthermore, it is almost devoid of side effects.[20]

NUTRITIONAL HEALING PLAN: Glucosamine Sulfate

Dosage: 500 mg of glucosamine sulfate 3 times daily

Trial Period

Results are expected within eight weeks.

S-Adenosyl-Methionine

S-adenosyl-methionine is another beneficial sulfur-containing compound. It reduces pain and inflammation and stimulates the manufacture of proteoglycans. On the basis of clinical trials on more than 22,000 patients, investigators have concluded that S-adenosyl-methionine is as effective as the NSAIDs, but without their side effects.[21]

NUTRITIONAL HEALING PLAN: S-Adenosyl-Methionine

Dosage: 1200 mg of S-adenosyl-methionine daily

Trial Period

four weeks

Superoxide Dismutase

Like vitamins C and E, superoxide dismutase (SOD) is an important *anti-oxidant*. (An antioxidant combats the unstable and potentially harmful free radicals that are released in various situations and can damage cells.) Administration of this enzyme directly into the involved joint is an effective treatment for an osteoarthritic joint. Oral administration, however, has been controversial because, in the past, oral preparations have failed to be absorbed from the gut.[22,23]

Recently, an unpublished study showed that a wheat sprout-derived, enteric-coated preparation (that is, one formulated not to dissolve in the stomach) containing a combination of SOD and catalase (another enzyme) raised serum SOD levels. In an unpublished open trial, the same preparation was effective for 90 percent of osteoarthritics; they noted decreased pain and demonstrated increased joint movement and decreased swelling. Since similar results were achieved in osteoarthritic dogs, it is unlikely that people improved only on the basis of suggestion (the placebo effect).[24,25,26]

NUTRITIONAL HEALING PLAN: Superoxide Dismutase

Preparation

superoxide dismutase with catalase (SOD/CAT, Biotic Food Corp., Hawaii)

Initial Dosage: 6 to 12 400 mg tablets daily, one hour before breakfast

Maintenance Dosage: one-half of the dose required to obtain improvement

Trial Period

two to four weeks

Botanical Extract: Devil's Claw (Harpagophytum)

The anti-inflammatory effects of the herb devil's claw appear to be equal to those of the NSAIDs. Adverse side effects, however, seem limited to the rare occurrence of slight digestive discomfort.[27]

In an open trial, almost 90 percent of people given the herb had reduced pain and increased movement in their affected joints. Moreover, morning stiffness wore off more rapidly.[28]

NUTRITIONAL HEALING PLAN: Devil's Claw

Preparation

harpagophytum (Arkocaps, Arkopharma, London & NY)

Dosage: 1.5 g daily

Trial Period

eight days

Tissue Extracts

New Zealand Green-Lipped Mussel Extract

In a double-blind study, an extract of the New Zealand green-lipped mussel was found to be effective for people with severe osteoarthritis who were not responding to standard medications and were awaiting joint surgery. Side effects were minimal. It is not known why the extract appears to help.[29]

NUTRITIONAL HEALING PLAN: New Zealand Green-Lipped Mussel

Preparation

Seatone (McFarland Labs, Auckland, NZ)

Initial Dosage: 1050 mg daily

Maintenance Dosage: 700 to 1050 mg daily

Trial Period

Three to 18 weeks.

Shark Cartilage Extract

Cartilade™ is an extract of shark cartilage. Although controlled studies of this extract have not been published, it was effective in treating osteoarthritic dogs. Also, in an open trial, six people who had failed to benefit from treatment with NSAIDs received the preparation. Their joint inflammation decreased, pain was reduced, and they became able to walk more easily. There were no side effects.[30,31]

NUTRITIONAL HEALING PLAN: Shark Cartilage Extract

Preparation

Cartilade™ (740 mg capsules) (Cartilage Technologies, U.S.)

Dosage: 4 capsules 4 times daily

Trial Period

Improvement usually begins by the end of the third week.

CHOOSING A PERSONAL PLAN

A trial of a food-elimination diet is suggested for everyone. It is especially recommended if your arthritic symptoms vary greatly from day to day or week to week, or if you have other symptoms that have a pattern of remissions and exacerbations. Also, increase your intake of foods that are good sources of boron.

Since vitamin E is one of the best proven Nutritional Healing plans, and since it has so many other potentially beneficial effects, I would suggest that you try it first. It would be a good idea to make it part of a broader antioxidant treatment plan, which would also include vitamin C and SOD/CAT. (You may wish to keep taking antioxidants even if they do not relieve your symptoms because it is possible that they will retard the progression of the disease.)

The other Nutritional Healing plans are best tried separately so that you can discover which ones are effective for you. Since glucosamine sulfate and S-adenosyl-methionine are the best-validated of the remaining plans, try them first if they are available.

Osteoporosis

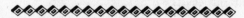

See also: KIDNEY STONES, PERIODONTAL DISEASE.

Osteoporosis, a condition marked by decreased density of the bones, develops when bone is being broken down faster than it is being formed. It affects one out of 4 women over age 65, making them vulnerable to collapse of the vertebrae of the spine and to fractures of the ribs and hips. Men are less vulnerable to developing osteoporosis, yet about 8 percent develop it during their lifetime.

DIETARY FACTORS

In industrialized societies, the amount of protein in the diet is often excessive. A high amount of protein increases calcium loss from the body; therefore protein should be limited to a moderate level of intake. Since fatty acids form calcium soaps in the gut that interfere with calcium absorption, the amount of fat in the diet should be restricted.[1,2]

When foods are burned, the ash that remains is either acid or alkaline. Acid ash-producing foods promote the loss of calcium from the body and are believed to cause increased bone loss; thus a diet biased toward foods that produce an alkaline ash may be preferable. Such foods include fruits (except for cranberries and plums), vegetables (except for corn and lentils), and dairy products (except for cheese). Meat and other high protein foods as well as most cereal grains and other starches produce an acid ash.[3]

Long-term avoidance of meat is associated with decreased loss of minerals from bones and a decreased risk of osteoporosis. Vegetarians may benefit from their lower intake of protein and fat, as well as from such factors as their higher intake of calcium and boron and lower intake of phosphorus.[4]

Table sugar (sucrose) should be restricted as it may cause excessive loss of calcium in the urine. Table salt may do the same. In post-menopausal women, the excessive loss of calcium in the urine adversely affects the balance of calcium in the body, causing calcium to be mobilized from its storage in the bones and thereby promoting osteoporosis.[5,6]

Alcoholics lose bone density substantially faster. Whether this is due to a direct effect of alcohol or to the many nutritional inadequacies of the alcoholic's diet is unknown. In any case, heavy alcohol consumption should be avoided. Since caffeine increases calcium loss in both the urine and the feces, its use should also be avoided.[7,8]

THE HEALING DIETS

1. Follow the Vegetarian Healing diet as described in Appendix A.
2. Follow the Alkaline Ash diet as described in Appendix A.
3. Minimize caffeine intake.

NUTRITIONAL HEALING PLANS

Vitamins

Vitamin C Deficiency

Adequate amounts of vitamin C are necessary for the activity of an important enzyme needed for the synthesis of *collagen,* a major component of bone; therefore osteoporosis can be caused by a vitamin C deficiency. Although the possibility that a marginal vitamin C deficiency contributes to osteoporosis has not been proven, vitamin C supplementation is so safe that it seems worthwhile to take it "just in case."[9]

NUTRITIONAL HEALING PLAN: Vitamin C Deficiency

Dosage: 500 mg of vitamin C daily

Vitamin D

Since vitamin D is necessary for the absorption of calcium in the gut, a deficiency of the active form of the vitamin (calcitriol) is a cause of osteoporosis, especially in the elderly. However, since too much vitamin D encourages bone resorption and the optimal supplemental dosage has yet to be established, my general recommendation would be to concentrate on making your own vitamin D: Go outside as regularly as possible to expose your body to sunlight or use full-spectrum lighting (which simulates sunshine) in your home or office.[10]

Minerals

Boron

Boron is a trace element whose potential importance in osteoporosis is just becoming recognized. In postmenopausal women, boron supplementation markedly reduces the urinary excretion of calcium and magnesium—two minerals whose conservation is important in preventing osteoporosis. Moreover, boron markedly elevates the concentration of the most biologically active form of estrogen (estradiol-17-beta) in the blood. Since estrogen administration has been proven to be effective for slowing calcium loss from bone in postmenopausal women, this finding may be of particular importance.[11]

At the present time, I do not recommend boron supplements. The human requirement for boron is not yet established, long-term toxicity studies have yet to be reported, and we lack proof that boron supplementation prevents osteoporosis. However, you can substantially increase your boron intake by increasing the amount of certain healthy foods in your diet (see Appendix D for a list of foods that are rich sources of boron).

Calcium

Since 99 percent of the body's calcium is in the bones, the relationship between calcium metabolism and bone density has been extensively studied. A high calcium intake (more than 500 mg daily), particularly during childhood and adolescence, is believed to reduce the risk of osteoporosis, and a very high calcium intake during breastfeeding (more than 1600 mg daily) may minimize bone loss in the mother.[12,13]

There is some controversy, however, over whether postmenopausal women require higher levels of dietary calcium than younger women to minimize their risk of osteoporosis. Calcium balance studies have found that women need to ingest more calcium after age 35 to avoid a negative calcium balance, most likely due to a reduced ability to absorb calcium. (Women over age 35 who ingest less than 1 g daily of calcium before menopause, or less than 1.5 g daily after menopause, are in negative calcium balance.) However, calcium balance studies are subject to inaccuracies, and at best can only suggest the possibility that a negative calcium balance may foster osteoporosis.

There are two types of bone in the body: *cortical* and *trabecular.* Cortical (compact) bone constitutes 80 percent of the skeleton and is found primarily in the limbs. Trabecular (spongy) bone is found primarily in the spinal vertebrae, although a relatively small percentage of the bone in the limbs is trabecular bone.

Sites that consist primarily of trabecular bone are more prone to osteoporosis because 40 percent of trabecular bone is dissolved and reformed each year, compared to only 10 percent of cortical bone. Calcium supplementation appears to be more effective in preventing the loss of cortical bone, which means that it may not be very effective in preventing bone loss in the limbs and consequently in preventing hip fractures due to osteoporosis. In addition, dietary calcium is not always well absorbed, as shown by a frequent lack of change in serum calcium levels after supplementation. The lack of efficacy of calcium supplementation in some studies may be due to poor absorption.[14]

NUTRITIONAL HEALING PLAN: Calcium Deficiency

Preparation

calcium citrate

Dosage: 500 mg of calcium daily; for postmenopausal women: 1000 mg daily

Note: This dosage assumes that some of your daily calcium needs are being met by your diet.

Fluorine

Clinical studies suggest that sodium fluoride is one of the most potent agents for increasing trabecular bone density. However, it decreases cortical bone, increases skeletal fragility, and frequently produces significant side effects, including damage to the stomach lining. For these reasons, it is not generally recommended.[15,16,17]

Magnesium Deficiency

The more magnesium in your diet, the higher your bone mineral density. Magnesium is required for the activation of alkaline phosphatase, an enzyme involved in forming calcium crystals in bone and in converting vitamin D into its active form. It also influences bone density by maintaining proper levels of parathyroid hormone, which stimulates the resorption of calcified bone.[18]

People with osteoporosis may have reduced bone magnesium content, and evidence of magnesium deficiency is common. Perhaps the best way your doctor can discover a magnesium deficiency is by doing a magne-sium-loading test; a test for the magnesium level in white blood cells could also be helpful.[19]

NUTRITIONAL HEALING PLAN: Magnesium Deficiency

Dosage: 500 mg of magnesium daily

Other Minerals

Many other minerals are involved in bone formation and breakdown, such as copper, iron, manganese, phosphorus, and zinc. Though inadequate levels of these minerals may contribute to osteoporosis, supplementary dosages have yet to be proven beneficial. For now, the best way to ensure an adequate mineral intake is to eat a wide variety of healthy foods and to follow the dietary advice given above.

CHOOSING A PERSONAL PLAN

Everyone concerned about osteoporosis should follow the principles of the Healing diet outlined above. Adequate calcium nutrition is important even when it cannot by itself fully protect you against osteoporosis. Be sure to guard against deficiencies of vitamin D, boron, and magnesium.

ADDITIONAL SUGGESTIONS

Inactivity promotes bone loss, whereas studies have found that gentle weight-bearing exercise reduces bone loss, and may even increase bone density. Consider, for example, taking a walk as part of your daily routine, or speak to your doctor about an exercise program.[20]

Pain

See also: MENSTRUAL CRAMPS, MIGRAINE HEADACHE, MUSCLE CRAMPS, PREMENSTRUAL TENSION SYNDROME (PMS).

Though pain can serve to warn us to avoid activities that are potentially damaging to our bodies, often it serves no useful purpose. Chronic pain is generally defined as pain lasting six months or longer. In contrast to acute pain, a person suffering from chronic pain is more likely to have become depressed, and their depression often makes chronic pain more difficult to treat.

DIETARY FACTORS

Food sensitivities may be a cause of pain. Many people are known to be intolerant to milk sugar (lactose) because they are deficient in the enzyme (lactase) that breaks it down in the gut so that it can be absorbed. Lactose intolerance has long been suspected as a cause of recurrent abdominal pain, and several pilot studies have suggested that a lactose-free diet may benefit lactose malabsorbers.

However, *Pediatrics* has published a controlled study suggesting that lactose elimination may not be beneficial for abdominal pain. Lactase deficiency was found to be as common in normals as it was in people with recurrent abdominal pain. Moreover, after a group of people with recurrent abdominal pain were followed for one year, those who were lactose malabsorbers did no better by following a lactose-free diet than did those who were able to absorb lactose normally, whether or not the normal absorbers followed the same diet.[1]

Besides abdominal pain, many other pains have been attributed to food sensitivities, including pains in the muscles, joints, and teeth. Pains that appear to be food-related remit on a food-elimination diet and return when particular foods are re-introduced. However, these reports have not been confirmed by studies using scientific research methods.

In the following case, food sensitivities were found to be the cause of various pains:

> For 20 years a 42-year-old woman had pain between the shoulders, in the hands, wrists, and elbows and left hip that gradually worsened and eventually forced her to discontinue work as a waitress. In addition, she was constantly fatigued. Frequent and at times prolonged bed rest was ineffectual. She had experienced sick headaches all of her life, three or four during the previous year, and she had occasionally suffered from hives. On examination, she had pain and soreness when she moved various joints. Allergy skin testing was negative.
>
> She was placed on a fruit- and cereal-free elimination diet and the pains disappeared in ten days. In three months she had no distress or discomfort even when doing physical work. During eight years of follow-up, her relief continued with the elimination of fruits, fish, and condiments from her diet, and restriction of wheat, milk, and eggs.[2]

Outside of the possibility of food sensitivities, coffee is the only food that appears to affect pain sensitivity. Researchers have found coffee, both regular and decaffeinated, to have powerful opiate receptor-binding activity. Since binding of the opiate receptors interferes with the body's ability to respond to its own pain-relieving compounds (endorphins), coffee consumption may theoretically make you more pain-sensitive, although this hypothesis has yet to be adequately tested. A substantial reduction in caffeine intake has been reported to decrease breast pain in women with fibrocystic breast disease; their pain reduction, however, could be due to remission of the disease.[3,4]

THE HEALING DIET

1. Avoid those foods found on testing to provoke symptoms. *See Appendix B for information about diagnosing food sensitivities.*
2. Avoid coffee.

NUTRITIONAL HEALING PLANS

Vitamins

Vitamin B Complex

Thiamine (vitamin B_1), vitamin B_6, and vitamin B_{12}—all members of the vitamin B complex—have been given together for the treatment of pain. When tested together, these vitamins have been shown to suppress pain at the level of the spinal cord. In a double-blind study of 376 people with acute pain due to disease of the lumbar spine, diclofenac, a nonsteroidal anti-inflammatory drug, was given to everyone, while some people were also given the vitamin combination. The combination significantly increased pain relief for those people who were complaining of severe pain.[5,6]

Thiamine (Vitamin B_1)

Massive doses of thiamine suppress the transmission of impulses along the nerve fibers that innervate the muscles. If supplemental doses of thiamine suppress the transmission of impulses along nerve fibers that carry pain messages, it may have some value in pain control. This could explain the results of an open trial in which 133 people in pain who had previously failed to benefit from pain medications or physical therapy were given high supplemental doses of thiamine. Seventy-three percent said that thiamine reduced their pain, including people with headaches, pains of the spine and joints, and neuralgia (nerve pain).[7,8]

NUTRITIONAL HEALING PLAN: Thiamine

Dosage: 1–4 g of thiamine daily

WARNING

Such a massive supplemental dose of thiamine should be taken only under medical supervision.

Vitamin B_6

Vitamin B_6 may affect pain through its influence on *serotonin,* a neurotransmitter that modulates our perception of pain. Serotonin is made from *tryptophan,* an amino acid in the diet. This conversion of tryptophan to serotonin requires vitamin B_6.

Because people with chronic pain have decreased serotonin levels, it may be possible to reduce pain by boosting serotonin levels through supplementation with vitamin B_6 along with adequate tryptophan. According to a review article published in the *Annals of the New York Academy of Science,* B_6 appears to be particularly beneficial in helping people to get off of pain medications and in the treatment of pain due to temporomandibular joint (jaw) dysfunction (TMJ).[9]

NUTRITIONAL HEALING PLAN: Vitamin B_6

Preparation

pyridoxine

Dosage: 50 mg daily

Vitamin B_{12}

When tested on rats, oral supplementation with vitamin B_{12} was found to have a pain-relieving effect; the higher the dosage, the greater the pain relief. When tested on humans, daily injections of massive doses of vitamin B_{12} reduced pain in all but 10 of a group of 400 people with pain and sensory disturbances due to disease of their spinal vertebrae. Similarly, 60 percent of a group of people suffering from pain due to cancer reported relief after 2 weeks of daily B_{12} injections.[10,11,12]

Though vitamin B_{12} is available for oral use in various forms, there is so far no evidence that it is effective for relieving pain when taken orally. Therefore, if you wish to try it, you need to arrange for your physician to give you injections.

NUTRITIONAL HEALING PLAN: Vitamin B_{12}

Preparation

hydroxycobalamin

Dosage: 5–10,000 IU daily by intramuscular injection

Vitamin C

Supplementation with megadoses of vitamin C has repeatedly been shown to reduce pain, although the reason it works is unknown. Improvement has been reported in people with pain from advanced cancer, bone disease, and dental and low back problems. In an open trial, women with breast cancer who no longer responded to the usual pain relievers sometimes became pain-free when their medication was administered together with a large intravenous dose of vitamin C.[13,14,15,16,17]

> ### NUTRITIONAL HEALING PLAN: Vitamin C
>
> *Dosage:* 5–10 g of vitamin C daily
>
> Note: Higher doses can be given by your doctor intrave-
> nously.
>
> ---
>
> **WARNING**
> Reduce the dosage if you develop abdominal discomfort or
> diarrhea.

Mineral Deficiencies

Copper Deficiency

Enkephalins are morphinelike compounds made by the body that, like
morphine, reduce pain. Copper deficiency has been shown to reduce
enkephalin levels, thus impairing our natural ability to control pain.[18]

Though diagnosing and correcting a deficiency may thus be beneficial
for patients in chronic pain, there is no evidence that copper supplementation is otherwise indicated. In fact, excess copper is potentially harmful; if
you wish to consider trying copper supplementation, I advise you to ask
a nutritionally trained physician to evaluate you for copper deficiency.

Selenium Deficiency

People who are developing a selenium deficiency may start to complain
of pain in their muscles. The results of a Swedish study suggest that,
among people with chronic muscle pains, a marginal selenium deficiency
may not be uncommon. In this study of middle-aged women with chronic
back and shoulder pains, their average serum selenium level was found to
be low. Moreover, those with relatively higher levels or whose serum
selenium increased with supplementation responded better than the rest
of the group to a program of physical therapy. Perhaps people with muscle
pains and low selenium levels may be less able to respond to physical
therapy because a marginal selenium deficiency is maintaining their
pain.[19,20]

Further evidence for an association between chronic muscle pain and
marginal selenium deficiency comes from a study of 81 people complaining of chronically disabling muscular pain and stiffness. When they were
given selenium along with vitamin E, serum levels of glutathione peroxidase (an important selenium-containing enzyme) increased in three-
fourths of them, suggesting that their selenium status before supplementa-

tion was less than optimal. Compared to those whose glutathione peroxidase levels failed to rise, the average reduction in pain of those whose
levels rose after supplementation was significantly greater.[21]

NUTRITIONAL HEALING PLAN: Selenium Deficiency

Suggested Use

chronic muscle pain

Preparation

organic selenium

Dosage: 200 mcg daily

Essential Amino Acids

D-Phenylalanine

Whereas a copper deficiency reduces enkephalin levels, D-phenylalanine
reduces pain by inhibiting the breakdown of enkephalins. One double-
blind crossover study found it to be effective; another similar study, however, had disappointing results, leaving its efficacy as a single treatment for
chronic pain in question.[22,23]

However, both human and animal studies have found that D-phenylalanine makes acupuncture more effective for reducing pain. Moreover,
D-phenylalanine may be a valuable adjunct to morphine for people in
severe pain. In a study using rats as experimental animals, supplementation with D-phenylalanine made morphine more powerful, made its effect
last longer, and retarded the development of drug addiction.[24,25,26]

NUTRITIONAL HEALING PLAN: D-phenylalanine

Dosage: 250 mg of D-phenylalanine

WARNING

not to be taken by phenylketonurics.

Instructions

1. Take 15 to 30 minutes before meals.
2. If you do not have pain relief within three weeks, double the
   dosage for an additional three-week trial.

L-Tryptophan

Tryptophan is converted in the body into serotonin, a neurotransmitter that modulates pain perception. In controlled studies, tryptophan supplementation has been shown to reduce the level of pain caused by both acute and chronic illnesses and to increase a person's ability to tolerate pain.[27,28]

Tryptophan acts as a mild pain reliever; it is roughly as potent as aspirin or acetaminophen. It can be taken together with a nonnarcotic pain-relieving drug to achieve greater pain relief than that provided by the drug alone.[29]

NUTRITIONAL HEALING PLAN: L-Tryptophan

Dosage: 2–4 g of L-tryptophan daily in divided doses

Trial Period

up to one month

Additional Instructions

1. Avoid protein for 90 minutes before and after ingestion.
2. Take with a carbohydrate (such as fruit juice).

Note: Since tryptophan supplements may not be currently available (see Introduction), you may wish to try foods with a high tryptophan to protein ratio (see Appendix A).

Botanical Extract: Capsaicin

Capsaicin is an alkaloid present in hot peppers that, when applied to the skin at the site of the pain, stimulates and then blocks certain pain fibers by depleting them of the neurotransmitter "substance p."[30]

The application of capsaicin cream may be effective for various localized types of pain, even if the pain is severe. Shingles (herpes zoster), for example, is a viral infection characterized by an acute rash that follows the route of a nerve. The rash disappears after several days, but the area where the rash appeared sometimes becomes extremely painful and hypersensitive to touch, a condition known as postherpetic neuralgia. Although postherpetic neuralgia is difficult to treat, capsaicin, in a double-blind study, provided substantial pain relief for people suffering from this chronic painful condition. There is also preliminary evidence that capsaicin may be effective in reducing chronic pain following amputation of a limb or of a breast, as well as for pain due to neuritis (inflammation of nerves).[31,32,33,34]

NUTRITIONAL HEALING PLAN: Capsaicin

Dosage: 0.025 percent capsaicin cream

Instructions: Apply to the painful area four times daily.

Note: Since capsaicin may be irritating before it becomes effective, it should be used under your physician's direction.

CHOOSING A PERSONAL PLAN

See for yourself if coffee affects your pain by avoiding it for a few days and then drinking two or more cups. Trying a food-elimination diet makes the most sense if your pain is not adequately explained by diagnosed structural abnormalities in your body.

The combination of tryptophan and vitamin B_6 is a logical one, since both supplements foster the production of serotonin. For chronic muscle pain, give selenium supplementation an adequate trial. Consider asking your doctor to evaluate your copper and selenium levels to make sure that you are not marginally deficient.

If you are receiving acupuncture, phenylalanine supplementation may make your sessions more effective, and if you require narcotics for pain relief, ask your doctor about adding phenylalanine. You may even wish to try phenylalanine on its own, despite the fact that its efficacy when given alone is uncertain.

Vitamin B_{12} and vitamin C may be effective, even for the treatment of severe pain. Massive doses of thiamine may also be effective, but more studies are needed to confirm its safety as well as its efficacy. Finally, the application of capsaicin cream to the skin appears to be effective in an increasing number of painful conditions, although the possibility of it increasing pain, at least temporarily, should be kept in mind.

ADDITIONAL SUGGESTIONS

Nutrition is one of many natural healing methods that influence pain. The others include:

▶ Physical therapy, including manipulation, massage, hot or cold packs, etc.

▶ Life style changes that improve your mood, since your emotional state can have a profound effect on pain. Sometimes counseling or psychotherapy is very helpful.

▶ Aerobic exercise under your doctor's direction. Just as certain Nutritional Healing plans can improve your body's ability to reduce pain by stimulating the endorphin system, regular aerobic exercise is an excellent stimulus for endorphin release.

▶ Relaxation training, perhaps assisted by biofeedback or hypnosis, reduces pain by several mechanisms. You can reduce muscle pain by learning to decrease muscle tension, while relaxation or hypnotic techniques help to "take the hurt out of the pain" and sometimes can even eliminate it.

Parkinson's Disease

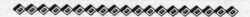

Parkinson's disease is a chronic, progressive disorder of the nervous system that affects about 1 percent of people over 50 years of age. It results from the degeneration of certain brain cells (in the substantia nigra and locus ceruleus) that produce the neurotransmitter *dopamine*. The disease commonly starts with a tremor of one arm that occurs only when the arm is at rest. As the disease progresses, movements gradually become rigid, the face becomes frozen, and there is progressive difficulty in performing simple tasks.

DIETARY FACTORS

L-*Dopa* (L-dihydroxy-phenylalanine) is the amino acid from which the neurotransmitter dopamine is derived. Since supplementation with L-dopa restores deficient brain dopamine levels and thereby decreases the symptoms of Parkinson's disease, it has become central to the medical treatment of this disease.

L-dopa is one of several amino acids that must compete with one another to be transferred from the bloodstream into the brain. Since protein is made up of amino acids linked together, restricting dietary protein would seem to be a logical method of reducing the competition from other amino acids, especially since the Western diet tends to be too high in protein.

Indeed, several studies have found that protein restriction makes L-dopa supplementation more effective. One common problem with L-dopa therapy is that people receiving it do better at certain times in the day than others. (This is called the *on-off* effect.) Protein restriction is particularly effective for reducing these daily fluctuations.[1]

WARNING

L-dopa should be administered only under close medical supervision because of its potential for side effects.

THE HEALING DIET

1. Restrict the daily intake of protein to the U.S. RDA of 0.8 g per kg (0.12 oz per lb) of body weight.
2. Serve 90 percent of the daily protein intake with the evening meal.

NUTRITIONAL HEALING PLANS

Vitamins

Folic Acid Deficiency

Parkinson's disease may occasionally be caused by a deficiency of folic acid (folate). Folate deficiency can cause anemia, but nonanemic people may still be folate-deficient. Therefore, to rule out folate deficiency, your doctor will need to do special laboratory tests for folate nutrition. If you are deficient, supplementation with folate should stop the progression of the disease.[2,3]

Niacin Deficiency

Despite an adequate intake of niacin in the diet, older people may become marginally niacin-deficient. In fact, oral niacin supplementation may not fully protect them from biochemical evidence of niacin deficiency. Moreover, treatment with L-dopa, particularly when given concurrently with a *decarboxylase inhibitor* (such as carbidopa or benserazide), further increases the risk that a marginal niacin deficiency will develop. (Decarboxylase inhibitors make L-dopa more effective by inhibiting its breakdown.) Conversely, niacin supplementation may prolong the length of time that brain dopamine levels are elevated after L-dopa supplementation is given.[4,5,6]

In the body, L-dopa is made from the amino acid *tyrosine*. Without adequate *NADH*, a coenzyme formed from niacin, the conversion of tyrosine to L-dopa cannot take place. Though it is not known whether niacin supplementation can reduce the symptoms of Parkinson's disease, one group of investigators tried giving 34 patients NADH by injection, and

found that two-thirds of them had a greater than 30 percent improvement
in their amount of disability. Scientific studies are needed to confirm the
efficacy of NADH, to determine whether niacin injections are equally
effective, and to establish whether oral supplementation is of value.[7]

NUTRITIONAL HEALING PLAN: Niacin Deficiency

Dosage: 100 mg of niacin daily

Vitamin B_6

The enzyme necessary to convert dopa to dopamine requires vitamin B_6,
which despite adequate intake and oral supplementation is often marginally deficient in elderly people. Moreover, treatment with the combination
of L-dopa and a decarboxylase inhibitor may cause a marginal vitamin B_6
deficiency.

In pilot studies, supplementation with pyridoxine (a form of vitamin
B_6) appeared to reduce the clinical signs of Parkinson's disease in people
who were not taking L-dopa. It remains to be seen if controlled studies will
confirm this finding, and whether supplementation works by restoring
low vitamin B_6 levels to normal.[8,9]

NUTRITIONAL HEALING PLAN: Vitamin B_6

Preparation

pyridoxine

Dosage: 50 mg daily

WARNING

Vitamin B_6 supplementation should not be taken along with
L-dopa unless you are also taking a decarboxylase inhibitor.

Vitamin C

The effects of vitamin C supplementation alone on Parkinson's disease
have not been reported. However, in a double-blind study, six people
receiving L-dopa supplementation had a modest improvement in their
ability to function following the addition of the vitamin.[10] The following
case is a typical example:

*A 62-year-old male who had stopped L-dopa because of intolerable
nausea and excessive salivation tried it again in combination with*

vitamin C. After four weeks, his ability to move his head increased, his excessive salivation decreased, and both his speech and handwriting improved considerably. In fact, his hand coordination improved so much that he began to play the organ for the first time in several years.

Several times, without his knowledge, a placebo was substituted for vitamin C. Each time he was switched to placebo, both he and the investigator (who also did not know when he was switched to placebo) noted that his condition would deteriorate until he was switched back to vitamin C.[11]

NUTRITIONAL HEALING PLAN: Vitamin C

Special Use

to enhance the benefits of L-dopa

Dosage: 1 g of vitamin C twice daily

Vitamin E

The development of Parkinson's disease appears to be associated with a low intake of vitamin E-rich foods in early life, suggesting that a higher intake of vitamin E early in life may protect against the eventual development of the disease.[12]

The efficacy of vitamin E alone once Parkinson's disease has developed remains to be studied, although a single case report suggests that the disease can develop despite long-term vitamin E supplementation.[13]

Since both vitamin C and vitamin E are powerful *antioxidants* (substances that combat the destruction of cells by harmful free radicals), and it is believed that Parkinson's disease may be one of the many degenerative diseases that antioxidants could combat, the two vitamins were given together in a pilot study. Compared to unsupplemented patients, 15 patients with mild Parkinson's symptoms who took vitamins C and E were able to delay starting standard drug treatment for an additional two and a half years, suggesting that the combined supplementation may delay the progression of the disease.[14]

NUTRITIONAL HEALING PLAN: Vitamin E

Dosage: 3200 IU of vitamin E daily

Instructions

1. Start with 400 IU daily and, with your physician's approval, gradually increase the dosage as tolerated.
2. Combine with 3000 mg of vitamin C daily.

Minerals

Iron

The conversion of tyrosine to dopa requires iron to activate the enzyme responsible for the reaction. The activity of this enzyme, which is reduced in Parkinson's disease, can be stimulated by iron supplementation. When ten patients with advanced symptoms of immobility despite L-dopa treatment received an iron complex intravenously, all improved remarkably; seven of them were able to reduce or discontinue L-dopa. In addition, there were no side effects. The effects of a single injection lasted one to two days.[15]

Despite this promising study, the use of iron supplementation is questionable, since people with Parkinson's disease have elevated iron levels in a portion of the substantia nigra (the part of the brain which is most affected by the disease) and it is possible that increased iron at this location promotes the progress of the disease. Moreover, long-term occupational exposure to iron appears to increase the risk of Parkinson's disease. Further studies are therefore needed before the safety of iron supplementation is established.[16,17,18]

Manganese Toxicity

Excessive manganese exposure increases the risk of Parkinson's disease as a result of the depletion of dopamine and the production of neurotoxins. Though manganese toxicity is usually due to occupational exposure, excessive doses of supplemental manganese may be equally dangerous:[19,20]

A woman with symptoms suggestive of early Parkinson's disease reported taking 1500 mg of manganese daily as a nutritional supplement for the past 6 months. Hair mineral analysis revealed 30 times the normal manganese level.[21]

Other Nutritional Factors

L-Methionine

L-*Methionine* is an essential amino acid. About three weeks after a group of people with untreated Parkinson's disease received L-methionine, most of their symptoms improved. The authors noted that L-methionine seemed to be as effective as L-dopa.[22]

Other investigators then gave L-methionine a more difficult test. For their study group they selected people with Parkinson's disease who had already been treated with L-dopa and other standard treatments, and who had already shown the maximum improvement standard treatments could provide.

After two months, two-thirds of their subjects showed further improvement. These additional improvements were in activity level, ease of movement, rigidity, difficulty in performing voluntary movement, mood, sleep, attention span, muscular strength, concentration, and voice. Tremor and drooling were unimproved. Hopefully, controlled studies will confirm these early reports.[23]

NUTRITIONAL HEALING PLAN: L-Methionine

Instructions

Start with 1 g daily of L-methionine and increase the dosage, as tolerated, to 2.5 g twice daily.

Trial Period

two months

Octacosanol

Octacosanol, a long-chain alcohol extracted from wheat germ oil, was given to people with mild to moderate Parkinsonian symptoms in a small double-blind crossover study. Octacosanol administration was associated with a small but statistically significant improvement in self-ratings of "activities of daily living" and "mood." Thirty percent of the subjects were significantly improved on octacosanol, while none worsened.[24]

The following case is an example of dramatic improvement with octacosanol:

> *When a man with Parkinson's disease received standard medical therapy, he needed hospitalization due to side effects of hallucinations and disorientation. He was placed on octacosanol, and within six weeks dramatic improvements began to be noted in his strength,*

appetite, and ability to get around. His improvements was so remark-
able that his neurologist had never before seen a Parkinsonian pa-
tient improve so much from treatment.[25]

Additional studies are needed to further clarify the efficacy of octacosanol.

NUTRITIONAL HEALING PLAN: Octacosanol

Dosage: 1–2 mg of octacosanol daily

Trial Period

six weeks

Omega-6 Fatty Acids

Evening primrose oil is a source of omega-6 fatty acids and a particularly
rich source of *gamma-linolenic acid,* a key intermediary in omega-6 fatty
acid metabolism. When a group of people with Parkinson's disease suffering from tremors received evening primrose oil, 55 percent of them became less tremulous. The results of controlled studies to prove the efficacy
of evening primrose oil have yet to be reported.[26]

NUTRITIONAL HEALING PLAN: Omega-6 Fatty Acids

Special Use

reduce tremor

Preparation

evening primrose oil

Dosage: 1 g 3 times daily

D-Phenylalanine

An essential amino acid, D-*phenylalanine* (**not** L-phenylalanine) is an
antagonist of drug-induced Parkinson's disease in animals. When a group
of people with Parkinson's disease who were not receiving medical treatment began to take D-phenylalanine, their movements became less rigid,
they walked and talked more easily, and their mood improved. Their
tremors, however, failed to improve. Controlled studies are needed to
confirm these early results.[27,28]

NUTRITIONAL HEALING PLAN: D-Phenylalanine

Dosage: 100–250 mg of D-phenylalanine twice daily

WARNING

Not to be taken by phenylketonurics.

Instructions

D-phenylalanine supplements should be taken as far apart as possible from L-dopa, with which it competes for transport from the bloodstream into the brain.

Trial Period

four weeks

L-Tryptophan

Tryptophan, like phenylalanine, is a large, neutral amino acid competing with L-dopa for transport from the bloodstream to the brain. Because of this competition, L-dopa supplementation may cause side effects by reducing brain serotonin (which is derived from dietary tryptophan). These side effects can be prevented by adding tryptophan supplementation whenever L-dopa is prescribed.

Compared to L-dopa alone, the addition of L-tryptophan appears to improve mental symptoms, reduces *on-off* fluctuations in the efficacy of L-dopa, and improves the ability to function.[29,30,31]

NUTRITIONAL HEALING PLAN: L-Tryptophan

Special Use

in combination with L-dopa

Dosage: 2 g of L-tryptophan 3 times daily

Additional Instructions

1. Avoid protein for 90 minutes before and after ingestion.
2. Take with a carbohydrate (such as fruit juice).

Note: Since tryptophan supplements may not be currently available (see Introduction), you may wish to try foods with a high tryptophan to protein ratio (see Appendix A).

L-Tyrosine

L-*Tyrosine,* derived in the body from phenylalanine, is the amino acid from which dopa is made. Like L-dopa, L-tyrosine readily crosses over from the bloodstream into the brain, where it appears to improve the function of dopaminergic neurons.[32]

This raises the question of how L-tyrosine compares to L-dopa for the treatment of Parkinson's disease. After three years of following people supplemented with L-tyrosine, one group of investigators concluded that for some of the subjects L-tyrosine supplementation was associated with better clinical results and many fewer side effects than L-dopa. Though further studies are needed before the two supplements can be fully compared, these results suggest that L-tyrosine may be a rational substitute for L-dopa when L-dopa produces side effects.[33]

NUTRITIONAL HEALING PLAN: L-Tyrosine

Special Use

a substitute for L-dopa

Dosage: 100 mg/kg (45.5 mg/lb) of L-tyrosine daily

Heavy Metal Toxicity

Aluminum

Long-term occupational exposure to aluminum may increase the risk of developing Parkinson's disease. Moreover, aluminum is present in the substantia nigra of Parkinsonian brains. Evidence that the presence of aluminum is not solely due to degeneration of neurons has increased the suspicion that aluminum exposure promotes the development of the disease.[34,35]

Mercury

Blood and urine levels of mercury, but not hair mercury levels, have been shown to be excellent predictors of the risk of Parkinson's disease, suggesting that mercury is another heavy metal whose presence may foster the development of the disease.[36]

CHOOSING A PERSONAL PLAN

Since supplementation with L-dopa is standard treatment, your choice of a personal plan depends on whether your doctor has already placed you on L-dopa with or without a decarboxylase inhibitor to inhibit it from breaking down. Choose Nutritional Healing plans according to your situation:

1. If you are receiving L-dopa, but wish to make it more effective, try the Healing diet along with niacin, vitamin C, and/or L-methionine.
2. If you are receiving L-dopa, but are suffering from its side effects, try L-tryptophan along with niacin, pyridoxine, and vitamin C.
3. If you wish to rule out a nutritional cause, ask your doctor to perform laboratory tests to evaluate your folic acid, manganese, aluminum, and mercury levels.
4. If you wish to try alternative nutritional treatments to L-dopa, try L-methionine, D-phenylalanine, or L-tyrosine, along with niacin, pyridoxine, vitamin C, and vitamin E, under your doctor's guidance.
5. If you have a tremor for which treatment has been ineffective, try evening primrose oil.

Peptic Ulcers

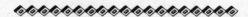

See also: HEARTBURN.

Peptic ulcers, the most common form of gastrointestinal ulceration, are localized erosions in the stomach or, more commonly, the duodenum (the part of the intestines just below the stomach). These organs have a lining that protects them from the otherwise destructive effect of stomach acid upon the delicate tissues; when the protective lining breaks down, a peptic ulcer is formed. Symptoms include stomach pain and nausea. Sometimes bleeding occurs, which, if untreated, can be dangerous. Peptic ulcers are a common disorder; perhaps one man in 10 and one woman in 20 will develop one during their lifetimes.

DIETARY FACTORS

Many of the traditional treatments for peptic ulcer, such as bland diets and frequent small meals, were never proven to be effective and are now largely discarded. Milk, formerly central to an ulcer diet, has been found to neutralize stomach acid only briefly—acid secretion subsequently rises higher than before, making the ulcers less likely to heal.[1,2]

Though a low-fiber diet was formerly recommended for the treatment of peptic ulcer disease, its value is also unproven. In fact, more recently the question has been whether increasing dietary fiber is beneficial. We do know that soluble dietary fiber, by thickening the stomach contents, slows gastric emptying. Although increasing dietary fiber has not been shown to promote the healing of peptic ulcers, fibers from whole grains and vegetables may help to prevent the ulcers from recurring.[3,4]

Alcohol, caffeine, and even decaffeinated coffee may exacerbate peptic ulcers by increasing acid secretion. Also, the more refined sugar in your diet, the greater your risk of developing peptic ulcers, probably because sugar also stimulates stomach acid secretion.[5,6,7,8,9]

Typically, people awaken at around 1 or 2 A.M. with ulcer pain. Investigators have found that the secretion of gastric acid during the night can be reduced by eating an early dinner. Less gastric acid secretion should mean less ulcer pain in the middle of the night and perhaps faster healing.[10]

Food sensitivities, including atopic allergies, are common among patients and appear to contribute to the development of peptic ulceration. Back in 1942, a research team showed that reactive foods slowed down stomach emptying and caused severe swelling and redness in the stomach lining. Further evidence that foods can promote the development of peptic ulcers has been accumulating ever since.[11,12,13]

In one study, for example, 98 percent of people with X-ray evidence of peptic ulcer also had respiratory tract allergies, suggesting that peptic ulceration may be an allergic manifestation. Biopsies from the edges of ulcers show evidence of a localized allergic reaction. When 30 people with scientifically proven food allergies had those food allergens directly applied to the stomach lining with a special instrument, obvious reactions such as swelling, erosions, and bleeding in the stomach lining were seen, although the usual skin and blood tests for allergy were positive only for those foods half of the time. Avoiding the implicated foods may improve healing and prevent recurrence.[14,15,16,17]

A 46-year-old woman with X-ray evidence of a gastric ulcer and a history of migraines failed to respond to a high-milk diet. She was placed on a five-day lamb, pear, and bottled spring water diet. Initially she experienced the worst migraine of her life which suggested that she was withdrawing from foods to which she was sensitive. When foods were reintroduced, she reacted to cow's milk products; by avoiding these, she experienced a rapid clearing of her ulcer symptoms and subsequently remained asymptomatic.[18]

THE HEALING DIET

1. Follow the Basic Healing diet as described in Appendix A.
2. Avoid caffeine (found in coffee, tea, and soft drinks).
3. Avoid foods found in testing to provoke ulcer symptoms. *See Appendix B for information about diagnosing food sensitivities.*
4. Eat an early dinner.

NUTRITIONAL HEALING PLANS

Vitamins

Vitamin A

Vitamin A appears to both protect against peptic ulceration and to promote healing. In an animal study, supplementation with vitamin A prevented the development of duodenal ulcers resulting from excessive stomach acid. In one controlled study, people with chronic gastric ulcers received either antacids or antacids plus high doses of vitamin A. After four weeks, the addition of vitamin A to antacid treatment resulted in the healing of twice the percentage of ulcers, and the remaining ulcers were smaller.[19,20]

NUTRITIONAL HEALING PLAN: Vitamin A

Dosage: 100,000 IU of vitamin A daily

WARNING

Because such high doses of vitamin A may occasionally cause side effects, it should be taken only under medical supervision.

Vitamin C Deficiency

The lower the levels of vitamin C in the blood and urine as well as in the stomach fluid, the greater the risk of peptic ulceration. Moreover, vitamin C levels are lower in people with bleeding peptic ulcers than in people with nonbleeding ones. Evidence that a vitamin C deficiency may cause peptic ulcers comes from an animal study. When guinea pigs were fed a vitamin C-deficient diet, they developed peptic ulcerations.[21,22,23,24,25]

The results of two pilot studies suggest that vitamin C supplementation may be an effective treatment. In a French study, treatment of gastric and duodenal ulcers with intravenous vitamin C appeared to be at least as effective as other intravenous therapies. A Japanese study reported that the combination of vitamin C and ferrous sulfate (an iron preparation) increased the healing of gastric, although not of duodenal, ulcers. Although it appears that people with peptic ulcers and low levels of vitamin C may benefit from supplementation, more studies are needed to clarify the efficacy of vitamin C supplementation for people with normal vitamin C levels.[26,27]

NUTRITIONAL HEALING PLAN: Vitamin C Deficiency

Preparation

potassium ascorbate

  Dosage: 0.5 g before meals and at bedtime

Vitamin E

Lipid peroxides are the products of the chemical damage done by oxygen free-radicals to the fatty components of cell membranes. Vitamin E, the major antioxidant of the cell membranes, plays an important role in protecting these membranes from damage. Recent Russian work suggests that peptic ulcer disease may be associated with both an enhancement of lipid peroxidation and a deficit of vitamin E. This deficit may be a result of lipid peroxidation, because in the process of combating cellular damage, vitamin E appears to be consumed.[28,29]

Animal and human studies have found that vitamin E supplementation protects against stomach ulcers, and early Russian studies have suggested that vitamin E supplementation may aid in the healing of peptic ulcers of both the stomach and the duodenum. Controlled studies are needed to confirm these findings.[30,31,32,33]

NUTRITIONAL HEALING PLAN: Vitamin E

  Dosage: 400–800 IU of vitamin E daily

Minerals

Aluminum

Aluminum hydroxide, an aluminum salt, has been shown to enhance the healing of peptic ulcers. The use of aluminum salts has been questioned recently because of growing evidence that aluminum exposure may promote the development of Alzheimer's dementia. Aluminum hydroxide, however, is believed to be unabsorbable, and the evidence is that the use of aluminum-containing antacids does not increase the risk of developing Alzheimer's dementia.[34,35]

The known problem with the long-term use of aluminum salts is a different one. Aluminum hydroxide has been shown to bind to phosphorus and thus interfere with its absorption. If taken regularly over a period of time, a phosphorus deficiency could develop, leading to osteomalacia (softening of the bones) and other adverse effects.[36]

NUTRITIONAL HEALING PLAN: Aluminum Salts

Preparation

aluminum hydroxide gel

Dosage: 5–30 ml daily

Bismuth

Bismuth inhibits the growth of *Campylobacter pylori* (a microorganism recently found to be associated with peptic ulcer disease) and has been shown to be as effective as the newest class of medications (the H_2-receptor [histamine] blocking agents) but with a lower relapse rate. However, because of the suspicion that chronic use could cause damage to the nervous system, a course of bismuth treatment should be limited to a maximum of six to eight weeks, with an eight-week interval between a further course of treatment.[37,38]

NUTRITIONAL HEALING PLAN: Bismuth

Dosage: 120 mg of bismuth 4 times daily before meals and at bedtime

---

Calcium

Calcium carbonate is a potent but inexpensive antacid. However, its ingestion is followed by increased gastric acid secretion, and regular ingestion of large doses over a period of time may occasionally cause nausea, headaches, and weakness, symptoms of the milk-alkali syndrome which can be harmful to the kidney. It is therefore not recommended for the treatment of peptic ulcers.[39]

Magnesium

Magnesium hydroxide is a potent and effective antacid when prescribed as a liquid formulation. Like aluminum hydroxide, it is unabsorbable and may interfere with phosphorus absorption. Because magnesium salts usually produce loosening of the stools, they are often combined with aluminum hydroxide (which is constipating).[40,41]

NUTRITIONAL HEALING PLAN: Magnesium

Preparation

magnesium hydroxide

Dosage: 15 to 30 ml 4 times daily (varies depending on the frequency and intensity of the pain and upon changes in bowel function)

Zinc

Animal studies have shown that zinc can prevent the release of chemical agents that weaken the stomach lining, predisposing it to ulceration. Under double-blind conditions, zinc supplementation has been shown to speed the healing of peptic ulcers in people who exhibit no evidence of zinc deficiency.[42,43,44]

NUTRITIONAL HEALING PLAN: Zinc

Dosage: 50 mg of zinc 3 times daily with meals

Instructions: Take with 2 mg of copper daily.

WARNING

High doses of zinc may occasionally elevate cholesterol; take only under medical supervision.

Botanical Extracts

Deglycyrrhizinated Licorice

Licorice root appears to be an effective treatment for peptic ulcers, but first its content of glycyrrhetinic acid has to be removed; otherwise with regular use it may elevate the blood pressure. In a controlled study, deglycyrrhizinated licorice (DGL) has been shown to be at least as effective as the newest class of anti-ulcer medications (the H_2-receptor [histamine] blocking agents) in speeding healing of gastric and duodenal ulcerations. DGL also appears to protect against aspirin-induced damage to the gastric mucosa. Animal research suggests that it promotes regeneration of the ulcerated lining by increasing the number of mucus-secreting glands as well as the number of mucus-secreting cells in each gland.[45,46,47,48]

NUTRITIONAL HEALING PLAN:
Deglycyrrhizinated Licorice

Preparation

chewable tablets

Initial Dosage: 760–1520 mg 3 times daily between meals

Maintenance Dosage: 760 mg 2 to 3 times daily

S-Methylmethionine ("Vitamin U")

Found in trace amounts in certain raw foods—particularly green vegetables—the administration of S-methylmethionine appears to speed the healing of peptic ulcers. When a group of 26 people with peptic ulcers received concentrated cabbage juice, a rich source of S-methylmethionine, 92 percent of them showed X-ray evidence of healing after 3 weeks, as compared to only 32 percent of a group of 19 similar people with ulcers who had not been treated. (Cabbage juice is also rich in glutamine, an amino acid that may also have contributed to its benefits.)[49]

The following case is a typical example of the benefits of cabbage juice for peptic ulcers:

A man was informed by his physician that X-rays showed that his old peptic ulcer had returned and a new one had formed. The pain ceased almost as soon as he started drinking five glasses of raw cabbage juice daily. After one week, he decreased the cabbage juice to three glasses daily. When, two months later, he was re-examined, both ulcers had healed.[50]

NUTRITIONAL HEALING PLAN: S-Methylmethionine

Preparation

raw cabbage juice

Dosage: one liter daily

CHOOSING A PERSONAL PLAN

Everyone who has, or has recovered from, a peptic ulcer should follow the principles of the Basic Healing diet. Mineral antacids are the best proven and most widely accepted of the Nutritional Healing plans. Magnesium hydroxide should be tried alone; if stools become too loose, you may need to combine it with aluminum hydroxide. Bismuth salts are indicated when your doctor has reason to believe that your ulcers are related to an infection with *Campylobacter pylori*. Since bismuth is accumulated in the tissues, the salts should be used cautiously and under medical supervision.

Deglycyrrhizinated licorice is the next best proven plan, and the fact that it repeatedly has been shown to be at least as effective as the new histamine-blocking medications is impressive. It appears to be a good alternative to the unabsorbable antacids.

Though S-methylmethionine may not be available, cabbage certainly is, and you may wish to make your own cabbage juice to give it a trial. Although there is evidence from scientific studies of the value of vitamin A and zinc, because of the potential for adverse effects at these high doses they should be taken only under medical supervision.

There are reasons to suspect that marginal deficiencies of vitamins C and E may promote the development of peptic ulcers. Also, it is possible, but not well proven, that supplementation with these vitamins promotes healing, not only in people with marginal deficiencies but in everyone suffering from peptic ulcers. If your doctor has no objection, since the supplemental doses are generally safe, you may wish to take them regularly.

ADDITIONAL SUGGESTIONS

Stress and psychological conflicts are known to promote the development of peptic ulcer disease. Moreover, there is evidence suggesting that the recurrence of symptoms can be prevented if life style changes are made to reduce stress and conflict.

Periodontal Disease

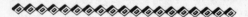

The *periodontal tissues* consist of the gums (gingiva), the bone into which the teeth are embedded, and the *periodontal ligament,* a thin layer of tissue between the teeth and the bone. Disease of these tissues is common, especially among older adults, and is responsible for about 10 percent of dental extractions. It progresses over a period of years until the supporting structures for the teeth are destroyed.

DIETARY FACTORS

It is well known that sugar ingestion promotes tooth decay, but not many people realize that sugar also promotes periodontal disease. One way in which it does this is by increasing the accumulation of *plaque,* a sticky combination of bacteria and their products that forms on the teeth within hours of cleaning. As plaque accumulates, it promotes the development of inflammation of the gums, or *gingivitis.* In experimental gingivitis, sugar has been shown to directly increase gingival inflammation. It also promotes periodontal disease by reducing the ability of the white blood cells to destroy harmful bacteria.[1]

THE HEALING DIET

Minimize the intake of sugar and brush your teeth and use dental floss as soon as possible after eating sugar.

NUTRITIONAL HEALING PLANS

Vitamins

Folic Acid

Folic acid has been shown in several scientific studies to be an effective treatment for periodontal disease. Though it can be swallowed, using a mouthwash that contains folic acid appears to give better results. The reason it works is unknown; even though blood levels of folic acid are usually normal in periodontal disease, there may be a deficiency of folic acid in the gums.[2,3,4]

NUTRITIONAL HEALING PLAN: Folic Acid

Preparations and Dosages

▶ A 0.1 percent solution of folate mouthwash. Rinse mouth with one tbsp twice daily, **or**
▶ 1 mg of folic acid. Take orally one daily.

Vitamin C

People with scurvy, a disease that results from vitamin C deficiency, have bleeding gums because collagen, the major protein of connective tissue, is poorly formed. Even in the absence of evidence of scurvy, people who are low in vitamin C are prone to develop periodontal disease. This appears to be due, at least in part, to a weakening of the immune system's ability to defend against the bacteria present in plaque.

For people who are not deficient in vitamin C, the value of vitamin C supplementation in fighting periodontal disease has yet to be well proven. There is early evidence that megadoses of vitamin C may be beneficial; however, not all studies have found it to be effective.[5,6]

NUTRITIONAL HEALING PLAN: Vitamin C

Dosage: 1 g of vitamin C twice daily

Minerals: Calcium Deficiency

Calcium deficiency is associated with loss of the bone underlying the teeth, leading to the loss of teeth. For people who have suffered from loss of bone structure, calcium supplementation, perhaps in combination with vitamin D, may reduce or prevent further bone loss.[7,8]

Less clear is the effect of calcium supplementation on gingival health, even among people whose diets are inadequate in calcium. One study found that people whose diets were inadequate in calcium had reduction in the size of periodontal inflammatory pockets after taking calcium supplements; however, when other investigators studied another group of similar people and compared calcium supplementation with a placebo, they failed to find that calcium had any advantage.[9,10]

NUTRITIONAL HEALING PLAN: Calcium Deficiency

Preparation

calcium citrate

Dosage: 750 mg daily

Instructions

Consider adding 400 IU of vitamin D daily if there are no other supplemental sources of vitamin D in your diet.

Other Nutritional Factors

Coenzyme Q_{10}

Coenzyme Q_{10} (CoQ_{10}) is a vitaminlike substance that, in periodontal disease, may be deficient both in the gingiva and in the white blood cells. A review of 7 studies found that 70 percent of a total of 332 people with periodontal disease responded to supplementation.[11,12]

In one of these studies, for example, 18 people were given either CoQ_{10} or a placebo. After 21 days, the severity of periodontal disease before and after treatment was rated by dentists who did not know who had received the real supplement. They rated all eight people who had received CoQ_{10} as improved, while they rated only three of the ten who had received the placebo as improved.[13]

The following case is a typical example of the benefits of COQ_{10} for periodontal disease:

An elderly woman had severe periodontal disease (desquamative gingivitis) which caused pain that was so severe she was unable to eat solid foods for months. She was placed on coenzyme Q_{10} and within two weeks, her pain diminished and she started to eat solid foods. Three months later, her gums were a healthy pink and the disease was almost completely reversed.[14]

NUTRITIONAL HEALING PLAN: Coenzyme Q$_{10}$

Dosage: 25 mg of coenzyme Q$_{10}$ twice daily

Botanical Extracts

Sanguinaria (bloodroot)

The plant extract *sanguinaria* has been successfully used to treat periodontal disease both as a mouthwash and as an ingredient in toothpaste, usually in combination with zinc. Scientific studies have found improvement in both plaque and gingival inflammation following regular use. One of these studies compared sanguinaria with and without the addition of zinc; the results suggested that zinc only mildly enhances the effectiveness of sanguinaria.[15,16]

NUTRITIONAL HEALING PLAN: Sanguinaria

Preparations

► mouthwash (dilute the extract in water)
► toothpaste

Dosage: depends upon the specific preparation

Other Factors

Metal Toxicity

Mercury, which comprises about 50 percent of silver amalgam fillings, is a toxic metal. Though silver amalgam fillings have not been proven to cause periodontal disease, people with amalgams appear to be more likely to have diseases of the mouth. Moreover, after the removal of all amalgams, symptoms of diminished oral health may be reduced or even eliminated. One possibility is that dental amalgam fosters periodontal disease by adversely affecting the ability of the immune system to combat the effects of plaque-forming bacteria.[17,18,19]

Hydrochloric Acid Deficiency

Reduced gastric acidity is associated with resorption of the bone beneath the teeth, most likely because calcium absorption from the gut is decreased when the stomach is unable to release enough hydrochloric acid. If your dentist has found that the supporting bone beneath your teeth is being resorbed, supplementation with a safe form of hydrochloric acid may be indicated.[20,21]

NUTRITIONAL HEALING PLAN: Hydrochloric Acid Deficiency

Preparation

10-gr capsules of betaine or glutamic HC1

Instructions: See Appendix C for detailed instructions.

CHOOSING A PERSONAL PLAN

Minimizing sugar in the diet and brushing and flossing as soon as possible after eating sugar are wise steps toward periodontal health. I suggest regular use of a mouthwash or toothpaste containing folic acid and/or sanguinaria extract, if available. Supplementation with coenzyme Q_{10} may also be tried. Given the safety of vitamin C, everyone with evidence of periodontal disease should take supplements, even though it is not yet known whether it is effective for people who are not deficient.

If you have evidence of bone resorption, consider supplemental calcium with vitamin D as well as hydrochloric acid. A nutritionally knowledgeable physician can best evaluate whether these supplements are indicated.

ADDITIONAL SUGGESTIONS

Nutritional healing methods are not a substitute for proper dental hygiene! Brush your teeth and floss after every meal to physically remove the plaque that promotes periodontal disease.

Premenstrual Tension Syndrome (PMS)

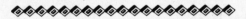

Dr. Guy Abraham has divided premenstrual tension syndrome (PMS) into four categories:[1]

1. **Premenstrual Anxiety.** Characterized by elevated blood estrogens and low progesterone. Symptoms are:

   ► anxiety
   ► irritability
   ► insomnia
   ► depression (just before menses)

2. **Premenstrual Craving.** Characterized by evidence of reactive hypoglycemia. Symptoms are:

   ► craving for sweets
   ► increased appetite
   ► headache
   ► palpitations
   ► fatigue or fainting

3. **Premenstrual Depression.** Characterized by elevated progesterone levels later in the menstrual cycle, and a possible increase in male hormones (androgens). Sometimes there is evidence of chronic lead intoxication. Symptoms are:

   ► depression
   ► forgetfulness
   ► confusion
   ► lethargy

4. **Premenstrual Hyperhydration.** Associated with salt retention and possibly elevated aldosterone (an adrenal hormone that affects fluid retention). Symptoms are:

- weight gain above 1.4 kg (3 lb)
- breast congestion
- abdominal bloating
- swelling of face and extremities

DIETARY FACTORS

PMS is associated with an increased intake of refined carbohydrates and, specifically, a greatly increased intake of sugar. Since carbohydrates improve mood by enhancing the synthesis of the neurotransmitter serotonin, women feeling "blue" premenstrually may unconsciously increase their intake of dietary carbohydrates in order to feel better.[2,3,4]

On the other hand, eating large amounts of sugar can cause premenstrual fluid retention, and refined carbohydrates (such as white flour and sugar) promote the hypoglycemic-like symptoms seen in premenstrual craving. Moreover, dietary sugar increases the loss of magnesium in the urine, and a marginal magnesium deficiency appears to be an important cause of PMS.[5,6,7]

Controlled trials of low-refined-carbohydrate diets in the treatment of PMS are needed to prove their efficacy. Until they are performed, however, it appears reasonable to restrict your intake of refined carbohydrates.

Dietary fiber reduces the influence of estrogen by increasing its binding and excretion. Since the estrogen to progesterone ratio is elevated in premenstrual anxiety, increasing dietary fiber would theoretically be beneficial in treating PMS. However, controlled trials of high-fiber diets are needed to confirm this.[8]

If you suffer from premenstrual fluid retention, it may result from the excessive retention of sodium by the kidney. Restricting salt in your diet before your period should help premenstrual craving, but for a different reason. Premenstrual craving may be caused by reactive hypoglycemia, which can result from the overproduction of insulin. By increasing the absorption of sugar (glucose) from the gut, salt stimulates the pancreas to produce more insulin.[9,10,11]

Alcohol, another stimulant of insulin release, should be entirely avoided in the second half of your cycle. In addition, heavy caffeine intake repeatedly has been found to be associated with PMS. Because caffeine increases nervous tension, it should particularly be avoided if you suffer from premenstrual anxiety.[12,13]

A low-fat diet (15–20 percent of calories from fat) is an effective treatment for premenstrual fluid retention. Not only do women report that their symptoms are reduced after following the diet; also, when examined they have less breast swelling, tenderness, and lumpiness.[14,15]

THE HEALING DIET

Follow the Basic Healing diet as described in Appendix A. To relieve specific symptoms, you might also try the following special diets:

1. For cravings, fluid retention, and magnesium deficiency, try the Low-Refined-Carbohydrate and Sugar-free diets.
2. For cravings and fluid retention, try the Low-Salt diet.
3. For fluid retention, try the Low-Fat diet.
4. For anxiety, try the High-Fiber diet.
5. For cravings, try avoiding alcohol.
6. For anxiety, try avoiding caffeine.

NUTRITIONAL HEALING PLANS

Vitamins

Vitamin B_6

PMS is not associated with evidence of a vitamin B_6 deficiency. However, supplementation with vitamin B_6 has been found to be an effective treatment in a number of double-blind studies. It appears to have some efficacy for all four categories of PMS.[16]

Even when vitamin B_6 is not deficient, intracellular magnesium levels may be deficient, and vitamin B_6 supplementation can bring these levels up to normal. Since decreased intracellular magnesium levels may be related to manifestations of premenstrual syndrome, this effect of the vitamin could be the explanation of its efficacy.[17]

NUTRITIONAL HEALING PLAN: Vitamin B_6

Preparation

pyridoxine

Dosage: **40 mg daily**

Vitamin E

Even when serum vitamin E levels are normal, vitamin E supplementation has been proven effective in double-blind studies. All categories of PMS except fluid retention appear to benefit.[18,19]

NUTRITIONAL HEALING PLAN: Vitamin E

Dosage: 300 IU of vitamin E twice daily

Minerals

Calcium

Women with premenstrual anxiety consume more calcium than normal women, and the ratio of calcium to magnesium in their diets is higher than it is for both normal women and women with the other three categories of PMS. Moreover, hair calcium levels tend to be elevated, suggesting a metabolic disturbance in calcium regulation.[20,21,22]

In a double-blind crossover study, supplementation with calcium was found to reduce symptoms both premenstrually and during the menstrual period. Depression and fluid retention were reduced premenstrually, while pain (perhaps another manifestation of fluid retention) was reduced both premenstrually and during menses.[23]

The efficacy of calcium supplementation suggests that the tendency of women with PMS to consume extra calcium may be an attempt to compensate for a disturbance in calcium metabolism. Since calcium supplementation impairs magnesium absorption, and magnesium deficiency may contribute to PMS, magnesium should be supplemented along with calcium, but at a level lower than that of calcium.[24]

NUTRITIONAL HEALING PLAN: Calcium

Preparation

calcium citrate

Dosage: 1000 mg daily

Instruction: Take with 400 mg of magnesium daily.

Magnesium Deficiency

The level of magnesium in the red blood cells is frequently reduced in PMS, whereas the magnesium level in the fluid portion of the blood is usually normal. In one study, for example, 45 percent of 105 women with PMS were found to have red blood cell magnesium levels that were below the normal range.[25]

Controlled trials of magnesium supplementation for PMS have not been undertaken. However, in a pilot study of 192 women with PMS who received magnesium supplements, nervous tension was relieved in 89 percent, breast pain in 96 percent, weight gain in 95 percent, and headaches in 43 percent. Moreover, in a controlled study of women with reactive hypoglycemia (closely related to premenstrual craving) and reduced magnesium levels, 50 percent of 14 women felt better after magnesium supplementation, compared to 25 percent of women on placebos.[26,27]

Since magnesium has many important functions, the correction of a magnesium deficit could improve PMS through any of several mechanisms. A magnesium deficiency causes changes in the adrenal gland that could promote premenstrual fluid retention. Premenstrual anxiety is believed to be associated with a relative depletion of the neurotransmitter dopamine in the brain, caused by the increase in estrogen levels in the latter part of the menstrual cycle. Magnesium deficiency may foster further dopamine depletion both directly and, by reducing estrogen excretion, indirectly. Finally, because magnesium may reduce glucose-induced insulin secretion, a deficiency would favor the development of premenstrual craving.[28,29,30,31,32]

The benefits of magnesium supplementation are shown by the following case:

A 40-year-old woman had a 10-year history of severe premenstrual fluid retention and irritability, with a 6 to 7 lb weight gain in the week prior to her period. Treatment with a diuretic drug was of only temporary benefit. Her serum magnesium was below the normal range. The fluid retention responded to a very-low-salt diet and worsened if she consumed salty foods or ate foods containing wheat.

She was given magnesium supplementation along with a specialized multivitamin/multimineral supplement (Optivite). As her serum magnesium normalized, her premenstrual fluid retention and irritability decreased, and she was able to stop the diuretic. Stopping her oral contraceptive (which tends to antagonize vitamin B₆) helped clear her symptoms completely.[33]

NUTRITIONAL HEALING PLAN: Magnesium Deficiency

Dosage: 400 mg of magnesium daily

Other Nutritional Factors

Omega-6 Fatty Acids

Omega-6 fatty acids are essential fatty acids; that is, they are necessary for our normal function and must come from our diets. Dietary linoleic acid is metabolized (converted) through a series of steps into a *prostaglandin*, a hormone-like chemical with important functions.

In a study of 42 women with PMS, their levels of linoleic acid were significantly elevated, while their levels of all its metabolites were significantly reduced, suggesting a block in the conversion of linoleic acid to gamma-linolenic acid, its first metabolite. As these differences were seen throughout the phases of the menstrual cycle, they have been postulated to cause PMS by making tissues hypersensitive to changes in sexual hormones in the premenstrual phase.[34]

Evening primrose oil, a rich source of gamma-linolenic acid, has been administered under double-blind conditions to women with PMS in several studies. Most studies showed evidence of benefit, even in women with treatment-resistant symptoms.[35] The following case is a typical example:

> *A woman complained of irritability or depression starting several days prior to menses. Progesterone was ineffective. Evening primrose oil, however, along with vitamin B₆ (which helps to promote its metabolism) relieved all her symptoms.*[36]

NUTRITIONAL HEALING PLAN: Omega-6 Fatty Acids

Preparation

evening primrose oil

Dosage: 1.5 g twice daily

Botanical Extracts

Ginkgo Biloba

Fifteen women with premenstrual fluid retention were studied. All were found to have leaky small blood vessels (capillaries), which permitted fluid to escape from the bloodstream into their tissues. They were given *Ginkgo biloba* extract either orally or by intravenous injection. Not only did their PMS respond, but repeat testing showed that their capillaries no longer tended to leak.[37]

NUTRITIONAL HEALING PLAN: Ginkgo Biloba

Preparation

solid extract

    Dosage: 40 mg of Ginkgo biloba 3 times daily

Other Factors: Lead Toxicity

Chronic lead intoxication prevents estrogen from performing properly by preventing it from binding to its receptors. Since decreased peripheral estrogen increases *monoamine oxidase levels* and increased monoamine oxidase levels are associated with depression, lead toxicity may hypothetically cause depression by increasing monoamine oxidase levels.[38,39,40]

In a study of 56 women with PMS and 14 normal women, hair lead levels were 34 percent higher in the women with PMS. Moreover, two women with severe premenstrual depression had hair lead levels that were 11.3 and 14 times the levels of the normal women.[41]

Magnesium blocks the absorption of lead and increases its urinary excretion. Therefore a magnesium deficiency, which is not uncommon in PMS, can promote the development of lead intoxication.[42,43]

CHOOSING A PERSONAL PLAN

It may be helpful to follow the principles of the Basic Healing diet, especially during the second half of your menstrual cycle. Alternatively, you may elect to follow just those parts of the diet that are applicable to the category of PMS that describes your specific symptoms.

The combination of vitamin B_6 and magnesium supplementation is recommended, as is the combination of vitamin E and evening primrose oil—or all four supplements can be tried together. Calcium supplementation would be indicated if you suffer from premenstrual depression or fluid retention, whereas *Ginkgo biloba* would be specifically indicated for premenstrual fluid retention, either alone or in combination with the other supplements.

Prostate Enlargement

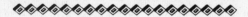

Though rare under age 40, 85 percent of men have some enlargement (*benign hyperplasia*) of their prostate by their eighth decade; the enlargement is associated with an increased concentration of a male hormone within the gland. Since the prostate surrounds the exit by which the urine leaves the bladder, prostate enlargement constricts the urinary passageway. This causes troublesome symptoms such as: a frequent need to urinate, even throughout the night; an inability to fully empty the bladder; difficulty or pain in urinating, a disorder known as *dysuria;* and a slow, diminished urinary stream.

NUTRITIONAL FACTORS

Minerals

Zinc

Zinc levels are higher in the prostate than in any other organ, probably because this mineral is required for the metabolism of male hormones within the prostate. When the prostate is enlarged, the binding of zinc to the cells of the prostate is decreased. Therefore, even though prostatic zinc levels may be elevated and blood zinc levels are normal, the prostatic cells may actually be zinc-deprived.[1]

In a few pilot studies, zinc supplementation successfully reduced the size of the prostate, along with the associated symptoms, in the majority of men. As hopeful as these early findings are, no investigations have been done since the 1970's to confirm them.[2,3]

The following case illustrates the benefits of zinc supplementation for prostate enlargement:

A 67-year-old man with urinary urgency and frequency, dysuria, and reduced size of urinary stream could pass only a small amount of urine at a time. His bladder always seemed full and there was a continual dull ache across his lower abdomen. His sleep was disturbed due to the need to urinate five or six times nightly. When dietary analysis showed an extremely low zinc intake, he was placed on 30 mg of zinc daily. Within a month, his condition began to improve; after six months, he was asymptomatic.[4]

NUTRITIONAL HEALING PLAN: Zinc

Dosage: 50 mg of zinc daily

Other Nutritional Factors

Amino Acids

Several studies, some of which were controlled, have found the combination of three amino acids—L-glutamic acid, L-alanine, and glycine—to be an effective treatment. Both shrinkage of the prostate and symptomatic improvement have been reported.[5,6]

NUTRITIONAL HEALING PLAN: Amino Acids

Preparation

L-glutamic acid, L-alanine, and glycine

Dosage: 250 mg of each 3 times daily for two weeks
followed by 125 mg of each 3 times daily

Essential Fatty Acids

When *testosterone,* a male hormone, enters the prostate cell, it stimulates growth of the gland. Simultaneously, it stimulates the release of hormone-like chemicals called prostaglandins which, in turn, prevent unrestrained growth by inhibiting further testosterone binding to the prostate. With aging, prostaglandin synthesis could decline, causing increased testosterone binding and unrestrained growth of prostatic cells. If so, supplementation with the essential fatty acids that are the nutritional precursors of the prostaglandins may stop the disorder from progressing.[7]

Unfortunately, the only research exploring this possibility is an unpublished pilot study whose results were reported in 1941. Several weeks after 19 men with prostatic hyperplasia received a combination of linoleic, linolenic, and arachidonic acids, all showed a reduction in the size of the prostate, an increase in the force of the urinary stream, and a diminution of residual urine in the bladder after urination. Twelve of the men no longer had residual urine and 13 no longer had to awaken at night to urinate. Controlled studies using specific essential fatty acids are needed before rational recommendations can be made concerning fatty acid supplementation.[8]

Botanical Extracts

Pollen

A double-blind study employing 60 men with prostatic hyperplasia confirmed the results of several early trials of *Cernilton,* an extract of flower pollen produced by A.B. Cernelle, Sweden. After 6 months, 69 percent of the men who had received pollen extract versus 30 percent of the men who had received placebos reported improvement. Men who had received pollen extract also displayed a significant decrease in residual urine and, as determined by ultrasound, in prostate size.[9]

The efficacy of pollen extract (Cernilton) has been compared to that of amino acids (L-glutamic acid, L-alanine, and glycine) under double-blind conditions. The investigators concluded that the two treatments were equally effective.[10]

NUTRITIONAL HEALING PLAN: Pollen Extract

Preparation

Cernilton

Dosage: **2 tablets 3 times daily**

Trial Period

three months

Pygeum Africanum

Pygeum is a tropical African evergreen tree. An extract made from its bark has been proven effective in several European studies. For example, in a German study employing 263 men with prostatic hyperplasia, urinary symptoms improved in 66 percent of the men given pygeum compared to 31 percent of the men given a placebo, although two men had to discontinue treatment due to gastrointestinal side effects.[11]

NUTRITIONAL HEALING PLAN: Pygeum Africanum

Preparation

extract made from the bark

> *Dosage:* 50 mg twice daily

Trial Period

two months

Saw Palmetto (Serenoa Repens)

The extract made from the berries of the saw palmetto palm tree, *Serenoa repens,* has been shown repeatedly in double-blind studies to reduce urinary symptoms caused by benign prostate enlargement. Moreover, when directly compared to pygeum, the berry extract was more effective and free of the gastrointestinal side effects noted with pygeum.[12,13]

The following case is an example of the benefits of *Serenoa repens* supplementation for prostate enlargement:

> *A 55-year-old man complained of nocturia (excessive urination at night), slight hesitancy on urination, and slightly reduced strength of the urinary stream. The condition had been present for several years and had gradually progressed. Rectal examination showed mild prostatic enlargement.*
>
> *He was treated with a liposterolic extract of 160 mg of saw palmetto berries daily. Within two days, there was considerable improvement in all of his symptoms. Several attempts to discontinue treatment were followed by a return of the previous symptoms within two days that resolved on restarting the treatment.*[14]

NUTRITIONAL HEALING PLAN: Saw Palmetto

Preparation

liposterolic berry extract

> *Dosage:* 160 mg twice daily

Trial Period

three months

Metal Toxicity: Cadmium

A research team has found prostatic cadmium levels in prostatic hyperplasia to be considerably higher than in normal prostates, with the cadmium level directly related to the level of dihydrotestosterone. Although another investigator failed to confirm these findings, prostatic hyperplasia has been produced in animals by injecting cadmium directly into the prostate. Moreover, in the test tube, cadmium stimulates the growth of human prostatic tissue.[15,16,17,18]

CHOOSING A PERSONAL PLAN

Because of the close relationship between prostatic function and zinc, I suggest you start a daily zinc supplement and continue it, whether or not you wish to try additional treatment plans. Of the other Nutritional Healing plans, saw palmetto berry extract is my first choice for a therapeutic trial. At least six out of seven double-blind studies have found this extract to be a safe and effective treatment; it has also been shown to be superior to pygeum, another herbal preparation that has been proven effective.

Pygeum extract and the amino acid regimen (L-glutamic acid, L-alanine, and glycine) have been equally well studied; either would be a logical choice if serenoa repens fails, although it is not known whether these Nutritional Healing plans are effective when serenoa repens has proven to be ineffective. Flower pollen extract (Cernilton), though less well studied, is also worth a therapeutic trial. Since we cannot assume that all pollen extracts are equally effective, make sure to get Cernilton, the specific preparation that was studied.

No matter which of the Nutritional Healing plans you select, remember that improvement may take up to three months to occur.

Psoriasis

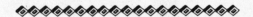

Psoriasis, a chronic, recurrent, scaling skin rash with a distinctive pattern, affects 1 to 2 percent of Caucasians at some point during their lives. It varies from small, almost insignificant patches on the knees and elbows to a massive eruption covering most of the body. Though the cause of psoriasis is unknown, heredity plays a role in determining who develops it.

DIETARY FACTORS

Pilot studies dating from early in the century have found that a low-protein diet may cause the lesions to regress. Striking improvement has also been reported for people on the rice diet originally developed by Dr. Walter Kempner at Duke University—a diet that contains very little protein. A vegetarian diet, low in protein and fat, has also been reported to be effective. Since a very low-fat diet may also be effective, the low fat content of these diets probably contributes to their efficacy.[1,2,3,4]

Alcohol abuse in men, but apparently not in women, increases the risk of psoriasis; however, we do not know whether abstention from alcohol affects the course of the disease. Food sensitivities may promote the development of lesions in predisposed people, since some people improve on food-elimination diets.[5,6]

THE HEALING DIET

1. Follow the Low-Protein diet combined with the Low-Fat diet or, alternatively, the Basic Vegetarian diet as described in Appendix A.
2. Avoid alcohol.
3. Avoid foods found on testing to provoke the rash or itching. *See Appendix B for information about diagnosing food sensitivities.*

NUTRITIONAL HEALING PLANS

Vitamins

Vitamin A

Psoriasis may be associated with a reduced level of vitamin A in the blood serum. Because of concerns about the side effects of supplementing people with large doses of vitamin A, *etretinate,* a synthetic vitamin A analog, has been used with some success not only in treating psoriasis but also in treating the arthritis that sometimes accompanies the skin rash. However, there are significant and possibly serious side effects, and an exacerbation of psoriasis may occur when treatment is stopped.[7,8]

With its potential for side effects, etretinate, which is available by prescription, is indicated only for people suffering from a severe case of psoriasis that has not responded to other treatments.

Vitamin B$_{12}$

Though pilot trials of a long series of daily intramuscular injections of vitamin B$_{12}$ have reported good results, a double-blind study failed to find evidence that B$_{12}$ was any better than a placebo.[9,10]

Vitamin B$_{12}$ has also shown promise when injected directly into the lesions. Though injections with salt water had no effect, lesions injected with B$_{12}$ regressed in six out of eight patients. There is no evidence that taking vitamin B$_{12}$ supplements orally is beneficial.[11]

Vitamin D

Calcitriol, the active form of vitamin D, plays an important role in the generation of cells in the skin's outer layer, and in advanced psoriasis its blood level may be reduced. In pilot studies, both oral and topical application of calcitriol have been found to be effective treatment. They are available by prescription.[12,13]

The following case illustrates the benefits of calcitriol supplementation for psoriasis:

A woman first developed psoriasis at age 14, and it worsened during her sophomore year in college. When initially examined, she had extensive lesions scattered all over her body except her face.

She was treated with calcitriol along with supplemental magnesium (to prevent the development of magnesium deficiency), and her serum calcium levels (which can become elevated with treatment) were monitored. Two months later, there was no improvement; however, after another six months, her psoriasis was nearly gone.[15]

In a Spanish study of more than 600 psoriatics, four out of five improved when treated with vitamin D combined with vitamin A. However, there were occasional side effects, especially headaches and gastrointestinal complaints.[14]

Minerals

Selenium

Selenium is required for the activation of an enzyme (glutathione peroxidase) that reduces inflammation. Although psoriasis may be associated with reduced blood selenium levels, oral supplementation does not increase skin selenium levels and is ineffective. Selenium may be effective, however, when it is applied directly to the skin as a salve.[16,17]

NUTRITIONAL HEALING PLAN: Selenium

Preparation

selenium sulfide salve

    Instruction: Apply regularly directly to the rash.

Other Nutritional Factors

Essential Fatty Acids

Fish oils are a good source of *eicosapentaenoic acid* (EPA), an omega-3 essential fatty acid. In several pilot studies, fish oil supplements were found to promote regression of the lesions, and one research team found that improvement tended to correlate with the level of EPA in the skin. Moreover, in a double-blind study, fish oil treatment reduced itching, redness, and scaling.[18,19,20]

Fish oil has also been applied as a salve directly on the skin lesions with considerable success. In one study, 8 out of 11 patients had greater improvement with a salve to which fish oil was added than with the salve alone.[21]

Arachidonic acid, a fatty acid that promotes inflammation, is increased in skin cells within psoriatic lesions. EPA, which tends to reduce inflammation, can substitute for it in cell membranes. Surprisingly, however, the application of an arachidonic acid salve, rather than causing a worsening of the rash, has been shown under double-blind conditions to produce improvement or complete resolution of the lesions in about half of the people who try it.[22,23]

NUTRITIONAL HEALING PLAN: Essential Fatty Acids

Fish Oil Oral Supplementation

Preparation

MaxEPA™ (manufactured by R. P. Scherer, U.S.) fish oil capsules containing 180 mg EPA per g

Dosage: 10 g daily

Fish Oil Salve

Preparation

MaxEPA™ 10 percent salve

Instructions: Apply regularly directly to the rash.

Arachidonic Acid Salve

Preparation

arachidonic acid 1 percent salve

Instructions: Apply regularly directly to the rash.

Fumaric Acid

Fumaric acid is formed in the skin upon exposure to ultraviolet rays, and people suffering from psoriasis appear to suffer from a biochemical defect in producing adequate fumaric acid. Controlled studies have reported improvement in psoriasis following supplementation with salts of fumaric acid, usually in combination with the application of a fumaric acid salve to the skin, fumaric acid baths, and a special diet. Because the protocol is complicated and because fumaric acid therapy may cause serious side effects, the treatment must be medically supervised. The Clinique Beau Reveil, CH1854, Leysin, Switzerland specializes in fumaric acid compound therapy for psoriasis, as described in the following case:[24,25]

A 28-year-old woman had pustular psoriasis for 3 years, during which period she was hospitalized 12 times for treatment, with limited improvement. Her body was totally covered with lesions, and she was in pain from the cracking and itching of the skin. She went to the Clinique Beau Reveil in Switzerland for fumaric acid compound therapy; the morning after starting treatment with fumaric acid pills, ointment, baths, and a special diet, her face was 95 percent cleared; within 3 days it was completely cleared. Within 2 weeks she noted dramatic improvement in the rash covering the rest of her body, and she was 98 percent cleared when she returned home 2 1/2 months later. [26]

Botanical Extracts

Capsaicin

Capsaicin is a substance derived from red peppers. Under double-blind conditions, the application of capsaicin salve to psoriasis lesions successfully reduced both scaling and redness. Initially, nearly half of the people in the study noted burning, stinging, itching, and increased redness; however, these side effects diminished or vanished with continued application of the salve. [27]

NUTRITIONAL HEALING PLAN: Capsaicin

Preparation

capsaicin salve

> *Instructions:* Apply regularly directly to the rash.

WARNING

Capsaicin may cause initial burning, stinging, itching, and redness.

Trial Period

three to six weeks

CHOOSING A PERSONAL PLAN

Anyone suffering from psoriasis should give a Healing diet a reasonable trial of perhaps a couple of months. A trial of an elimination diet is worth considering, especially if you have other symptoms that may be food-related.

Fish oil, both as an oral supplement and as a salve to apply directly to the rash, is the nutritional treatment I would recommend trying first. Salves containing arachidonic acid or selenium would be my next choice, whereas I would save a trial of the capsaicin salve for last as it is the salve most likely to initially cause an increase in symptoms.

The remaining Nutritional Healing plans need to be administered by your physician. Both fumaric acid compound therapy and etretinate (vitamin A analog) treatment have potentially serious side effects but are reasonably well proven to be effective. Although vitamin B_{12} therapy is generally safe, intramuscular injections have not been proven effective, and injections directly into the lesions may not be practical when you have many lesions.

Finally, local treatment with vitamin D appears safe but has not been proven effective, whereas taking vitamin D orally is probably the least preferable plan because it is both unproven and may have side effects.

ADDITIONAL SUGGESTION

When Dr. R. N. Shore, a physician at Johns Hopkins University School of Medicine, removed a bandage that his patient had left on for three weeks, he discovered that the scaly plaque beneath the dressing had totally cleared. On testing various types of bandage tapes, he found that a waterproof dressing left on for at least one week helps in most cases. Since then, other researchers have confirmed his observation.[28,29]

Rheumatoid Arthritis

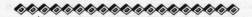

See also: PAIN.

A disease mediated by the immune system, *rheumatoid arthritis* is a degenerative joint disease characterized by overgrowth of the joint lining and infiltration of that lining by cells belonging to the immune system. Usually, its manifestations are chronic and progressive, with periods of exacerbation and remission. Three times as many women are affected as men, and the prevalence of the disease increases with age.

DIETARY FACTORS

Malnutrition is commonly associated with the disease. Since the nutritional status of people with rheumatoid arthritis relates more closely to the severity of the disease than to their diet, malnutrition is believed to be primarily due to difficulty in absorbing nutrients. (Your doctor can evaluate you for malnutrition.)

Dietary fat, especially saturated fat, appears to have an adverse effect. Obese people with active rheumatoid arthritis have experienced long-term remissions within days of going on a low-calorie, fat-free, weight-control formula diet; one or two days after return to high-fat foods or vegetable oils, they had exacerbations.[1]

Numerous studies have found food sensitivities to play a role in disease activity. In addition to feeling better, objective measures of disease activity may show improvement once people are placed on a proper elimination diet. Conversely, if these people eat the foods they are sensitive to, an exacerbation of the disease may occur.[2] The following case illustrates how food sensitivities can contribute to disease activity:

> *A woman with a 25-year history of active rheumatoid arthritis was gradually getting worse despite all treatments. When she was tested, corn (which was the filler in both of her medications) appeared to be her major food allergen. She improved dramatically after one week on a corn exclusion diet; however, after six weeks she had a severe exacerbation following her inadvertent ingestion of corn as corn-flour thickening in gravy. Afterward, she improved again and began to regain weight. She was able to discontinue all medications, and now feels and looks better than she has for more than 20 years.[3]*

Nonsteroidal anti-inflammatory drugs (NSAIDs) are often used to treat rheumatoid arthritis. There is evidence suggesting that these drugs may make it easier for food antigens to penetrate the gut lining and enter the bloodstream; they may thus promote the development of food sensitivities.[4]

THE HEALING DIET

1. Follow the Low-Fat diet as described in Appendix A for a trial period of three months (although relief may start within days).
2. In case of malnutrition, increase food intake.
3. Avoid foods found to exacerbate symptoms. *See Appendix B for information about diagnosing food sensitivities.*

NUTRITIONAL HEALING PLANS

Vitamins

Pantothenic Acid

The blood level of pantothenic acid tends to be lower in people with rheumatoid arthritis than in people without the disease; the more severe the disease, the lower the level. In a double-blind study, supplementation was followed by significant reductions in pain, disability, and the duration of morning stiffness, whereas similar patients given an inactive pill that looked identical failed to improve.[5,6]

NUTRITIONAL HEALING PLAN: Pantothenic Acid

Dosage: 500 mg of pantothenic acid daily

Instructions: Start with 500 mg daily and gradually increase to 500 mg 4 times daily by day 10.

Trial Period

two months

Vitamin C

Even despite a normal vitamin C intake, the levels of vitamin C in people with rheumatoid arthritis may be so inadequate as to cause spontaneous bruising on the forearms as well as hemorrhages in the skin. These symptoms disappear promptly with vitamin C supplementation. Since bioflavonoids (which are generally found in nature wherever vitamin C is found) are known to strengthen capillary walls, they should be combined with vitamin C at an equal dosage.[7,8]

NUTRITIONAL HEALING PLAN: Vitamin C

Dosage: 1 g of vitamin C daily

Instructions: Take with 1 g of citrus bioflavonoids daily.

Minerals

Copper

In rheumatoid arthritis, copper levels increase in both the blood serum and the joint linings, while the levels decrease in the liver. Though the meaning of these changes is unknown, copper supplementation does appear to have therapeutic value as an anti-inflammatory agent.[9,10,11]

For example, the wearing of copper bracelets is an old folk remedy that was recently studied with modern research techniques. When people were given both a copper and an imitation copper bracelet to wear—one at a time in either order—and not told which they were given, those who noted a difference found the copper bracelet to be more effective for reducing their symptoms. Moreover, people who had been wearing copper bracelets at the start of the study found that their arthritis worsened when they switched to the imitation copper bracelets. There was even evidence that copper was absorbed: while being worn in the study, the copper content of each bracelet declined.[12]

Copper, when combined with aspirin to form copper salicylate, appears to be more effective than aspirin alone in combating arthritic pain and inflammation, and short-term treatment may bring about long-lasting remissions. Copper complexes appear to fight inflammation in two ways. They combat unstable, destructive free radicals that are released in the process and activate receptors in the brain that reduce the perception of pain.[13,14]

NUTRITIONAL HEALING PLAN: Copper

Preparation

copper salicylate

Dosage: 60 mg once to twice daily

Instructions: Take at mealtimes with fluids.

Alternative: 2–4 mg of copper amino acid-chelate daily

Trial Period

Restrict a trial period to ten days.

Zinc

Like copper, serum zinc levels are reduced in rheumatoid arthritis, whereas the levels in the joint spaces are increased. The results of studies with zinc supplementation suggest that supplementation is most likely to be beneficial if zinc is deficient. The frequent appearance of white spots on your fingernails suggests zinc deficiency; a nutritionally oriented physician can evaluate you further to determine your zinc status.[15]

NUTRITIONAL HEALING PLAN: Zinc

Preparation

zinc sulfate

Dosage: 220 mg 3 times daily

Instructions: Take with meals.

Trial Period

six weeks

Other Nutritional Factors

Omega-3 Fatty Acids

Members of both families of essential fatty acids (the omega-3 and the omega-6 series), with their well-known anti-inflammatory effects, have been shown to be beneficial in a number of studies. Double-blind studies have found that the administration of fish oils that are rich in omega-3 fatty acids may produce improvement in such symptoms as the number of tender joints, morning stiffness, and grip strength, although there is no evidence that they will slow the progress of the disease.[16]

NUTRITIONAL HEALING PLAN: Omega-3 Fatty Acids

Preparation

MaxEPA™ (manufactured by R. P. Scherer, U.S.) (Each capsule contains 0.18 grams of eicosapentaenoic acid.)

Dosage: 10–12 capsules daily

Trial Period

two to three months

Botanical Extract: Bromelain

A substance derived from the stem of the pineapple, *bromelain* is an enzyme with anti-inflammatory properties. In a pilot study, 25 people received bromelain that was enteric-coated to escape digestion in the stomach. Almost one-third had excellent results, while almost one-half had good results. Most had a significant reduction in joint swelling and an increase in joint mobility. There were no adverse side effects, and those who were on steroids seemed to need lower steroid dosages during bromelain therapy.[17]

NUTRITIONAL HEALING PLAN: Bromelain

Dosage: varies with each preparation

Instructions: Take 3 to 4 times daily between meals.

Trial Period

three weeks minimum

Mollusk Extract: New Zealand Green-Lipped Mussel

In a double-blind study, an extract of the New Zealand green-lipped mussel was found by one group of investigators to be effective for people with severe arthritis who were not responding to NSAIDs and were awaiting joint surgery. Adverse side effects were minimal. It is not known why the extract appears to help, and more studies are needed to confirm these exciting findings.[18]

NUTRITIONAL HEALING PLAN: New Zealand Green-Lipped Mussel

Preparation

Seatone (manufactured by McFarland Labs, Auckland, NZ)

Initial Dosage: 1050 mg daily

Maintenance Dosage: 700–1050 mg daily

Trial Period

Results are seen in 3 to 18 weeks.

CHOOSING A PERSONAL PLAN

Lowering the amount of fat you eat, especially the saturated fat, makes good sense. If, however, you have any evidence of being malnourished, replace those fat calories with calories from other foods such as starches. (If you are malnourished, it would be a good idea to consider seeing a dietitian for assistance in designing a high-calorie diet.) Also, since food sensitivities may be contributing to your symptoms, you should investigate that possibility through a proper evaluation.

Of all the Nutritional Healing plans, the efficacy of increasing dietary omega-3 fatty acids has been best proven. You may therefore wish to try it first. Eating fish that are rich in omega-3 fatty acids should be equally beneficial if you would rather eat fish frequently (at least two times a week) than take the fish oil supplement. *(See Appendix D for a list of fish rich in omega–3 fatty acids.)*

If available, copper salicylate may prove to be an excellent substitute for a nonsteroidal anti-inflammatory drug. If it is not available, you may wish to try another form of copper supplementation. Zinc supplementation is most likely to be beneficial if you are zinc-deficient; however, because copper decreases zinc absorption, anybody who takes copper should also take zinc.

Both pantothenic acid and bromelain are quite safe and well worth trying. Since bromelain supplements vary in potency, ask for the highest potency brand available. Though the research on the New Zealand green-lipped mussel needs to be confirmed, that treatment also appears worthy of a trial.

Finally, if you suffer from spontaneous bruising or hemorrhages into the skin, try vitamin C along with bioflavonoids.

ADDITIONAL SUGGESTIONS

Rheumatoid arthritis appears to be affected by stress. Therefore, anything you can do to reduce stress in your life may be beneficial. You may also wish to try relaxation exercises in order to learn to calm your body down.

APPENDIX A

How to Plan
Your Healing Diet

❖❖❖❖❖❖❖❖❖❖❖❖❖❖❖❖❖❖❖❖

Your diet will have an effect on your body's ability to heal, no matter what your illness may be. Do not make the mistake of taking nutritional supplements as a substitute for a healthy diet. Unless you are following a special Healing diet, two general Healing diets are suggested: the Basic Healing diet and the Vegetarian diet. (Detailed information about different aspects of these diets are given in the discussions of the Special Healing diets.)

GENERAL HEALING DIETS

The Basic Healing Diet

1. Eat a variety of foods.
2. Emphasize ample portions of fruits and vegetables (especially uncooked) and whole-grain foods.
3. Limit total fat intake to a maximum of 30 percent of your daily calories. *(If you eat a typical Western diet, you should reduce your fat intake by at least one-quarter.)*
4. Limit saturated fat intake to less than 10 percent of your daily calories. *(If you eat a typical Western diet, this is a mild to moderate reduction.)*
5. Target total mono- and polyunsaturated fat intake to be about 10 percent of your daily calories. Nuts, seeds, and olives are good food sources. The following chart lists good oil sources of these fats.

OILS RICH IN MONO- OR POLYUNSATURATES

canola
corn
cottonseed
olive
safflower
sesame
soybean
sunflower

6. Limit cholesterol intake to less than 300 mg daily. *(If you eat a typical Western diet, you will need to reduce your intake by about one-third.)*

HIGH-CHOLESTEROL FOODS

eggs: 272 mg each
beef liver (fried): 147 mg/oz
shrimp (boiled): 56 mg/oz
spare ribs (pork): 35 mg/oz
cheese (cheddar): 30 mg/oz

7. If you eat red meat, fish or fowl, limit a serving to 4 oz.
8. Restrict refined sugars.
9. Use salt in moderation; add as little as possible to foods and choose less salty foods.
10. Limit alcohol to a maximum of two drinks a day.
11. Minimize consumption of salt-cured, salt-pickled, smoked, and charcoal-broiled foods.
12. Eat as much food as you need to achieve or maintain a desirable body weight. *(If you follow this diet, your weight will tend to normalize over time.)*

The Vegetarian Healing Diet

This diet follows the principles of the Basic Healing diet, but it excludes foods made from the bodies of animals. These include:

► beef
► fish
► lamb
► mollusks
► pork
► shellfish

In contrast to a vegan diet, this diet does **not** exclude milk or eggs or any of the food products made from them.

SPECIAL HEALING DIETS

The following diets are designed for specific therapeutic purposes. In general, they need not be followed strictly but should be used as general guides for meal planning. Applications of these diets, as they relate to specific disorders, are included in the individual chapters of this book. Refer to the appropriate chapter for detailed information. Also, consider seeing a professional trained in dietetics for more specific help in planning nutritious meals based on the principles of the specific diet you plan to follow.

The Low-Fat Diet

In the usual Western diet, 35 to 40 percent of calories come from fat. It is well established that this is too high a percentage of fat, but there is some disagreement as to how low the percentage of fat should be. The major medical organizations generally suggest a maximum of 30 percent of calories from fat. Though this is an improvement, it appears that a diet containing 20 percent of calories from fat is even healthier and yet not too difficult to follow.

Dietary fat can be divided into saturated, monounsaturated, and polyunsaturated fats, and further divided into the specific fatty acids that distinguish these fats from one another. Though we now know that it is not entirely accurate to blame the saturated fats for the unhealthy effects of high-fat diets (in part because different specific saturated fatty acids have different properties), it is simpler for diet planning to focus on minimizing saturated fats.

SOURCES OF SATURATED FAT

butter
cheese
cream
gravies
ice cream
lard
meat fats and drippings (including chicken skin)
fatty meats

—bacon	—sausage
—hot dogs	—lunch meats
—ribs	—hamburger
—salami	—bologna

whole milk
hydrogenated oils:
  —solid shortenings
  —stick margarines
  —nondairy creamers (some)
  —pastries (some commercial)

The High-Fiber Diet

Dietary fiber consists of the insoluble fibers (cellulose, hemicellulose, and lignin) and the soluble, or gel-forming, fibers (pectin, gums, mucilage). By absorbing water, insoluble fibers (especially cellulose and hemicellulose) increase the size of the stool and normalize its transit time through the bowel to combat both constipation and diarrhea. There is evidence that they may protect against diverticulosis, colon cancer, hemorrhoids, and varicose veins.

Soluble fibers (and lignin) bind with bile acids, decreasing fat absorption and lowering cholesterol levels. Soluble fibers also delay glucose absorption, helping to control blood sugar fluctuations in diabetics.

The typical Western diet today contains about 19 g of dietary fiber. Many experts believe that the intake of dietary fiber should be doubled, or even tripled, for optimum health. Since fiber fills your stomach and satisfies your appetite without adding calories, increasing your fiber intake not only gives you the direct benefits of fiber and of the healthy foods that contain it, but it will tend to reduce your intake of other foods, many of which are far less healthy. If you are overweight, you may even discover yourself losing weight without dieting.

Increase your intake of the foods shown in the following charts to make your diet high in fiber.

FOODS THAT CONTAIN CELLULOSE AND HEMICELLULOSE

apples
green beans
wax beans
beets
bran
broccoli
brussels sprouts
cabbage
carrots
eggplant
whole-grain flour
pears
peas
peppers
radishes

FOODS THAT CONTAIN LIGNIN

green beans
bran
breakfast cereals
eggplant
pears
radishes
strawberries

FOODS THAT CONTAIN PECTIN, GUMS, AND MUCILAGE

apples
bananas
green beans
cabbage
cauliflower
carrots
citrus fruits
grapes
oatmeal
potatoes
sesame seeds
strawberries
squash

The High-Complex-Carbohydrate Diet

Complex carbohydrates are starches. Emphasize dishes rich in the following foods:

▶ grains
▶ fruits
▶ vegetables
▶ nuts
▶ seeds

Try to eat these natural foods in as unprocessed a form as possible. Examples of unprocessed or lightly processed foods are:

▶ breakfast cereals
▶ juices
▶ salads
▶ fruit salads

Snacks such as fresh fruit, carrots, or a "trail mix" of nuts, seeds, and raisins are all recommended. More highly processed (refined) foods that are rich in complex carbohydrates (but low in sugar) include:

▶ pizza
▶ bread
▶ cheese sandwich
▶ pretzels
▶ vegetarian casseroles

Main courses should emphasize vegetables. If you wish to eat meat, keep portions small.

The Low-Refined-Carbohydrate Diet

Refined carbohydrates have been processed so that some of the healthy ingredients that are contained in the foodstuff in its raw state have been removed. The Low-Refined-Carbohydrate diet is **not** a low-carbohydrate diet. It should follow the principles of the Basic Healing diet, except for minimizing the intake of all refined carbohydrates. Refined carbohydrates include:

▶ refined sugars, such as cane, beet, and corn sugar
▶ white (bleached, enriched) wheat flour
▶ white (polished) rice

The Sugar-Free Diet

This diet removes all sources of refined sugar from the diet. Sugar in its natural form is not excluded unless it is highly concentrated.

EXCLUDED FOODS

cakes
hard candies
chocolates
soft drinks
honey
pies
maple sugar
table sugar

FOODS NOT EXCLUDED

fruit
milk (contains sugar as lactose)

The High- and Low-Protein Diets

In general, high-protein foods come from animals; thus the High-Protein diet usually emphasizes meat, fish, and eggs. The Low-Protein diet is also a high-carbohydrate diet. In addition to restricting meat, fish, and eggs, it is healthiest if it follows the principles of the High-Complex-Carbohydrate diet.

Experts believe that a healthy diet should contain roughly 0.8 g/kg (0.36 g/lb) of protein per day. However, in the Western industrialized countries, the usual diet contains twice that amount of protein, which makes it a high-protein diet.

HIGH-PROTEIN FOODS

beef
cheese (including cottage cheese)
eggs
fish
lamb
pork
shellfish

The Low-Tryptophan Diet

1. Restrict foods with a high tryptophan to protein ratio, such as

   ► soya beans
   ► dairy products
   ► eggs
   ► fish
   ► meat

2. Emphasize vegetables, root vegetables, and tryptophan-poor cereals such as rye, corn, and buckwheat.
3. Exclude serotonin-rich foods such as bananas, tomatoes, and walnuts.
4. There is no restriction on fat or sugar, but remember that these may be bad for your health in other ways.

The Alkaline Ash Diet

The following charts show alkaline- and acid-forming foods.

ALKALINE ASH-FORMING FOODS

fruits (except cranberries and plums)
milk
molasses
certain nuts (almonds, chestnuts, coconuts)
vegetables (except corn and lentils)

ACID ASH-FORMING FOODS

buckwheat
cheese
cranberries
grains (including wheat, corn, rye, barley, and rice)
lentils
meat (including fish, poultry, shellfish, and eggs)
plums (and prunes)
sugar (refined)

The charts above should only be used as a general guide to aid you in shifting your diet toward a higher alkaline ash-forming content. Foods listed as producing an acid ash should not be strictly excluded just for the purpose of this diet, because specific prepared foods vary greatly in the acidity of their ash. (For example, wheat germ has a markedly acid ash, whereas whole-wheat bread produces only a slightly acid ash.) Also, since this list is unrelated to nutritional considerations, a strict alkaline ash diet should be attempted only under the supervision of a dietitian or other specially trained health professional.

You may wish to consider switching to a vegetarian diet. In addition to its other benefits, a vegetarian diet is significantly more alkaline.

APPENDIX B

How to Diagnose Food Sensitivities

Elimination of suspected foods from the diet is the direct method of diagnosing food sensitivities; if the eliminated foods contributed to your illness, improvement will occur. Foods must be eliminated for a minimum of five days to allow for the removal of their remains from the gastrointestinal tract and to provide time for the effects of their absorption into the body to dissipate. As some of these effects may be protracted, a longer period of food exclusion, ranging from two to six weeks, may sometimes produce results when a shorter period fails to relieve symptoms.

Foods you select to remain in the diet should be those that are least suspected of causing symptoms. Most definitive, but most severe and potentially unhealthful, is a five-day *water-only fast*. An *elemental diet*, consisting of a liquid mixture in which as few of the ingredients as possible are food-derived, provides basic nourishment but is difficult to tolerate. A *two-food diet*, such as the lamb and pear diet, consists of one protein- and fat-rich food and one carbohydrate-rich food. If you wish to try any of these limited diagnostic diets or similar ones, you should be in reasonably good health and under your physician's supervision.

A *common food-elimination diet* is often the most practical. In this diet, only foods (such as wheat, dairy products, yeast, and corn) that are normally eaten more often than twice a week are eliminated. This diet minimizes your inconveniences and provides a wide enough variety of foods to usually ensure nutritional adequacy. However, to be absolutely sure that your personal elimination diet is nutritionally balanced, I suggest you review it with a dietitian or nutritionist.

For accurate results, you must restrict yourself to foods whose ingredients are not on your elimination list. For example, bread (which is usually a combination of wheat, milk, sugar, salt, and baking soda or yeast) should be avoided if you are eliminating any one of those foods. Similarly, ketchup should be avoided if you are eliminating any one of its many ingredients or if you do not know what those ingredients are.

Medications, nutritional supplements, and toothpaste may be sources of eliminated foods that could possibly reduce the diagnostic value of the diet. (Baking soda can be substituted for toothpaste.) Of course, medications should not be discontinued without your physician's approval.

Sometimes only one food, or a few foods, need be eliminated. Occasionally specific foods have been linked to certain illnesses, such as gluten (which is found in wheat, oats, rye, and barley) in the case of celiac disease. Though this theory is unproven, an unusually strong craving for a particular food is believed to suggest that you are sensitive to that food. Since eliminating only suspicious foods is the easiest elimination diet to follow, it can be tried first, and a more extensive elimination diet can be tried later if your symptoms fail to improve.

Some people initially feel worse, usually starting 12 to 24 hours after beginning the diet. Their usual symptoms may worsen, or they may experience new symptoms, such as headaches or a flulike syndrome. The onset of new symptoms after starting an elimination diet is believed to increase the likelihood that you are sensitive to one or more of the eliminated foods and that you will feel better if you continue to follow the diet.

If you do improve while following a food-elimination diet, reintroduce the eliminated foods one at a time in order to identify the specific foods to which you are sensitive. Ideally, since food reactions may sometimes be delayed for 72 hours, one food should be introduced every 3 days.

When many foods have been eliminated, these food challenges may take a month or longer. They can be done at closer intervals—daily, for example—but sometimes identification of inciting foods becomes difficult when delayed reactions overlap, and it may take several days before you return to your baseline state.

During the elimination period, and especially during this testing period, keep a food diary. One column can be used to record the time each food was ingested, while in another column you can record changes in signs and symptoms. A particular symptom can be rated on a scale, and ratings at the end of each day can be averaged to provide a comparison over time.

Individualized elimination diets can be based on the results of blood testing. Several types of blood tests for food sensitivities are available. They may evaluate cellular damage when blood cells are exposed to a food (*cytotoxic tests*) or immune reactions to a food (*IgE or IgG RAST; IgG immune complexes; ELISA/ACT™*). Much of their appeal is due to their convenience, which is counterbalanced by their cost.

Despite improvements in recent years, different types of blood testing yield different results; some even yield quite different results when repeated. At best, blood tests for food sensitivities indicate only an abnormal response to a food; they are unable to tell whether that food is contributing to an illness or whether it eventually produces symptoms if it continues to be consumed.

Even with their limitations, elimination diets based on blood testing may be effective in reducing symptoms. However, when such a diet has proven ineffective, you should still consider a standard elimination diet.

Skin testing is another diagnostic method. Prick and scratch tests, which test only for atopic allergic reactions, are of very limited value for diagnosing food sensitivities, while provocative testing may be a more suitable technique. In provocative testing, various dilutions of each food are placed into or under the skin or under the tongue, and both you and your doctor look for changes in signs or symptoms within the next ten minutes. The attraction of provocative testing is that it is not only diagnostic but may also be therapeutic. However, though experienced clinicians report excellent results with this method, its efficacy is highly controversial.

FOR FURTHER INFORMATION

Brostoff J., Gamlin L. *The Complete Guide to Food Allergy and Intolerance*. London, Bloomsbury Publishing, Ltd., 1989.

Faelten, S. *The Allergy Self-Help Book*. Emmaus, Penn., Rodale Press, 1983.

APPENDIX C

A Brief Guide to Hydrochloric Acid (HCl) Supplementation

Before you consider supplementation with hydrochloric acid (HCl), I suggest that you have your level of stomach acid tested. In the past this procedure was an uncomfortable one, as samples of fluid were removed from the stomach through a thick tube that was pushed down the nose into the stomach.

Doctors now have far more comfortable methods of testing the level of stomach acid. All you need to do is swallow a small capsule. One type of capsule (the Heidelberg pH capsule) is a small radiotransmitter that relays data on acid levels directly from the stomach. Another type (the Gastro-Test capsule) contains a specially coated string, one end of which is held outside the mouth while the capsule is swallowed. After a few minutes, the string is gently pulled out and treated with a chemical; it then turns a color that indicates the degree of stomach acidity.

Whichever method is used, the test should be done after acid production has been stimulated. The less acidic the gastric juice after stimulation, the greater the dosage of HCl needed. Supplementation is generally in the form of either betaine or glutamic HCl, preferably as 10-gr capsules. Between one and five capsules are swallowed immediately following meals, depending on your degree of HCl deficiency and the size of the meal.

If testing is unavailable and if your doctor approves, you could try supplementation by starting with a single capsule after each meal and, unless improvement occurs, slowly increasing the dosage to 5 capsules. In the event that there is any discomfort such as burning after taking the supplement, stop taking it until a few days after the symptom goes away; then you may cautiously try a smaller dosage. **Irritation of the stomach**

lining and even ulceration can result if these precautions are not followed.

If HCl supplementation is effective, you may have prompt relief of gastrointestinal symptoms that were due to insufficient hydrochloric acid, although it may be weeks before you feel the full therapeutic benefits from normalizing your stomach acid.

APPENDIX D
Food Sources of Nutrients

◇◇◇◇◇◇◇◇◇◇◇◇◇◇◇◇◇◇◇◇◇◇◇◇◇

FISH RICH IN OMEGA-3 FATTY ACIDS

herring
mackerel
salmon
shark
sturgeon
tuna
turbot

FOODS RICH IN VITAMIN B$_6$

bananas
avocados
whole grain cereals
wheat germ
soybeans
prunes
raisins
potatoes
walnuts
peanuts
meat:
  turkey
  chicken
  beef liver
  pork
fish:
  mackerel
  tuna
  swordfish
  salmon

FOODS RICH IN VITAMIN C

Fruits

        oranges
        grapefruit
        papayas
        kiwi
        cantaloupe
        strawberries

Vegetables

        green and red peppers
        broccoli
        cauliflower
        cabbage
        peas
        potatoes

FOODS RICH IN BETA-CAROTENE

Fruits

        cantaloupe
        peaches

Vegetables

        dark green leafy vegetables
        winter squash (deep orange)
        broccoli
        carrots
        tomatoes
        beets
        spinach
        parsley

FOODS RICH IN BORON

Vegetables, Especially

alfalfa
cabbage
lettuce
peas
snap beans
soy

Fruits, Especially

apples
dates
prunes
raisins

Nuts, Especially

almonds
hazel nuts
peanuts

FOODS RICH IN MAGNESIUM

dried apricots
cereals
fish
nuts
green vegetables
whole wheat (including wheat bran and wheat germ)

FOODS RICH IN POTASSIUM

Fruits (Especially When Dried)

apricots
bananas
cantaloupe
figs
grapes (raisins)
peaches
plums (prunes)

Seeds

pumpkin
squash

Nuts

almonds
peanuts
soybeans

Vegetables

avocados
beet greens
beets
lima beans
potatoes
spinach
squash
swiss chard
tomatoes

Wheat

wheat bran
wheat germ

Others

Brewer's yeast
skim milk

FOODS RICH IN SODIUM

dill pickles
pretzels
sauerkraut
soy sauce

Processed Meat

Canadian bacon
dried beef
ham

Soups

beef and chicken broth
black bean
chicken gumbo
cream of potato
Manhattan clam chowder

Processed Fish

canned sardines
canned tuna
kippered herring
smoked salmon

APPENDIX E

The U.S. RDA: What Does It Mean?

◈◈◈◈◈◈◈◈◈◈◈◈◈◈◈◈◈◈◈◈◈

The term *RDA* commonly refers to one of the Recommended Dietary Allowances formulated in the United States by the Food and Nutrition Board of the National Research Council, whose members are drawn from the councils of the National Academy of Sciences, the National Academy of Engineering, and the Institute of Medicine. First formulated in 1941, and periodically revised since then, the RDAs became the basis for establishing guidelines for the nutritional labeling of foods in the United States in 1968. These guidelines are called the *U.S. Recommended Daily Allowances.*

The RDA is defined as the level of intake of an essential nutrient that is judged by the Food and Nutrition Board to be adequate to meet the known nutrient needs of practically all healthy persons. In other words, so long as you are healthy, it is the amount of an essential nutrient you require in order to avoid developing the illness caused by a deficiency of that nutrient. (You can avoid getting Pellagra, for example, by consuming the RDA of niacin.)

The RDA does not apply to individuals with special nutritional needs. Therefore, if you are suffering from an illness, consuming the RDA of a nutrient may not necessarily protect you from developing that nutrient's deficiency disease. Also, the RDA is not meant to suggest what the optimal intake of a nutrient may be. Since the RDAs were first formulated, a huge amount of scientific data has accumulated showing that, when people consume nutrients at levels well above their RDAs, these nutrients have an important additional function: they prevent and combat many common illnesses.

In summary, the RDA is a valuable tool to assist in the prevention and treatment of nutrient deficiency diseases. It fails to suggest, however, the level of a nutrient that provides us with its optimal benefits for health and healing.

Notes

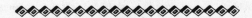

Acne

1. Lobitz, W. C. The structure and function of the sebaceous glands. *Arch Dermatol* 76:162–71, 1957.
2. Ibid.
3. Ringsdorf, W. M. Jr., Cheraskin, E. Diet and dermatosis. *South Med J* 69(6):732, 734, 1976.
4. Cornbleet, T., Gigli, I. Should we limit sugar in acne? *Arch Dermatol* 83:968, 1961.
5. Kaufman, W. F. The diet and acne. Letter to the Editor. *Arch Dermatol* 119(4):276, 1983.
6. Anderson, P. C. Foods as a cause of acne. *Am Fam Physician* 3(3):102–3, 1971.
7. Kligman, A. M., et al. Oral vitamin A in acne vulgaris. *Int J Dermatol* 20(4):278–85, 1981.
8. Anderson, J. A. D., Stokoe, I. H. Vitamin A in acne vulgaris. *Br Med J* 2:294–6, 1963.
9. Ayres, S. Jr., Mihan, R. Acne vulgaris and lipid peroxidation: New concepts in pathogenesis and treatment. *Int J Dermatol* 17:305, 1978.
10. Bushnell, D. E., et al. The retinoids in acne. *Am Fam Physician* 29(3):221–6, 1984.
11. Heel, R. C., et al. Vitamin A acid: A review of its pharmacological properties and therapeutic use in the topical treatment of acne vulgaris. *Drugs* 14:401–9, 1977.
12. Snider, B. L., Dieteman, D. F. Pyridoxine therapy for premenstrual acne flare. Letter to the Editor. *Arch Dermatol* 110:130–31, 1974.
13. Michaëlsson, G., Edqvist, L. Erythrocyte glutathione peroxidase activity in acne vulgaris and the effect of selenium and vitamin E treatment. *Acta Derm Venereol (Stockh)* 64(1):91–14, 1984.
14. Pohit, J., et al. Zinc status of acne vulgaris patients. *J Appl Nutr* 37(1):18–25, 1985.
15. Michaëlsson, G., Ljunghall, K. Patients with dermatitis herpetiformis acne, psoriasis and Darier's disease have low epidermal zinc concentrations. *Acta Derm Venereol (Stockh)* 70(4):304–8, 1990.

16. Lidén, S., et al. Clinical evaluation of acne. *Acta Derm Venereol Suppl (Stockh)* Suppl 89:49–52, 1980.
17. Cunliffe, W. J., et al. A double-blind trial of a zinc sulphate/citrate complex and tetracycline in the treatment of acne vulgaris. *Br J Dermatol* 101(3):321–5, 1979.
18. Lidén, et al, op. cit.
19. Michaëlsson, G., et al. Serum zinc and retinol-binding protein in acne. *Br J Dermatol* 96(3):283–86, 1977.
20. Morello, A. M., Downing, D. T., Strauss, J. S. Octadecadienoic acids in the skin surface lipids of acne patients and normal subjects. *J Invest Dermatol* 66:319–23, 1976.
21. Hubler, W. R. Unsaturated fatty acids in acne. *Arch Dermatol* 79:644, 1959.
22. Abdel, K. M., et al. Glucose tolerance in blood and skin of patients with acne vulgaris. *Ind J Dermatol* 22:139–49, 1977.
23. McCarty, M. High chromium yeast for acne? *Med Hypotheses* 14:307–10, 1984.
24. Norris, J., et al. Azelaic acid really does work in acne—a double-blind national and international study. *Br J Dermatold* 32(Suppl):34, 1987.
25. Bassett, I. B., et al. A comparative study of tea-tree oil versus benzoyl peroxide in the treatment of acne. *Med J Aust* 153:455–8, 1990.

Alcoholism

1. Chalmers, T. C., Davidson, C. S. Survey of recent therapeutic measures in cirrhosis of the liver. *N Engl J Med* 240:449, 1949.
2. Register, U. D., et al. Influence of nutrients on intake of alcohol. *J Am Diet Assoc* 61(2):159–62, 1972.
3. Douglass, J., et al. Effects of a raw food diet on hypertension and obesity. *South Med J* 78(7):841, 1985.
4. Smith, R. F. Status report concerning the use of megadose nicotinic acid in alcoholics. *J Orthomol Psychiatry* 7(1), 1978.
5. Yunice, A. A., Lindeman, R. D. Effect of ascorbic acid and zinc sulphate on ethanol toxicity and metabolism. *Proc Soc Exp Biol Med* 154:146–50, 1977.
6. Watanabe, A., et al. Lowering of blood acetaldehyde but not ethanol concentrations by pantethine following alcohol ingestion: Different effects in flushing and non-flushing subjects. *Alcohol Clin Exp Res* 9:272, 1985.
7. Chen, M. F., et al. Effect of ascorbic acid on plasma alcohol clearance. *J Am Coll Nutr* 9(3):185–89, 1990.
8. Yunice, A. A., et al. Ethanol-ascorbate interrelationship in acute and chronic alcoholism in the guinea pig. *Proc Soc Exp Biol Med* 177(2):262–71, 1984.
9. DeLuzio, N. R. A mechanism of the acute ethanol-induced fatty liver and the modification of liver injury by antioxidants. *Lab Invest* 15:50–61, 1966.
10. Redetzki, J. E., et al. Amelioration of cardiotoxic effects of alcohol by vitamin E. *J Toxicol Clin Toxicol* 20(4):319–31, 1983.
11. Ward, R. J., et al. Reduced antioxidant status in patients with chronic alcoholic myopathy. *Biochem Soc Trans* 16:581, 1988.
12. Korpela, H., et al. Decreased serum selenium in alcoholics as related to liver structure and function. *Am J Clin Nutr* 42(1):147–51, 1985.
13. Leevy, C. M. Thiamin deficiency and alcoholism. *Ann N Y Acad Sci* 378:316–26, 1982.

14. Majumdar, S. K., et al. Vitamin A utilization status in chronic alcoholic patients. *Int J Vitam Nutr Res* 53(3):273–9, 1983.

15. Ward, R. J., et al. Reduced antioxidant status in patients with chronic alcoholic myopathy. *Biochem Soc Trans* 16:581, 1988.

16. Lieber, C. S. Biochemical and molecular basis of alcohol-induced injury to liver and other tissues. *N Engl J Med* 391(25):1639–50, 1988.

17. Garrett-Laster, M., et al. Impairment of taste and olfaction in patients with cirrhosis: The role of vitamin A. *Hum Nutr: Clin Nutr* 38C:203–214, 1984.

18. Lieber, op. cit.

19. Pitts, T. O., Thiel, D. H. Disorders of divalent ions and vitamin D metabolism in chronic alcoholism. *Recent Dev Alcohol* 4:357–77, 1986.

20. Pall, H. S., et al. Hypomagnesaemia causing myopathy and hypocalcaemia in an alcoholic. *Postgrad Med J* 63:665–67, 1987.

21. Norton, V. P. Interrelationships of nutrition and voluntary alcohol consumption in experimental animals. *Br J Addition* 72(3):205–12, 1977.

22. Eriksson, K., et al. The effects of dietary thiamin on voluntary ethanol drinking and ethanol metabolism in the rat. *Br J Nutr* 43(1):1–13, 1980.

23. Rogers, L. L., et al. Voluntary alcohol consumption by rats following administration of glutamine. *J Biol Chem* 220(1):321–3, 1956.

24. Rogers, L. L, Pelton, R. B. Glutamine in the treatment of alcoholism: A preliminary report. *Quart J Stud Alcohol* 18(4):581–87, 1957.

25. Ibid.

26. Glen, I., et al. Possible pharmacological approaches to the prevention and treatment of alcohol-related CNS impairment: Results of a double blind trial of essential fatty acids, in G. Edwards, J. Littleton, Eds. *Pharmacological Treatments for Alcoholism*. London, Croom, Helm, 1984:331–50.

27. Bates, C. *Essential Fatty Acids and Immunity in Mental Health*. Tacoma, WA, Life Sciences Press, 1987, p. 71.

28. Ikeda, H. Effects of taurine on alcohol withdrawal. Letter to the Editor. *Lancet* 2:509, 1977.

Allergy

1. Pastorello, E., et al. Evaluation of allergy etiology in allergic rhinitis. *Ann Allergy* 55:854–6, 1985.

2. Baumgardner, D. J. Persistent urticaria caused by a common coloring agent. *Postgrad Med* 85(6):265, 1990.

3. Bekier, E., Maslinski, C. Z. Antihistaminic action of nicotinamide. *Agents Actions* 4(3):196, 1974.

4. Daiñow, I. Recherches cliniques sur certaines propriétés anti-allergiques de la nicotinamide. *Z Vitamin-forsch* 15:245–50, 1944.

5. Martin, W. On treating allergic disorders. Letter to the Editor. *Townsend Letter for Doctors* Aug/Sept, 1991:670–1.

6. Williams, R. J. The expanding horizon in nutrition. *Texas Rep Biol Med* 19(2):245–58, 1961.

7. Crook, W. G. Letter to the Editor. *Ann Allergy* 49:45–46, 1987.

8. Folkers, K., et al. Biochemical evidence for a deficiency of vitamin B_6 in subjects reacting to monosodium-L-glutamate by the Chinese restaurant syndrome. *Biochem Biophys Res Commun* 100:972–77, 1981.

9. Bhat, N. K. Presentation at the 43rd Annual Meeting, American Academy of Allergy and Immunology, 1987.

10. Clemetson, C. A. Histamine and ascorbic acid in human blood. *J Nutr* 110(4):662–8, 1980.

11. Brown, E. A., Ruskin, S. The use of cervitaminic acid in the symptomatic and coseasonal treatment of pollinosis. *Ann Allergy* 7:65–70, 1949.

12. Fortner, B. R. Jr., et al. The effect of ascorbic acid on cutaneous and nasal response to histamine and allergen. *J Allergy Clin Immunol* 69(6):484–88, 1982.

13. Ahmad, K., Jahan, K. Studies on the preventive and curative action of ascorbic acid on the neurological toxicity of monosodium glutamate. *Food Nutr Bull* 7(4):51–3, 1985.

14. Bachert, C., et al. Decreased airway reactivity in allergic rhinitis after intravenous application of calcium. A study on the alteration of local airway resistance after nasal allergen provocation. *Arzneimmittelforsch* 40:984–7, 1990.

15. Utz, G., Hauck, A. M. [Oral application of calcium and vitamin D_2 in allergic bronchial asthma.] *MMW* 118(43):1395–8, 1976.

16. Durlach, J. Repports experimentaux et cliniques entre magnésium et hypersensibilite. *Rev Fr Allergo* 15:133–46, 1975.

17. Lee, T. H., Arm, J. P. Modulation of the allergic response by fish oil lipids and eicosatrienoic acid. *Prog Clin Biol Res* 297:57–69, 1989.

18. Manku, M. S., et al. Reduced levels of prostaglandin precursors in the blood of atopic patients: Defective delta-6-desaturase function as a biochemical basis for atopy. *Prostaglandins Leukotrienes Med* 9(6):615–28, 1982.

19. Galland, L. Increased requirements for essential fatty acids in atopic individuals: A review with clinical descriptions. *Am J Clin Nutr* 5:213–28, 1986.

Anxiety

1. Uhde, T. W., et al. Glucose tolerance testing in panic disorder. *Am J Psychiatry* 141(11):1461–3, 1984.

2. Boulenger, J. P., et al. Increased sensitivity to caffeine in patients with panic disorders: Preliminary evidence. *Arch Gen Psychiatry* 41:1067–71, 1984.

3. Bruce, M., Lader, M. Caffeine abstention in the management of anxiety disorders. *Psychol Med* 19:211–14, 1989.

4. King, D. S. Can allergic exposure provoke psychological symptoms? A double-blind test. *Biol Psychiatry* 16(1):3–19, 1981.

5. Mohler, H., et al. Nicotinamide is a brain constituent with benzodiazepine-like actions. *Nature* 278:563–65, 1979.

6. Wendel, O. W., Beebe, W. E. Glycolytic activity in schizophrenia, in D Hawkins and L Pauling, Eds. *Orthomolecular Psychiatry: Treatment of Schizophrenia*. San Francisco, W. H. Freeman, 1973.

7. Williams, R. D., et al. Induced thiamine (Vitamin B_1) deficiency in man; relation of depletion of thiamine to development of biochemical defect and of polyneuropathy. *Arch Intern Med* 71:38–53, 1943.

8. Keatinge, A. M. B., et al. Vitamin B_1, B_2, B_6 and C status in the elderly. *Irish Med J* 76:488–90, 1983.

9. Wick, H., et al. Thiamine dependency in a patient with congenital lactiacidaemia. *Agents Actions* 7(3):405–10, 1977.

10. Hoes, M., et al. Hyperventilation syndrome, treatment with L-tryptophan and pyridoxine; predictive values of xanthurenic acid excretion. *J Orthomol Psychiatry* 10(1):7–15, 1981.

11. Carlson, R. J. Longitudinal observations of two cases of organic anxiety syndrome. *Psychosomatics* 27(7):529–31, 1986.

12. Rudin, D. O. The major psychoses and neuroses as omega-3 essential fatty acid deficiency syndrome: Substrate pellagra. *Biol Psychiatry* 16(9):837–50, 1981.

13. Ibid.

14. Hoyse, S. E. Experiences with L-tryptophan in a child and family psychiatric department. *J Int Med Res* 10(3):157–9, 1982.

Asthma

1. Lindahl, O., et al. Vegan diet regimen with reduced medication in the treatment of bronchial asthma. *J Asthma* 22:45–55, 1985.

2. Pelikan, Z., et al. Bronchial asthma due to food allergy. Paper presented at the XII International Congress of Allergy and Clinical Immunology, Washington, D.C., October, 1985.

3. Hoj, L., et al. A double-blind controlled trial of elemental diet in severe, perennial asthma. *Allergy* 36:257–62, 1981.

4. May, C. Objective clinical and laboratory studies of immediate hypersensitivity reactions to foods in asthmatic children. *J Allergy Clin Immunol* 58:500–512, 1978.

5. Burney, P. G., et al. Response to inhaled histamine and 24 hour sodium excretion. *Br Med J* 292:1483–6, 1986.

6. Javaid, A., et al. Effect of dietary salt on bronchial reactivity to histamine in asthma. *Br Med J* 297:454, 1988.

7. Delport, R., et al. Vitamin B_6 nutritional status in asthma: The effect of theophylline therapy on plasma pyridoxal-5¹-phosphate and pyridoxal levels. *Int J Vitam Nutr Res* 58(1):67–72, 1988.

8. Collip, P. J., et al. Pyridoxine treatment of childhood bronchial asthma. *Ann Allergy* 35:93–97, 1975.

9. Reynolds, R. D., Natta, C. L. Depressed plasma pyridoxal phosphate concentrations in adult asthmatics. *Am J Clin Nutr* 41:684–88, 1985.

10. Wright, J. Vitamin B_{12}: Powerful protection against asthma. *Int Clin Nutr Rev* 9(4):185–8, 1989.

11. Simon, R. A., et al. Sulfite-sensitive asthma. *Res. Instit. of Scripps Clinic Scientific Report* 39:57–58, 1982–83.

12. Wright Jonathan, V. Vitamin B-12 and asthma. *Let's Live,* June, 1986, pp. 16 & 18.

13. Rozanov, E. M., et al. [Vitamin PP and C allowances and their correction in the treatment of bronchial asthma patients.] *Vopr Pitan* (6):21–24, 1987.

14. Schwartz, J., Weiss, S. T. Dietary factors and their relation to respiratory symptoms. The Second National Health and Nutrition Examination Survey. *Am J Epidemiol* 132(1):67–76, 1990.

15. Anah, C. O., et al. High dose ascorbic acid in Nigerian asthmatics. *Tropical Geograph Med* 32:132–37, 1980.

16. Schachter, E. N., Schlesinger, A. The attenuation of exercise-induced bronchospasm by ascorbic acid. *Ann Allergy* 49:146–50, 1982.

17. Clemetson, Ca. Histamine and ascorbic acid in human blood. *J Nutr* 110(4):662–8, 1980.
18. Haury, V. G. Blood serum magnesium in bronchial asthma and its treatment by the administration of magnesium sulfate. *J Lab Clin Med* 26:340–4, 1940.
19. Rolla, G., et al. Magnesium attenuates methacholine-induced bronchoconstriction in asthmatics. *Magnesium* 6(4):201–4, 1987.
20. Skobeloff, E. M., et al. Intravenous magnesium sulfate for the treatment of acute asthma in the emergency department. *JAMA* 262(9):1210–13, 1989.
21. Bray, G. W. The hypochlorhydria of asthma of childhood. *Quart J Med* 24:181–97, 1931.
22. Urge, G., et al. Effect of dietary tryptophan restrictions on clinical symptoms in patients with endogenous asthma. *Allergy* 38:211–12, 1983.
23. Becker, A. J., et al. The bronchodilator effects and pharmacokinetics of caffeine in asthma. *N Engl J Med* 310(12):743–6, 1984.
24. Gong, H. Jr., et al. Bronchodilator effects of caffeine in coffee. A dose-response study of asthmatic subjects. *Chest* 89(3):335–42, 1986.
25. Gaby Alan, R. Editorial: Asthma. *The Townsend Letter for Doctors,* April, 1987, p. 73.

Breast Disease

1. Boyd, N. F., et al. Effect of a low-fat high-carbohydrate diet on symptoms of cyclical mastopathy. *Lancet* 2:128–32, 1988.
2. Russell, L. C. Caffeine restriction as initial treatment for breast pain. *Nurse Pract* 14:36–40, 1989.
3. Minton, J. P., Aboud-Issa H. Nonendocrine theories of the etiology of benign breast disease. *World J Surg* 13(6):680–4, 1989.
4. Band, P. R., et al. Treatment of benign breast disease with vitamin A. *Prev Med* 13:549–54, 1984.
5. Ibid.
6. London, R. S., et al. Endocrine parameters and alpha-tocopherol therapy of patients with mammary dysplasia. *Cancer Res* 41 (9 Pt2):3811–13, 1981.
7. London, R. S., et al. Mammary dysplasia: Endocrine parameters and tocopherol therapy. *Nutr Res* 2:243–47, 1982.
8. London, R. S., et al. The effect of vitamin E on mammary dysplasia: A double-blind study. *Obstet Gyn* 65:104–06, 1985.
9. Meyer, E. C., et al. Vitamin E and benign breast disease. *Surgery* 107(5):549–51, 1990.
10. Bricklin, M., Ed. *Rodale's Encyclopedia of Natural Home Remedies.* Emmaus, PA, Rodale Press, 1982, p. 48.
11. Ghent, W. R., Eskin, B. A. Elemental iodine supplementation in clinical breast dysplasia. Abstract. *Proc Annu Meet Am Assoc Cancer Res* 27:189, 1986.
12. Eskin, B. and Ghent, W.—reported in *Med World News* January 11, 1988, p. 25.
13. Ibid.
14. Pashby, N. L., et al. *Br J Surg* 68:801, 1981.
15. Pye, J. K., et al. Clinical experience of drug treatments for mastalgia. *Lancet* 2:373–77, 1985.
16. Wright, J. V. *Dr. Wright's Guide to Healing with Nutrition.* Emmaus, PA, Rodale Press, 1984, pp. 260–77.

17. Dukes, M. N. Ginseng and mastalgia. Letter. *Br Med J* 1:1621, 1978.
18. Porrath, S.—quoted in *Am Med News*, January 27, 1984.

Cancer

1. National Academy of Sciences. *Diet, Nutrition and Cancer.* Washington, D.C., National Academy Press, 1982.
2. Hinds, M. W., et al. *Am J Clin Nutr* 37:192–3, 1983.
3. Hughes, R. E. Hypothesis: A new look at dietary fiber. *Hum Nutr Clin Nutr* 40C:81–6, 1986.
4. Greenward, P., Lanza, E. Dietary fiber and colon cancer. *Contemp Nutr* 11(1), 1986.
5. DeCosse, J. J., et al. Effect of wheat fiber and vitamins C and E on rectal polyps in patients with familial adenomatous polyposis. *J Natl Cancer Inst* 81(17):1290–7, 1989.
6. Colditz, G. A., et al. Increased green and yellow vegetable intake and lowered cancer deaths in an elderly population. *Am J Clin Nutr* 41(1):32–6, 1985.
7. Goldin, B. R., et al. Effect of diet and Lactobacillus acidophilus supplements on human fecal bacterial enzymes. *J Natl Cancer Inst* 64(2):255–61, 1980.
8. Barale, R., et al. Vegetables inhibit, in vivo, the mutagenicity of nitrite combined with nitrosable compounds. *Mutation Res* 120:145, 1983.
9. Nair, P. P., et al. Diet, nutrition intake, and metabolism in populations at high and low risk for colon cancer: Dietary cholesterol, beta-sitosterol, and stigmasterol. *Am J Clin Nutr* 40(4 suppl):927–30, 1984.
10. Santisteban, G. A., et al. Glycemic modulation of tumor tolerance in a mouse model of breast cancer. *Biochem Biophys Res Commun* 132(3):1174–9, 1985.
11. Seely, S., Horrobin, D. F. Diet and breast cancer: The possible connection with sugar consumption. *Med Hypotheses* 11(3):319–27, 1983.
12. Tuyns, A. J., et al. Colorectal cancer and the intake of nutrients: Oligosaccharides are a risk factor, fats are not. A case-control study in Belgium. *Nutr Cancer* 10:181–96, 1987.
13. Kruis, W., et al. Influence of diets high and low in refined sugar on stool qualities, gastrointestinal transit time and fecal bile acid excretion. *Gastroenterology* 92:-1483, 1987.
14. Garro, A., Lieber, C. Alcohol and cancer. *Ann Rev Pharmacol Toxicol* 30:219–49, 1990.
15. National Academy of Sciences, op. cit.
16. Pozniak, P. C. The carcinogenicity of caffeine and cancer: A review. *J Am Diet Assoc* 85(9):1127–33, 1985.
17. Norie, I. H., Foster, H. D. Water quality and cancer of the digestive tract: The Canadian experience. *J Orthomol Med* 4(2):59–69, 1989.
18. Borgman, R. F. Dietary factors in essential hypertension. *Prog Food Nutr Sci* 9:109–47, 1985.
19. Cantor, K. P., et al. Bladder cancer, drinking water source, and tap water consumption: A case-control study. *J Natl Cancer Inst* 79(6):1269–79, 1987.
20. Orr, J. W. Jr., et al. Nutritional status of patients with untreated cervical cancer. II. Vitamin assessment. *Am J Obstet Gynecol* 151(5):632–5, 1985.
21. Butterworth, C. E., et al. Improvement in cervical dysplasia associated with folic acid therapy in users of oral contraceptives. *Am J Clin Nutr* 35:73–82, 1982.

22. Heimburger, D. C., et al. Improvement in bronchial squamous metaplasia in smokers treated with folate and vitamin B_{12}: Report of a preliminary randomized, double-blind intervention trial. *JAMA* 259(10):1525–30, 1988.

23. Schmitt-Gräff, A., Scheulen, M. E. Prevention of adriamycin cardiotoxicity by niacin, isocitrate or N-acetyl-cysteine in mice. A morphological study. *Pathol Res Pract* 181(2):168–74, 1986.

24. Popov, A. I. [Effect of the nonspecific prevention of thrombogenic complications on late results in the combined treatment of bladder cancer.] *Med Radiol (Mosk)* 32(2):42–45, 1987.

25. Lippman, S. M., Meyskens, F. L. Jr. Vitamin A derivatives in the prevention and treatment of human cancer. *J Am Coll Nutr* 7(4):269–84, 1988.

26. Stich, H. F., et al. Use of the micronucleus test to monitor the effect of vitamin A, beta-carotene and canthaxantin on the buccal mucosa of betel nut/tobacco chewers. *Int J Cancer* 34(6):745–50, 1984.

27. Prior, F. Theoretical involvement of vitamin B_6 in tumor initiation. *Med Hypotheses* 16:421–8, 1985.

28. Ha, C., et al. The effect of B-6 on host susceptibility to Moloney Sarcoma Virus-induced tumor growth in mice. *J Nutr* 114:938–45, 1984.

29. Chrisley, B. M., et al. Vitamin B_6 status of a group of cancer patients. *Nutr Res* 6(9):1023–30, 1986.

30. Gey, K. F., et al. Plasma levels of antioxidant vitamins in relation to ischemic heart disease and cancer. *Am J Clin Nutr* 45(5 Suppl):1368–77, 1987.

31. Wagner, D. A., et al. Effect of vitamins C and E on endogenous synthesis of N-nitrosamino acids in humans: precursor-product studies with [15N]nitrate. *Cancer Res* 45:6519–22, 1985.

32. Prasad, K. N., et al. Sodium ascorbate potentiates the growth inhibitory effect of certain agents on neuroblastoma cells in culture. *Proc Natl Acad Sci USA* 76(2):829–32, 1979.

33. Gupta, S. Effect of radiotherapy on plasma ascorbic acid concentration in cancer patients. Unpublished thesis—summarized in Hanck A.B. Vitamin C and cancer. *Prog Clin Biol Res* 259:307–20, 1988.

34. Cameron, E., Pauling, L. Supplemental ascorbate in the supportive treatment of cancer: Reevaluation of prolongation of survival times in terminal human cancer. *Proc Nat Acad Sci USA* 75:4538–42, 1978.

35. Hoffer, A., Pauling, L. Hardin Jones biostatistical analysis of mortality data for cohorts of cancer patients with a large fraction surviving at the termination of the study and a comparison of survival times of cancer patients receiving large regular oral doses of vitamin C and other nutrients with similar patients not receiving those doses. *J Orthomol Med* 5(3):143–54, 1990.

36. Garland, C. F., et al. Serum 25-hydroxyvitamin D and colon cancer. Eight-year prospective study. *Lancet* 1178–8, 1989.

37. Colston, K. W., et al. Possible role for vitamin D in controlling breast cancer proliferation. *Lancet* 1:188–91, 1989.

38. Reichel, H., et al. The role of the vitamin D endocrine system in health and disease. *N Engl J Med* 320(15):980–91, 1989.

39. Knekt, P., et al. Serum vitamin E and risk of cancer among Finnish men during a 10–year follow-up. *Am J Epidemiol* 127(1):28–41, 1988.

40. Lathia, D., Blum, A. Role of vitamin E as nitrite scavenger and N-nitrosamine inhibitor: a review. *Int J Vitam Nutr Res* 59(4):430–8, 1989.

41. Bruce, W. R., Dion, P. W. Studies relation to a fecal mutagen. *Am J Clin Nutr* 33:2511–12, 1980.

42. Ura, H., et al. Effect of vitamin E on the induction and evolution of enzyme-altered foci in the liver of rats treated with diethylnitrosamine. *Carcinogenesis* 8:1595–1600, 1987.

43. London, R. S., et al. Breast cancer prevention by supplemental vitamin E. *J Am Coll Nutr* 4(5):559–64, 1985.

44. Shklar, G., et al. Prevention of experimental cancer and immunostimulation by vitamin E (immunosurveillance). *J Oral Pathol Med* 19:60–4, 1990.

45. Wood, L. Possible prevention of adriamycin-induced alopecia by tocopherol. *N Engl J Med* 312:1060, 1985.

46. Sorenson, A. W., et al. Calcium and colon cancer: A review. *Nutr Cancer* 11:135–45, 1988.

47. Lipkin, M., Newmark, H. Effect of added dietary calcium on colonic epithelial-cell proliferation in subjects at high risk for familial colonic cancer. *N Engl J Med* 313:1381–84, 1985.

48. Iakovleva, S. S. [Use of calcium salts in treatment of malignant tumors.] *Arkh Patol* 42(9):93–94, 1980.

49. Blondell, J. M. The anticarcinogenic effect of magnesium. *Med Hypotheses* 6:863–71, 1980.

50. Clark, L. C. The epidemiology of selenium and cancer. *Fed Proceed* 44:2584, 1985.

51. Watrach, A. M., et al. Inhibition of human breast cancer cells by selenium. *Cancer Lett* 25:41–7, 1984.

52. Barch, D. H. Esophageal cancer and microelements. *J Am Coll Nutr* 8(2):99–107, 1989.

53. Lippman, S. M., Meyskens, F. L., Jr. Vitamin A derivatives in the prevention and treatment of human cancer. *J Am Coll Nutr* 7(4):269–84, 1988.

54. Habib, F. K., et al. Metal-androgen interrelationships in carcinoma and hyperplasia of the human prostate. *J Endocrinol* 71(1):133–41, 1976.

55. Webber, M. M. Effects of zinc and cadmium on the growth of human prostatic epithelium in vitro. *Nutr Res* 6:35–40, 1986.

56. Feustel, A., Wennrich, R. Zinc and cadmium in cell fractions of prostatic cancer tissues of different histological grading in comparison to BPH and normal prostate. *Urol Res* 12(2):147–50, 1984.

57. Brohult, A., et al. Effect of alkoxylglycerols on the frequency of fistulas following radiation therapy for carcinoma of the uterine cervix. *Acta Obstet Gynecol Scand* 58(2):203–07, 1979.

58. Brohult, A., et al. Reduced mortality in cancer patients after administration of alkoxylglycerols. *Acta Obstet Gynecol Scand* 65(7):779–85, 1986.

59. Ziegler, R. B. A review of epidemiologic evidence that carotenoids reduce the risk of cancer. *J Nutr* 119:116–22, 1989.

60. Wald, N., et al. Serum beta-carotene and subsequent risk of cancer: Results from the BUPA study. *Br J Cancer* 57:428–33, 1988.

61. Tomita, Y., et al. Augmentation of tumor immunity against syngeneic tumors in mice by b-carotene. *JNCI* 78(4):679–81, 1987.

62. Stich, H. F., et al. A pilot beta-carotene intervention trial with Inuits using smokeless tobacco. *Int J Cancer* 36(3):321–27, 1985.

63. Prasad, K. N., Sinha, P. K. Effect of sodium butyrate on mammalian cells in culture: A review. *In Vitro* 12:125–32, 1976.

64. Whitehead, R. H., et al. Effects of short-chain fatty acids on a new human colon carcinoma cell line (LIM 1215). *Gut* 27:1457–63, 1986.

65. Langer, R., Murray, J. Angiogenesis inhibitors and their delivery systems. *Appl Biochem Biotechnol* 8(1):9–24, 1983.

66. Lee, A., Langer, R. Shark cartilage contains inhibitors of tumor angiogenesis. *Science* 221:1185–87, 1983.

67. Durie, B. G., et al. Antitumor activity of bovine cartilage (Catrix-S) in the human tumor stem cell assay. *J Biol Response Mod* 4(6):590–95, 1985.

68. Prudden, J. F. The treatment of human cancer with agents prepared from bovine cartilage. *J Biol Response Mod* 4(6):551–84, 1985.

69. Ibid.

70. Lee and Langer, op. cit.

71. Yamawaki, S., et al. *Jpn J Cancer Clin* 25:1081–86, 1979 (in Japanese).

72. Karmali, R. A. Eicosanoids in neoplasia. *Prev Med* 16(4):493–502, 1987.

73. Reich, R., et al. Eicosapentaenoic acid reduces the invasive and metastatic activities of malignant tumor cells. *Biochem Biophys Commun* 160:559–64, 1989.

74. Norman, A., et al. Antitumor activity of sodium linoleate. *Nutr Cancer* 11(2):107–15, 1988.

75. Carroll, K. K. Lipid oxidation and carcinogenesis. *Prog Clin Biol Res* 206:237–44, 1986.

76. van der Merwe, C. F., et al. Oral gamma-linoleic acid in 21 patients with untreatable malignancy. An ongoing pilot open clinical trial. *Br J Clin Pract* 41(9):907–15, 1987.

77. van der Merwe, C. F. The reversibility of cancer. *S Afr Med J* 65:712, 1984.

78. McIllmurray, M. B., Turkie, W. Controlled trial of gamma-linolenic acid in Dukes's C colorectal cancer. *Br Med J* 294:1260, 1987.

79. Maurer, H. R., et al. Bromelain induces the differentiation of leukemic cells in vitro: An explanation for its cytostatic effects? *Planta Med* 54(5):377–81, 1988.

80. Batkin, S., et al. Antimetastatic effect of bromelain with or without its proteolytic and anticoagulant activity. *J Cancer Res Clin Oncol* 114(5):507–8, 1988.

81. Horwitz, N. Garlic as a plat du jour: Chinese study finds it could prevent G.I. cancer. *Med Trib* August 12, 1981.

82. Kandil, O. M., et al. Garlic and the immune system in humans: Its effect on natural killer cells. *Fed Proc* 46(3):441, 1987.

83. Belman, S. Onion and garlic oils inhibit tumor promotion. *Carcinogenesis* 4(8):1063–5, 1983.

84. Taguchi, T. Clinical efficacy of lentinan on patients with stomach cancer. End point results of a four-year follow-up survey. *Cancer Detect Prev* (Suppl)1:333–49, 1987.

85. Kosaka, A., et al. [Effect of lentinan administration on adrenalectomized rats and patients with breast cancer.] *Gan To Kagaku Ryoho* 15(4 Pt 2-1):827–33, 1988 (in Japanese).

86. Gorbach, S. L. The intestinal microflora and its colon cancer connection. *Infection* 10(6):379–84, 1982.

Canker Sores

1. Wray, D., et al. Food allergens and basophil histamine release in recurrent aphthous stomatitis. *Oral Surg Oral Med Oral Pathol* 54(4):388–95, 1982.
2. Wray, D., et al. Recurrent aphthae: Treatment with vitamin B_{12}, folic acid, and iron. *Br Med J* 2:490–3, 1975.
3. Palopoli J., Waxman, J. Recurrent aphthous stomatitis and vitamin B_{12} deficiency. *South Med J* 83:475–7, 1990.
4. Wang, S. W., et al. [The trace element zinc and aphthosis.] *Rev Stomatol Chir Maxillofac* 87(5):339–43, 1986.
5. Merchant, H. W., et al. Zinc sulfate supplementation for treatment of recurring oral ulcers. *South Med J* 70(5):559–61, 1977.
6. Das, S. K., et al. Deglycyrrhizinated liquorice in aphthous ulcers. *J Assoc Physicians India* 37(10):647, 1989.
7. James, A. P. R. Common dermatologic disorders. *CIBA Clinical Symposia* 19(2):38–64, 1967.
8. Gertenrich, R. L., Hart, R. W. Treatment of oral ulcerations with Bacid (Lactobacillus acidophilus). *Oral Surg* 30(2):196–200, 1970.
9. Weekes, D. J. *N Y State J Med* 58(16), August 15, 1958.

Carpal Tunnel Syndrome

1. Ellis, J., et al. Therapy with vitamin B_6 with and without surgery for treatment of patients having the idiopathic carpal tunnel syndrome. *Res Commun Chem Path Pharm* 33(2):331, 1981.
2. Fuhr, J. E., et al. Vitamin B_6 levels in patients with carpal tunnel syndrome. *Arch Surg* 124:1329–30, 1989.
3. Driskell, J. A., et al. Effectiveness of pyridoxine hydrochloride treatment on carpal tunnel patients. *Nutr Reports Int* 34:1031–40, 1986.
4. Ibid.,
5. Folkers, K., et al. Biochemical evidence for a deficiency of vitamin B_6 in the carpal tunnel syndrome based on a crossover clinical study. *Proc Natl Acad Sci USA* 75(7):3410–2, 1978.
6. Folkers, K., et al. Enzymology of the response of the carpal tunnel syndrome to riboflavin and to combined riboflavin and pyridoxine. *Proc Natl Acad Sci U S A* 81(22):7076–8, 1984.
7. Deahl, M. P. Lithium-induced carpal tunnel syndrome. *Br J Psychiatry* 153:250–1, 1988.
8. Fisher, H. B_6: A solution to a painful problem. *Prevention* January, 1987, pp. 56–8.

Cataract

1. Couet, C., et al. Lactose and cataract in humans: A review. *J Am Coll Nutr* 10(1):79–86, 1991.
2. Prchal, J. T., et al. Association of presenile cataracts with heterozygosity for galactosaemic states and with riboflavin deficiency. *Lancet* 1:12–13, 1978.
3. Jacques, P. F., et al. Antioxidant status in persons with and without senile cataract. *Arch Ophthalmol* 106(3):337–40, 1988.

4. Varma, S. D., Richards, R. D. Light-induced damage to ocular lens cation pump: Prevention by vitamin C. *Proc Natl Acad Sci U S A* 76:3504–6, 1979.

5. Varma, S. A., et al. Photoperoxidation of lens lipids: prevention by vitamin E. *Photochem Photobiol* 36(6):623–36, 1982.

6. Bouton, S. M. Jr., Vitamin C and the aging eye. *Arch Intern Med* 63:930–45, 1939.

7. Muhlmann, V., et al. Vitamin C therapy of incipient senile cataract. *Arch Oftalmol B Aires* 14:552–75, 1939.

8. Atkinson, D. Malnutrition as an etiological factor in senile cataract. *Eye Ear Nose Throat Mon* 31:79–83, 1952.

9. Robertson, J. M., et al. Vitamin E intake and risk of cataracts in humans. *Ann N Y Acad Sci* 570:372–82, 1989.

10. Sydenstricker, U. of Georgia and U. of Georgia Hospital—reported in C. Gerras, et al., Eds. *The Encyclopedia of Common Diseases.* Emmaus, PA, Rodale Press, 1976, pp. 652–3.

11. Lerman, S. *Arch Ophthalmol* 65:181, 1961.

12. Hoffer, A. Cataracts and Orthomolecular treatment. *J Orthomol Med* 3(2):61–62, 1988.

13. Bhat, K. S. Plasma calcium and trace minerals in human subjects with mature cataract. *Nutr Rep Int* 37:157–63, 1988.

14. Chuistova, I. P., et al. [Experimental morphologic foundation for the usage of zinc in the treatment of cataract.] *Oftalmol Zh* 7:396, 1985.

15. Todd, G. P. *Nutrition, Health and Disease.* Norfolk, VA, The Donning Company, 1985, p. 175.

16. Todd, G. P.—interviewed in *Prevention* March, 1985, pp. 74–80.

17. Azar, R.—interviewed in *Prevention* July, 1983, pp. 99–103.

Cervical Dysplasia

1. Lindenbaum, J., et al. Oral contraceptive hormones, folate metabolism, and the cervical epithelium. *Am J Clin Nutr,* April, 1975:346–53.

2. Steiff, R. Folate deficiency and oral contraceptives. *JAMA* 214:105–8, 1970.

3. Butterworth, C. E., et al. Improvement in cervical dysplasia associated with folic acid therapy in users of oral contraceptives. *Am J Clin Nutr* 35:73–82, 1982.

4. Wylie-Rosett, J. A., et al. Influence of vitamin A on cervical dysplasia and carcinoma in situ. *Nutr Cancer* 6(1):49–57, 1984.

5. Palan, P. R., et al. Vaginal hydrolysis of retinyl acetate: increase in plasma retinol and retinol binding protein in women with cervical dysplasias. *Biochem Med Metab Biol* 40(3):282–90, 1988.

6. Meyskens, F. L. Jr., Surwit, E. S. Clinical experience with topical tretinoin in the treatment of cervical dysplasia. *J Am Acad Dermatol* 15(4 Pt 2):826–29, 1986.

7. Weiner, S. A., et al. A phase I trial of topically applied trans-retinoic acid in cervical dysplasia—clinical efficacy. *Invest New Drugs* 4(3):241–44, 1986.

8. Palan, P. R., et al. Plasma levels of antioxidant beta-carotene and alpha-tocopherol in uterine cervix dysplasias and cancer. *Nutr Cancer* 15:13–20, 1991.

9. La Vecchia, C., et al. Dietary vitamin A and the risk of invasive cervical cancer. *Int J Cancer* 34:319–22, 1984.

10. Wassertheil-Smoller, S., et al. Dietary vitamin C and uterine cervical dysplasia. *Am J Epidemiol* 114(5):714–24, 1981.

11. Romney, S. L., et al. Plasma vitamin C and uterine cervical dysplasia. *Am J Obstet Gynecol* 151(7):976–80, 1985.

12. Prasad, K., Ed. *Vitamins, Nutrition and Cancer.* New York, Karger, 1984.

13. Dawson, E., et al. Serum vitamin and selenium changes in cervical dysplasia. *Fed Proc* 43:612, 1984.

14. Wright, J. V. *Dr. Wright's Guide to Healing with Nutrition.* Emmaus, PA, Rodale Press, 1984, Chapter 19, pp. 220–9.

Colds

1. Beisel, W. R. Single nutrients and immunity. *Am J Clin Nutr* 35:417–68 (Suppl), 1982.

2. Eby, G. A., et al. Reduction in duration of common colds by zinc gluconate lozenges in a double-blind study. *Antimicrob Agents Chemother* 25(1):20–24, 1984.

3. Al-Nakib, W., et al. Prophylaxis and treatment of rhinovirus colds with zinc gluconate lozenges. *J Antimicrob Chemother* 20(6):893–901, 1987.

4. Farr, B. M., et al. Two randomized controlled trials of zinc gluconate lozenge therapy of experimentally induced rhinovirus colds. *Antimicrob Agents Chemther* 31(8):1183–7, 1987.

5. Ponte, L. The bugs that bug us: What you should know about colds. *Reader's Digest* October, 1987:85–9.

6. Jennings, L. C., Dick, E. C. Transmission and control of rhinovirus colds. *Eur J Epidemiol* 3(4):327–35, 1987.

7. Porte, op. cit.

8. Ibid.

Constipation

1. Taylor, R. Management of constipation: High fiber diets work. *Br Med J* 300:-1063–4, 1990.

2. Corinaldesi, F., et al. Dietary fibers and intestinal transit times. *Curr Ther Res* 31:173–80, 1983.

3. Graham, D. Y., et al. The effect of bran on bowel function in constipation. *Am J Gastroenterol* 77(9):599–603, 1982.

4. Gay, L. P. Gastrointestinal allergy. *J Missouri Med Assoc* 29:7–10, 1932.

5. Botez, M. I., et al. Neurologic disorders responsive to folic acid therapy. *Can Med Assoc J* 15:217, 1976.

6. Hanck, A. B., Goffin, H. Dexpanthenol (Ro 01–4709) in the treatment of constipation. *Acta Vitaminol Enzymol* 4(1–2):87–97, 1982.

7. *A. M. A. Drug Evaluations,* Fifth Edition. Chicago, American Medical Association, 1983.

8. Ibid.

9. Ibid.

10. Ibid.

11. Ibid.

12. Rettger, L. F., et al. *Lactobacillus Acidophilus: Its Therapeutic Application.* New Haven, CT, Yale U. Press, 1935.

Dementia (Senile)

1. Abalan, F. Alzheimer's disease and malnutrition: A new etiological hypothesis. *Med Hypotheses* 15:385–93.

2. Thomas, D. E., et al. Tryptophan and nutritional status of patients with senile dementia. *Psychol Med* 16(2):297–305, 1986.

3. Melamed, E., et al. Reversible central nervous system dysfunction in folate deficiency. *J Neurol Sci* 25:93–98, 1975.

4. Frank, O., et al. Superiority of periodic intramuscular vitamins over daily oral vitamins in maintaining normal vitamin titers in a geriatric population. *Am J Clin Nutr* 30:630, 1977.

5. Spivak, J. L., Jackson, D. L. Pellagra: an analysis of 18 patients and a review of the literature. *Johns Hopkins Med J* 140(6):295–309, 1977.

6. Thomas, et al., op. cit.

7. Gibson, G. E., et al. Reduced activities of thiamine-dependent enzymes in the brains and peripheral tissues of patients with Alzheimer's disease. *Arch Neurol* 45:836–40, 1988.

8. Geland, B. Presentation to the European College of Neuropsychopharmacology, reported in *Clin Psychiatry News,* September, 1989.

9. Abalan, F., Delile, J. M. Vitamin B_{12} deficiency in presenile dementia. Letter. *Biol Psychiatry* 20(11):1251, 1985.

10. Ikeda, T., et al. Vitamin B_{12} levels in serum and cerebrospinal fluid of people with Alzheimer's disease. *Acta Psychiatr Scand* 82(4):327–9, 1990.

11. Wright, J. V. *Dr. Wright's Guide to Healing with Nutrition.* Emmaus, PA, Rodale Press, 1984, Chapter 46, pp. 472–9.

12. Gronek, I., Kolomaznik, M. [Serum zinc levels in various mental disorders.] *Zh Nevropatol Psikhiatr* 90(10):126–7, 1989.

13. Corrigan, F. M., et al. Aluminium and Alzheimer's disease. Letter. *Lancet* 2:268–9, 1989.

14. Ward, N. I., Mason, J. A. Neutron activation analysis techniques for identifying elemental status in Alzheimer's disease. *J Radioanalyt Nucl Chem* 113(2):515–26, 1987.

15. Burnet, F. M. A possible role of zinc in the pathology of dementia. *Lancet* 1:186–88, 1981.

16. Constantinidis, J. [Alzheimer's disease and the zinc theory.] *Encephale* 16(4):231–9, 1990.

17. Dysken, M. A review of recent clinical trials in the treatment of Alzheimer's disease. *Psychiatric Annals* 17(3):178, 1987.

18. Thomas, et al, op. cit.

19. Lehmann, J., et al. Tryptophan malabsorption in dementia. Improvement in certain cases after tryptophan therapy as indicated by mental behaviour and blood analysis. *Acta Psychiatr Scand* 64(2):123–31, 1981.

20. Smith, D. F., et al. Lack of effect of tryptophan treatment in demented gerontopsychiatric patients. A double-blind, crossover-controlled study. *Acta Psychiatr Scand* 70(5):470–77, 1984.

21. Lehmann, J., et al. Tryptophan malabsorption in dementia. Improvement in certain cases after tryptophan therapy as indicated by mental behaviour and blood analysis. *Acta Psychiatr Scand* 64(2):123–31, 1981.

22. Michel, P. F. Chronic cerebral insufficiency and Gingko biloba extract, in A.

Agnoli, et al., Eds. *Effects of Ginkgo Biloba Extract on Organic Cerebral Impairment.* John Libbey Eurotext Ltd., 1985, pp. 71–76.

23. Taillandier, J., et al. [Ginkgo biloba extract in the treatment of cerebral disorders due to aging.] *Presse Med* 15(31):1583–7, 1986.

24. Candy, J. M., et al. Aluminosilicates and senile plaque formation in Alzheimer's disease. *Lancet* 1:354–7, 1986.

25. Martyn, C. N., et al. Geographical relation between Alzheimer's disease and aluminium in drinking water. *Lancet* 1:59–62, 1989.

26. Beal, M. F., et al. Neurochemical characteristics of aluminum-induced neurofibrillary degeneration in rabbits. *Neuroscience* 29(2):339–46, 1989.

27. Challem, J. J., Lewin, R. Beating Alzheimer's disease: How Tom Warren cured himself. *Let's Live* June, 1990, pp. 56–9.

Depression

1. Kreitsch, K., et al. Prevalence, presenting symptoms, and psychological characteristics of individuals experiencing a diet-related mood disturbance. *Behav Ther* 19:593–604, 1988.

2. King, D. S. Can allergic exposure provoke psychological symptoms? A double-blind test. *Biol Psychiatry* 16(1):3–19, 1981.

3. Brostoff, J., Gamlin, L. *The Complete Guide to Food Allergy and Intolerance.* London, Bloomsbury Publishing Ltd., 1989, p. 142.

4. Kitahara, M. Dietary tryptophan ratio and suicide in the United Kingdom, Ireland, the United States, Canada, Australia, and New Zealand. *Omega J Death Dying* 18:71–6, 1987.

5. Coppen, A., Wood, K. Tryptophan and depressive illness. *Psychological Med* 8:49–57, 1978.

6. Delgado, P. D., et al. Serotonin function and the mechanism of antidepressant action. *Arch Gen Psychiatry* 47:411–18, 1990.

7. Young, S. N. The clinical psychopharmacology of tryptophan, in R. J. Wurtman, J. J. Wurtman, Eds. *Nutrition and the Brain* Volume 7. New York, Raven Press, 1986:49–88.

8. van Praag, H. M., Lemus, C. Monamine precursors in the treatment of psychiatric disorders, in R.J. Wurtman, J.J. Wurtman, Eds. *Nutrition and the Brain,* Volume 7. New York, Raven Press, 1986.

9. van Praag, H. M. Studies in the mechanism of action of serotonin precursors in depression. *Psychopharmacol Bull* 20:599–602, 1984.

10. Sabelli, H. C., et al. Clinical studies on the phenylethylamine hypothesis of affective disorder: Urine and blood phenylacetic acid and phenylalanine dietary supplements. *J Clin Psychiatry* 47(2):66–70, 1986.

11. Ibid.

12. Heller, B. Pharmacological and clinical effects of D-phenylalanine in depression and Parkinson's disease, in Mosnaim, Wolf, Eds. *Noncatecholic Phenylethylamines, Part I.* New York, Marcel Dekker, 1978, pp. 397–417.

13. Beckmann, H., et al. DL-phenylalanine versus imipramine: A double-blind controlled study. *Arch Psychiat Nervenkr* 227:49–58, 1979.

14. Beckmann, H. Phenylalanine in affective disorders. *Adv Biol Psychiatry* 10:137–47, 1983.

15. Gibson, C. J., Gelenberg, A. Tyrosine for the treatment of depression. *Adv Biol Psychiatry* 10:148–59, 1983.
16. Subar, A. F., et al. Folate intake and food sources in the US population. *Am J Clin Nutr* 50:508–16, 1989.
17. Abou-Saleh, M. T., Coppen, A. The biology of folate in depression: Implications for nutritional hypotheses of the psychoses. *J Psychiatri Res* 20(2):91–101, 1986.
18. Godfrey, P. S. A., et al. Enhancement of recovery from psychiatric illness by methylfolate. *Lancet* 336:392–5, 1990.
19. Reynolds, E. H., et al. Methylation and mood. *Lancet* 2:196–8, 1984.
20. Botez, M. I., et al. Neuropsychological correlates of folic acid deficiency: Facts and hypotheses, in M. I. Botez, E. H. Reynolds, Eds. *Folic Acid in Neurology, Psychiatry and Internal Medicine.* New York, Raven Press, 1979.
21. Carney, M. W., et al. Thiamine, riboflavin and pyridoxine deficiency in psychiatric in-patients. *Br J Psychiatry* 141:271–72, 1982.
22. Williams, R. D., et al. Induced thiamine (B_1) deficiency in man: relation of depletion of thiamine to development of biochemical defect and of polyneuropathy. *Arch Intern Med* 71:38–53, 1943.
23. Brozek, J. Psychologic effects of thiamine restriction and deprivation in normal young men. *Am J Clin Nutr* 5(2):109–20, 1957.
24. Russ, C. S., et al. Vitamin B_6 status of depressed and obsessive-compulsive patients. *Nutr Rep Int* 27(4):867–73, 1983.
25. Carney, M., et al. Thiamin and pyridoxine lack in newly-admitted psychiatric patients. *Br J Psychiatry* 135:249–54, 1979.
26. Stewart, J. W., et al. Low B_6 levels in depressed outpatients. *Biol Psychiatry* 19(4):613–16, 1984.
27. Bermond, P. Therapy of side effects of oral contraceptive agents with vitamin B_6. *Acta Vitaminol Enzymol* 4(1–2):45–54, 1982.
28. Edwin, E., et al. Vitamin B_{12} hypovitaminosis in mental diseases. *Acta Med Scand* 177:689–99, 1965.
29. Bell, I., et al. Vitamin B_{12} and folate status in acute geropsychiatric inpatients: Affective and cognitive characteristics of a vitamin nondeficient population. *Biol Psychiatry* 27(2):125–37, 1990.
30. Ellis, F. R., Nasser, S. A pilot study of vitamin B_{12} in the treatment of tiredness. *Br J Nutr* 30:277–83, 1973.
31. Hodges, R. E., et al. Clinical manifestations of ascorbic acid deficiency in man. *Am J Clin Nutr* 24:432–3, 1971.
32. Kitahara, M. Insufficient ascorbic acid uptake from the diet and the tendency for suicide. *J Orthomol Med* 2(4):217–18, 1987.
33. Schorah, C. J., et al. Plasma vitamin C concentration in patients in a psychiatric hospital. *Hum Nutr Clin Nutr* 37C:447–52, 1983.
34. Leitner, Z. A., Church, I. C. Nutritional studies in a mental hospital. *Lancet* 1:565–7, 1956.
35. Milner, G. Ascorbic acid in chronic psychiatric patients: A controlled trial. *Br J Psychiatry* 109:294–99, 1963.
36. Parker, S. D. Depression and nutrition: Anemia and glucose imbalances. *Anabolism* Jan–Feb., 1984.
37. Hall, R. C. W., Joffe, J. R. Hypomagnesemia: physical and psychiatric symptoms. *JAMA* 224(13):1749–51, 1973.

38. Wester, P. Magnesium. *Am J Clin Nutr* 45:1305–12, 1987.

39. Webb, W. L., Gehi, M. Electrolyte and fluid imbalance: Neuropsychiatric manifestations. *Psychosomatics* 22(3):199–203, 1981.

40. Cox, J. R., et al. Changes in sodium, potassium and fluid spaces in depression and dementia. *Gerontology Clin* 13:232–45, 1971.

41. Webb and Gehi, op. cit.

42. Keuter, E. J. W. *Nutr Abstr Rev* 29:273, 1959.

43. Muldner VonH, Zoller, M. Antidepressive wirkung eines auf den wirkstoffkomplex hypericin standardisierten hypericum-extraktes. *Arzneim-Forsch* 34:918, 1984.

44. Ibid.

45. van Praag, op. cit.

46. Martinsen, E. W., et al. Effects of aerobic exercise on depression: A controlled study. *Br Med J* 291:109, 1985.

Diabetes

1. Anderson, J. W. Recent advances in carbohydrate nutrition and metabolism in diabetes mellitus. *J Am Coll Nutr* 8(Suppl):61S–67S, 1989.

2. Meyer, J. H., et al. Intragastric vs intraintestinal viscous polymers and glucose tolerance after liquid meals of glucose. *Am J Clin Nutr* 48:260–6, 1988.

3. Anderson, J. W., Gustafson, N. J. Dietary fiber in disease prevention and treatment. *Compr Ther* 13(1):43–53, 1987.

4. West, K. M., Kalbfleisch, J. M. Influence of nutritional factors on prevalence of diabetes. *Diabetes* 20:99–108, 1971.

5. Snowdon, D. A., Phillips, R. L. Does a vegetarian diet reduce the occurrence of diabetes? *Am J Public Health* 75(5):507–12, 1985.

6. Vandongen, R., et al. Hypercholesterolemic effect of fish oil in insulin-dependent diabetic patients. *Med J Aust* 148:141–3, 1988.

7. Glauber, H., et al. Adverse metabolic effect of omega-3 fatty acids in non-insulin-dependent diabetes mellitus. *Ann Intern Med* 108(5):663–8, 1988.

8. Houtsmuller, A. J., et al. Favourable influences of linoleic acid on the progression of diabetic micro and macroangiopathy. *Nutr Metab* 24:Suppl 1:105–18, 1980.

9. Heine, R. J., et al. Linoleic-acid-enriched diet: long-term effect on serum lipoprotein and apolipoprotein concentrations and insulin sensitivity in noninsulin-dependent diabetic patients. *Am J Clin Nutr* 49:448–56, 1989.

10. Wahlqvist, M. L., et al. Food variety is associated with less macrovascular disease in those with type II diabetes and their healthy controls. *J Am Coll Nutr* 8(6):515–23, 1989.

11. Avogaro, A., et al. Alcohol impairs insulin sensitivity in normal subjects. *Diabetes Res* 5:23–7, 1987.

12. O'Dea, K. Marked improvement in carbohydrate and lipid metabolism in diabetic Australian aborigines after temporary reversion to traditional lifestyle. *Diabetes* 33(6):596–603, 1984.

13. Vague, P. H., et al. Nicotinamide may extend remission phase in insulin-dependent diabetes. *Lancet* 1:619–20, 1987.

14. Wahlberg, G., et al. Protective effect of nicotinamide against nephropathy in diabetic rats. *Diabetes Res* 2:307, 1985.

15. Saito, N., et al. Blood thiamine levels in outpatients with diabetes mellitus. *J Nutr Sci Vitaminol (Tokyo)* 33(6):421–30, 1987.

16. Skelton, W. P. III, Skelton, N. K. Thiamine deficiency neuropathy: It's still common today. *Postgrad Med* 85(8):301–6, 1989.

17. Mirsky, Stanley. *Diabetes: Controlling it the Easy Way.* New York, Random House, 1981.

18. Ribaya-Mercado, J., et al. Vitamin B$_6$ deficiency elevates serum insulin in elderly subjects. *Ann N Y Acad Sci* 585:531–3, 1990.

19. Hollenbeck, C. B., et al. The composition and nutritional adequacy of subject-selected high carbohydrate, low fat diets in insulin-dependent diabetes mellitus. *Am J Clin Nutr* 38(1):41–51, 1983.

20. Rao, R. H., et al. Failure of pyridoxine to improve glucose tolerance in diabetics. *J Clin Endocrinol Metab* 50(1):198–200, 1980.

21. Coelingh Bennink, H. J. T., et al. Improvement of oral glucose tolerance in gestational diabetes by pyridoxine. *Br Med J* 3:13–15, 1975.

22. McCann, V. J., Davis, R. E. Serum pyridoxal concentrations in patients with diabetic neuropathy. *Aust N Z J Med* 8:259–61, 1978.

23. Jones, C. L., Gonzales, V. Pyridoxine deficiency: A new factor in diabetic neuropathy. *J Am Podiatry Assoc* 68(9):646–53, 1978.

24. Levin, E. R., et al. The influence of pyridoxine in diabetic peripheral neuropathy. *Diabetes Care* 4:606, 1981.

25. Bhatt, H. R., et al. Can faulty vitamin B$_{12}$ (cobalamin) metabolism produce diabetic neuropathy? Letter to the Editor. *Lancet* 2:572, 1983.

26. Sancetta, S. M., et al. The use of vitamin B$_{12}$ in the management of the neurological manifestations of diabetes mellitus, with notes on the administration of massive doses. *Ann Intern Med* 35:1028–48, 1951.

27. Cunningham, J., et al. Reduced mononuclear leukocyte ascorbic-acid content in adults with insulin-dependent diabetes mellitus consuming adequate dietary vitamin C. *Metabolism* 40:146–9, 1991.

28. Ginter, E. M., Chorvathova, V. Vitamin C and diabetes mellitus. *Nutr Health* 2:3–11, 1983.

29. Sandhya, P., Das, U. N. Vitamin C therapy for maturity onset diabetes mellitus: Relevance to prostaglandin involvement. *IRCS J Med Sci* 9(7):618, 1981.

30. Turley, S., et al. Role of ascorbic acid in the regulation of cholesterol metabolism and the pathogenesis of atherosclerosis. *Atherosclerosis* 24:1–18, 1976.

31. Kapeghian, J. C., Verlangieri, A. J. The effects of glucose on ascorbic acid uptake in heart endothelial cells: Possible pathogenesis of diabetic angiopathies. *Life Sci* 34(6):577–84, 1984.

32. Ginter, E., et al. Hypocholesterolemic effect of ascorbic acid in maturity-onset diabetes mellitus. *Int J Vitam Nutr Res* 48(4):368–73, 1978.

33. Cox, B. D., Butterfield, W. J. H. Vitamin C supplements and diabetic cutaneous capillary fragility. *Br Med J* 3:205, 1975.

34. Lubin, B., Machlin, L. Biological aspects of vitamin E. *Ann N Y Acad Sci* 1982, p. 393.

35. Vogelsang, A. Vitamin E in the treatment of diabetes mellitus. *Ann NY Acad Sci* 52:406, 1949.

36. Gisinger, C., et al. Vitamin E and platelet eicosanoids in diabetes mellitus. *Prostaglandins Leukot Essent Fatty Acids* 40:169–76, 1990.

37. Haylock, S. J., et al. Separation of biologically active chromium-containing complexes from yeast extracts and other sources of glucose tolerance factor (GTF) activity. *J Inorg Biochem* 18(3):195–211, 1983.

38. Liu, V. J., Abernathy, R. P. Chromium and insulin in young subjects with normal glucose tolerance. *Am J Clin Nutr* 25(4):661–7, 1982.

39. Freund, H., et al. Chromium deficiency during total parenteral nutrition. *JAMA* 241(5):496–8, 1979.

40. Martinez, O. B., et al. Dietary chromium and effect of chromium supplementation on glucose tolerance of elderly Canadian women. *Nutr Res* 5:609–20, 1985.

41. Mertz, W. Chromium occurrence and function in a biological system. *Physiol Rev* 49:163–230, 1969.

42. Jeejeebhoy, K. N., et al. Chromium deficiency, glucose tolerance, and neuropathy reversed by chromium supplementation, in a patient receiving long-term parenteral nutrition. *Am J Clin Nutr* 30(4):531–8, 1977.

43. Chatfield, K. Preventive medicine clinics: A case of diabetes. *Townsend Letter for Doctors* March, 1985, p. 105.

44. Klevey, L. M., et al. Diminished glucose tolerance in two men due to a diet low in copper. Abstract. *Am J Clin Nutr* 37:717, 1983.

45. Fields, M., et al. Accumulation of sorbitol in copper deficiency: Dependency on gender and type of dietary carbohydrate. *Metabolism* 38(4):371–5, 1989.

46. Cogan, D. G., et al. Aldose reductase and complications of diabetes. *Ann Intern Med* 101:82–91, 1984.

47. Durlach, J., Collery, P. Magnesium and potassium in diabetes and carbohydrate metabolism. Review of the present status and recent results. *Magnesium* 3(4–6):315–23, 1984.

48. Wen-gang, Z., et al. Hypomagnesemia and heart complications in diabetes mellitus. *Chin Med J* 100:719–22, 1987.

49. McNair, P., et al. Hypomagnesemia, a risk factor for diabetic retinopathy. *Diabetes* 27:1075–7, 1978.

50. Ditzel, J. Morphologic hemodynamic changes in small blood vessels in diabetes mellitus. *N Engl J Med* 250:541–6, 1954.

51. Paolisso, G., et al. Improved insulin response and action by chronic magnesium administration in aged NIDDM subjects. *Diabetes Care* 12:265–69, 1989.

52. Kosenko, L. G. *Klin Med* 42:113, 1964.

53. Wimhurst, J. M., Manchester, K. L. Comparison of ability of Mg and Mn to activate the key enzymes of glycolysis. *FEBS Letters* 27:321–6, 1972.

54. Baly, D., et al. Effect of manganese deficiency on insulin binding, glucose transport and metabolism of rat adipocytes. *J Nutr* 120:1075–9, 1990.

55. Rubenstein, A. H. Hypoglycemia induced by manganese. *Nature* 194:188–89, 1962.

56. DeFronzo, R. A., Lang, R. Hypophosphatemia and glucose intolerance: Evidence for tissue insensitivity to insulin. *N Engl J Med* 303(22):1259–63, 1980.

57. Ditzel, J. Oxygen transport impairment in diabetes. *Diabetes* 25(Suppl 2):832–38, 1976.

58. Ibid.,

59. Greene, D. A., et al. Correction of myo-inositol depletion in diabetic humans sural nerve by treatment with an aldose reductase inhibitor. Abstract. *Diabetes* 36(Suppl 1):86A, 1987.

60. Clements, R. S. Jr., et al. Dietary myo-inositol intake and peripheral nerve function in diabetic neuropathy. *Metabolism* 28:477, 1979.

61. Gregersen, G., et al. Oral supplementation of myoinositol: Effects on peripheral nerve function in human diabetics and on the concentration in plasma, erythrocytes, urine and muscle tissue in human diabetics and normals. *Acta Neurol Scand* 67:164–72, 1983.

62. Varma, S. D. Inhibition of aldose reductase by flavonoids: Possible attenuation of diabetic complications. *Prog Clin Biol Res* 213:343–58, 1986.

63. Jaspan, J., et al. Treatment of severely painful diabetic neuropathy with an aldose reductase inhibitor: Relief of pain and improved somatic and automatic nerve function. *Lancet* 2:758–62, 1983.

64. Gabor, M. Pharmacologic effect of flavonoids on blood vessels. *Angiologica* 9:355–74, 1972.

65. Clemetson, A. B. Ascorbic acid and diabetes mellitus. *Med Hypotheses* 2:193–4, 1976.

66. Lacombe, C., et al. Hemorheological improvement after Daflon 500 mg treatment in diabetes. *Int Angiol* 7(2 Suppl):21–24, 1988.

67. Jamal, G. A., et al. Treatment of diabetic neuropathy with gamma-linolenic acid (GLA) as evening primrose oil (Efamol). *J Am Coll Nutr* 6:86, 1987.

68. Offenbacher, E., Stunyer, F. Beneficial effect of chromium-rich yeast on glucose tolerance and blood lipids in elderly patients. *Diabetes* 29:919–25, 1980.

Eczema

1. Sampson, H. A. Food hypersensitivity as a pathogenic factor in atopic dermatitis. *N Engl Reg Allergy Prac* 7(6):511–19, 1986.

2. Pike, M. G., et al. Increased intestinal permeability in atopic eczema. *Int J Dermatol* 25(5):301–4, 1986.

3. Davies, S., Stewart, A. *Nutritional Medicine.* London, Pan Books, 1987, p. 279.

4. Kline, G. Presentation to the Annual Meeting, American Academy of Allergy and Immunology, 1989.

5. David, T. J., et al. Low serum zinc in children with atopic eczema. *Br J Dermatol* 111(5):597–601, 1984.

6. Wright, J. V. *Dr. Wright's Book of Nutritional Therapy.* Emmaus, PA, Rodale Press, 1979, p. 38.

7. Bjorneboe, A., et al. Effect of dietary supplementation with eicosapentaenoic acid in the treatment of atopic dermatitis. *Br J Dermatol* 117(4):463–69, 1987.

8. Morse, P. F., et al. Meta-analysis of placebo-controlled studies of the efficacy of Epogram in the treatment of atopic eczema: relationship between plasma essential fatty changes and treatment response. *Br J Dermatol* 121:75–90, 1989.

9. Allison, J. R. The relation of hydrochloric acid and vitamin B complex deficiency in certain skin diseases. *South Med J* 38:235–41, 1945.

10. Ayers, S. Gastric secretion in psoriasis, eczema and dermatitis herpetiformis. *Arch Dermatol Syph* 20:854–57, 1929.

11. Ibid.

12. Davies and Stewart, op. cit., pp. 280–1.

Epilepsy

1. Passmore, R., Eastwood, M. A. *Davidson and Passmore: Human Nutrition and Dietetics.* Edinburgh, Churchill Livingstone, 1986, pp. 471.

2. Baulac, M., Laplane, D. [Alcohol and epilepsy.] *Rev Prat* 40(4):307–11, 1990.

3. Marangos, P. J., et al. The benzodiazepines and inosine antagonize caffeine-induced seizures. *Psychopharmacology (Berlin)* 72(3):269–73, 1981.

4. De Vivo, D. C. How to use other drugs (steroids) and the ketogenic diet, in P. L. Morselli, C. E. Pippenger, and J. K. Penry, Eds. *Antiepileptic Drug Therapy in Pediatrics.* New York, Raven Press, 1983, pp. 283–92.

5. Passmore and Eastwood, op. cit., p. 471.

6. Egger, J., et al. Oligoantigenic diet treatment of children with epilepsy and migraine. *J Pediatr* 114:51–58, 1989.

7. Crayton, J. W., et al. Epilepsy precipated by food sensitivity: report of a case with double-blind placebo-controlled assessment. *Clin Electroencephalography* 12(4):192–98, 1981.

8. Smith, D. B., Obbens, E. A. M. T. Anti-folate-antiepileptic relationships, in M. I. Botez, E. H. Reynolds, Eds. *Folic Acid in Neurology, Psychiatry and Internal Medicine.* New York, Raven Press, 1979.

9. Drew, H. J., et al. Effect of folate upon phenytoin hyperplasia. *J Clin Periodontol* 14:350, 1987.

10. Bourgeois, B. F. D., et al. Potentiation of the antiepileptic activity of phenobarbital by nicotinamide. *Epilepsia* 24:238–44, 1983.

11. Hoffer, A. *Niacin Therapy in Psychiatry.* Springfield, IL, Charles C. Thomas, 1962.

12. Crowell, G. F., Roach, E. S. Pyridoxine-dependent seizures. *Am Fam Physician* 27(3):183–87, 1983.

13. Ibid.

14. Nightingale, G.—reported in C. Gerras, et al., Eds. *The Encyclopedia of Common Diseases.* Emmaus, PA, Rodale Press, 1976, pp. 638–9.

15. Sholer, A., Pfeiffer, C. C. Vitamin B_6 and the treatment of mental disease. *Int Clin Nutr Rev* 8(3), 1988.

16. Ogunmekan, A. O. Plasma vitamin E levels in normal children and in epileptic children with and without anticonvulsant therapy. *Trop Geog Med* 37:175–7, 1985.

17. Ogunmekan, A. O., Hwang, P. A. A randomised double blind, placebo-controlled, clinical trial of D-alpha-tocopherol acetate (vitamin E) as add-on therapy for epilepsy in children. *Epilepsia* 30(1):84–89, 1989.

18. Sorenson, J. R. J. Therapeutic uses of copper, in J. O. Nriagu, Ed. *Copper in the Environment. Part II: Health Effects.* New York, John Wiley & Sons, 1979:83–162.

19. Mëhes, K., Petrovicz, E. Familial benign copper deficiency. *Arch Dis Child* 57(9):716–18, 1982.

20. Hall, R. C. W., Joffe, J. R. Hypomagnesemia: physical and psychiatric symptoms. *JAMA* 224(13):1749–51, 1973.

21. Benga, I., et al. Plasma and cerebrospinal fluid concentrations of magnesium in epileptic children. *J Neurol Sci* 67(1):29–34, 1985.

22. Barnet, L. B. *J Clin Physiol* 1:25, 1959.

23. Gorges, L. F., Gücer, G. Effect of magnesium on epileptic foci. *Epilepsia* 19(1):81–91, 1978.

24. Papavasiliou, P. S., et al. Seizure disorders and trace metals: Manganese tissue levels in treated epileptics. *Neurology* 29:1466, 1979.

25. Pfeiffer, C. C., LaMola, S. Zinc and manganese in the schizophrenias. *J Orthomol Psychiatry* 12:215–34, 1983.

26. Tanaka, Y. Low manganese may trigger epilepsy. *JAMA* 238:1805, 1977.

27. Shoji, Y. Serum magnesium and zinc in epileptic children. *J Neurol Sci* 67(1):29–34, 1985.

28. Lewis-Jones, M. S., et al. Cutaneous manifestations of zinc deficiency during treatment with anticonvulsants. *Br Med J* 290:603–4, 1985.

29. Lankford, H. G. Zinc metabolism and chronic alcoholism. *Am J Clin Nutr* 17:57–72, 1965.

30. Sterman, M. B., et al. Zinc and seizure mechanisms, in J. Morley, M. B. Sterman, Eds. *Nutritional Modulation of Neural Function.* New York, Academic Press, 1988, pp. 307–19.

31. Roach, E. S., Carlin, L. N,N-dimethylglycine for epilepsy. Letter. *N Engl J Med* 307:1081–82, 1982.

32. Vaddadi, K. S. The use of gamma-linolenic acid and linoleic acid to differentiate between temporal lobe epilepsy and schizophrenia. *Prostaglandins Med* 6:375–79, 1981.

Fatigue

1. Weinberg, E. G., Tuchinda, M. Allergic tension-fatigue syndrome. *Ann Allergy* 31:209–11, 1973.

2. Costill, D. L., Dalsky, G. P., Fink, W. J. Effects of caffeine ingestion on metabolism and exercise performance. *Med Sci Sports* 1093):155–8, 1978.

3. Greden, J. F., et al. Anxiety and depression associated with caffeinism among psychiatric inpatients. *Am J Psychiatry* 135(8):963–6, 1978.

4. Estler, C. J., Ammon, H. P., Herzog, C. Swimming capacity of mice after prolonged treatment with psychostimulants. I. Effects of caffeine on swimming performance and cold stress. *Psychopharmacology (Berlin)* 58(2):161–6, 1978.

5. Hughes, J. R., et al. Caffeine self-administration, withdrawal, and adverse effects among coffee drinkers. *Arch Gen Psychiatry* 48:611–17, 1991.

6. Fox, A. Caffeine—unexpected cause of fatigue! *Let's Live* April, 1982, pp. 16–20.

7. Christensen, L. Psychological distress and diet—effects of sucrose and caffeine. *J Appl Nutr* 40(1):44–50, 1988.

8. Spring, B., et al. Psychobiological effects of carbohydrates. *J Clin Psychiatry* 50 Suppl:27–33, 1989.

9. Subar, A. F., et al. Folate intake and food sources in the US population. *Am J Clin Nutr* 50:508–16, 1989.

10. Botez, M. I. Neuropsychological correlates of folic acid deficiency: facts and hypotheses, in M. I. Botez, E. H. Reynolds, Eds. *Folic Acid in Neurology, Psychiatry and Internal Medicine.* New York, Raven Press, 1979.

11. Wright, J. V. A case of apathy and depression. *Prevention* June, 1984, pp. 113–18.

12. Ellis, F. R., Nasser, S. A pilot study of vitamin B_{12} in the treatment of tiredness. *Br J Nutr* 30:277–83, 1973.

13. Wright, J. V. A case of tiredness. *Prevention* September, 1979, pp. 68–72.

14. Cheraskin, E., et al. Daily vitamin C consumption and fatigability. *J Am Geriatr Soc* 2493):136–7, 1976.

15. Gerster, H. The role of vitamin C in athletic performance. *J Am Coll Nutr* 8(6):636–43, 1989.
16. Schultz, B. M., Freedman, M. L. Iron deficiency in the elderly. *Baillieres Clin Haematol* 1(2):291–313, 1987.
17. Buetler, E., et al. Iron therapy in chemically fatigued non anemic women: A double-blind study. *Ann Intern Med* 52:378, 1960.
18. Niederau, C., et al. Survival and causes of death in cirrhotic and noncirrhotic patients with primary hemochromatosis. *N Engl J Med* 313:1256–62, 1985.
19. Wright, J. V. A case of iron deficiency without anemia. *Prevention* November, 1984, pp. 67–71.
20. Snively, W. D., Westerman, R. L. *Minn Med* June, 1965.
21. Abdulla, M., et al. Dietary intake of potassium in the elderly. *Lancet* 2:562, 1975.
22. Judge, T. G., Cowan, N. R. Dietary potassium intake and grip strength in older people. *Gerontologia Clinica* 13:221–6, 1971.
23. Wright, J. V. A case of weak muscles. *Prevention* October, 1974, pp. 113–20.
24. Rude, R. K. Physiology of magnesium metabolism and the important role of magnesium in potassium deficiency. *Am J Cardiology* 63:31G–34G, 1989.
25. Krotkiewski, M., et al. Zinc and muscle strength and endurance. *Acta Physiol Scand* 116(3):309–11, 1982.
26. Prasad, A. Clinical manifestation of zinc deficiency. *Nutr Rev* 41(7):197, 1983.
27. Wright, J. V. The healing powers of zinc. *Let's Live* March, 1989, pp. 72–3.
28. Bakan, P. Confusion, lethargy and leukonychia. *J Orthomol Med* 5(4):198–202, 1990.
29. Gaby, A. R. Aspartic acid salts and fatigue. *Curr Nutr Therapeut* November, 1982.

Gallstones

1. Scragg, R. K., et al. Diet, alcohol, and relative weight in gall stone disease: A case-control study. *Br Med J* 288:1113–9, 1984.
2. Thornton, J. R. Gallstone disappearance associated with weight loss. Letter. *Lancet* 2:478, 1979.
3. Pixley, F., et al. Effect of vegetarianism on development of gall stones in women. *Br Med J* 291:11–12, 1985.
4. Thornton, J. R., et al. Diet and gallstones: Effects of refined carbohydrates on bile cholesterol saturation and bile acid metabolism. *Gut* 24:2–6, 1983.
5. Capron, J. P., et al. Meal frequency and duration of overnight fast: A role in gall-stone formation? *Br Med J* 283:1435, 1981.
6. Conter, R. L., et al. Carbohydrate diet-induced calcium bilirubinate sludge and pigment gallstones in the prairie dog. *J Surg Res* 40(6):580–7, 1986.
7. Scragg, op. cit.
8. Ibid.
9. Lillemoe, K. D., et al. Caffeine prevents cholesterol gallstone formation. *Surgery* 106(2):400–07, 1989.
10. Douglas, B. R., et al. Coffee stimulation of cholecystokinin release and gallbladder contraction in humans. *Am J Clin Nutr* 52:553–6, 1990.
11. Beardshall, K., et al. Saturation of fat and cholecystokinin release: implications for pancreatic carcinogenesis. *Lancet* 2:1008–10, 1989.
12. Sarles, H. Gallbladder contraction and type of fat. Letter. *Lancet* 2:1399, 1989.

13. Brennerman, J. C. Allergy elimination diet as the most effective gallbladder diet. *Ann Allergy* 26:83, 1968.

14. Wright, J. V. A case of gallbladder pain and allergy. *Prevention* September, 1980, pp. 67–71.

15. Ginter, E. Cholesterol: vitamin C controls its transformation to bile acids. *Science* 179(74):702–4, 1973.

16. Pedersen, L. Biliary lipids during vitamin C feeding in healthy persons. *Scand J Gastroenterol* 10(3):311–14, 1975.

17. Christensen, F., et al. *Acta Physiol Scand* 27:315, 1952.

18. Dam, H., et al. *Acta Physiol Scand* 36:329, 1956.

19. Dam, H., et al. *Acta Pathol Microbiol Scand* 30:256, 1952.

20. Saito, T., Tanimura, H. The preventive effect of vitamin E on gallstone formation. (3). A study of the biliary lipids in patients with gallstones. *Arch Jpn Chir* 56(3):276–88, 1987.

21. Duff, G. L., et al. *Am J Med* 11:92, 1951.

22. Nakumura-Yamanaka, Y., et al. Effect of dietary taurine on cholesterol 7 alpha-hydroxylase activity in the liver of mice fed a lithogenic diet. *J Nutr Sci Vitaminol (Tokyo)* 33(3):239–43, 1987.

23. Wang, W. Y., Liaw, K. Y. Effect of a taurine-supplemented diet on conjugated bile acids in biliary surgical patients. *JPEN J Parenter Enteral Nutr* 15(3):294–7, 1991.

24. Capper, W. M., et al. Gallstones, gastric secretion, and flatulent dyspepsia. *Lancet* 1:413–15, 1967.

25. Rappaport, E. M. Achlorhydria: Associated symptoms and response to hydrochloric acid. *N Engl J Med* 252:802–05, 1955.

Glaucoma

1. Berens, C., et al. Allergy in glaucoma. *Ann Allergy* 5:526–35, 1947.

2. Raymond, L. F. Allergy and chronic simple glaucoma. *Ann Allergy* 22:146–50, 1964.

3. Berens, et al, op. cit.

4. Higginbotham, E. J., et al. The effect of caffeine on intraocular pressure by glaucoma patients. *Ophthalmology* 96(5):624–26, 1989.

5. Asregadoo, E. R. Blood levels of thiamine and ascorbic acid in chronic open-angle glaucoma. *Ann Ophthalmol* 11(7):1095–1100, 1979.

6. Ibid.

7. Ibid.

8. Lee, P., et al. Aqueous humor ascorbate concentration and open-angle glaucoma. *Arch Ophthalmol* 95(2):308–10, 1977.

9. Linner, E. The pressure lowering effect of ascorbic acid. *Ann Ophthalmol (Copen)* 47:685–9, 1969.

10. Linner, E. Intraocular pressure regulation and ascorbic acid. *Acta Soc Med Upsal* 69:225–32, 1964.

11. Mehra, K. S. Relationship of pH of blood and aqueous with vitamin C. *Ann Ophthalmol* 10(1):83–92, 1978.

12. Stocker, F. W. New ways of influencing the intraocular pressure. *NY State J Med* 49:58–63, 1949.

Heartburn

1. Castell, D. O. Diet and the lower esophageal sphincter. *Am J Clin Nutr* 28:1296–98, 1975.
2. Ibid.
3. Babka, J. C., Castell, D. O. On the genesis of heartburn. The effects of specific foods on the lower esophageal sphincter. *Am J Dig Dis* 18(5):391–7, 1973.
4. Dennish, G. W., Castell, D. O. Caffeine and the lower esophageal sphincter. *Am J Digest Dis* 17:993–6, 1972.
5. Dubey, P., et al. Effect of tea on gastric acid secretion. *Dig Dis Sci* 29(3):202–6, 1984.
6. Hogan, W. J., et al. Ethanol induced acute esophageal sphincter motor dysfunction. *J Appl Physiol* 32:755–60, 1972.
7. Ippoliti, A. F., et al. The effect of various forms of milk on gastric-acid secretion. *Ann Intern Med* 84:286–9, 1976.
8. Lenz, H. J., et al. Wine and five percent ethanol are potent stimulants of gastric acid secretion in humans. *Gastroenterology* 85(5):1082–7, 1983.
9. Nebel, O. T., Castell, D. O. Kinetics of fat inhibition of the lower esophageal sphincter. *J Appl Physiol* 35:6, 1973.
10. Yudkin, J. Eating and ulcers. Letter. *Br Med J* February 16, 1980:483–4.

Heart Disease

1. McNamara, D. J. Effects of fat-modified diets on cholesterol and lipoprotein metabolism. *Annu Rev Nutr* 7:273–90, 1987.
2. Keys, A., et al. Lessons from serum cholesterol studies in Japan, Hawaii and Los Angeles. *Ann Intern Med* 43:83, 1958.
3. Renaud, S. Dietary fats and platelet function. *Proc Nutr Soc Aust* 10:1–13, 1985.
4. Fehily, A. M., et al. Dietary determinants of lipoproteins, total cholesterol, viscosity, fibrinogen, and blood pressure. *Am J Clin Nutr* 36(5):890–6, 1982.
5. Martin, W. Margarine (not butter) the culprit? Letter. *Lancet* 2:407, 1983.
6. Booyens, J., et al. The role of unnatural dietary trans and cis unsaturated fatty acids in the epidemiology of coronary heart disease. *Med Hypotheses* 25(3):175–82, 1988.
7. Keys, A., Parlin, R. W. Serum cholesterol response to changes in dietary lipids. *Am J Clin Nutr* 19:175, 1966.
8. Weisweiler, P., et al. Influence of polyunsaturated fat restriction on lipoproteins in humans. *Metabolism* 34(1):83–7, 1985.
9. Mensink, R. P., Katan, M. B. Effect of a diet enriched with monounsaturated or polyunsaturated fatty acids on levels of low-density and high-density lipoprotein cholesterol in healthy women and men. *New Engl J Med* 321(7):436–41, 1989.
10. Truswell, A. S. ABC of nutrition. Reducing the risk of coronary heart disease. *Br Med J* 291:1729–39, 1987.
11. Edington, J. D., et al. Serum lipid response to dietary cholesterol in subjects fed a low-fat, high-fiber diet. *Am J Clin Nutr* 50:58–62, 1989.
12. McNamara, D. J. The diet-heart question: How good is the evidence? *Contemp Nutr* 12(4), 1987.

13. Anderson, J. W., Tietyen-Clark, J. Dietary fiber: Hyperlipidemia, hypertension, and coronary heart disease. *Am J Gastroenterol* 81(10):907–19, 1986.

14. Jenkins, D. J. A., et al. Effect of pectin, guar gum, and wheat fiber on serum-cholesterol. *Lancet* 1:1116–7, 1975.

15. Hoagland, P. D., Pferrer, P. E. *J Agric Food Chem* May/June, 1987.

16. Anderson, J. W., et al. Serum lipid response of hypercholesterolemic men to single and divided doses of canned beans. *Am J Clin Nutr* 51:1013–19, 1990.

17. Ernst, E. Cardiovascular effects of garlic (Allium sativum): A review. *Pharmatherapeutica* 5(2):83–9, 1987.

18. Backon, J. Ginger: Inhibition of thromboxane synthetase and stimulation of prostacyclin: Relevance for medicine and psychiatry. *Med Hypotheses* 20:271, 1986.

19. Srivastava, K. C. Effects of aqueous extracts of onion, garlic and ginger on platelet aggregation and metabolism of arachidonic acid in the blood vascular system: In vitro study. *Prostagl Med* 13:227, 1984.

20. Thorogood, M., et al. Plasma lipids and lipoprotein cholesterol concentration in people with different diets in Britain. *Br Med J* 295:351–53, 1987.

21. Sacks, F. M., et al. Plasma lipoprotein levels in vegetarians. The effect of ingestion of fats from dairy products. *JAMA* 254(10):1337–41, 1985.

22. Hepner, G., et al. Hypocholesterolemic effect of yogurt and milk. *Am J Clin Nutr* 32(1):19–24, 1979.

23. Kilara, A.—reported in *Med World News* January 11, 1988:39.

24. Hepner, et al, op. cit.

25. Reiser, S. Effect of dietary sugars on metabolic risk factors associated with heart disease. *Nutr Health* 3:203–16, 1985.

26. Reiser, S., et al. Isocaloric exchange of dietary starch and sucrose in humans. I. Effects on levels of fasting blood lipids. *Am J Clin Nutr* 32(8):1659–69, 1979.

27. Yudkin, J. Effects of high dietary sugar. *Br Med J* 281:1396, 1980.

28. Kozlovsky, A. S., et al. Effects of diets high in simple sugars on urinary chromium losses. *Metabolism* 35:515, 1986.

29. Moore, R. D., Pearson, T. A. Moderate alcohol consumption and coronary artery disease. A review. *Medicine* 65(4):242–67, 1986.

30. Eichner, E. R. Alcohol versus exercise for coronary protection. *Am J Med* 79(2):231–40, 1985.

31. Davis, B. R., et al. Coffee consumption and serum cholesterol in the hypertension detection and follow-up program. *Am J Epidemiol* 128:124–36, 1988.

32. Forde, O. H., et al. The Tromso heart study: Coffee consumption and serum lipid concentrations in men with hypercholesterolaemia: A randomised intervention study. *Br Med J* 290:893–95, 1985.

33. Bonaa, K., et al. Coffee and cholesterol: Is it all in the brewing? The Tromso study. *Br Med J* 297:1103–04, 1988.

34. Haffner, S. M., et al. Coffee consumption, diet and lipids. *Am J Epidemiol* 122(1):1–12, 1985.

35. McCully, K. S., Wilson, R. B. Homocysteine theory of arteriosclerosis. *Atherosclerosis* 22:215–27, 1975.

36. Harker, L. A., et al. Homocystine-induced arteriosclerosis. The role of endothelial cell injury and platelet response in its genesis. *J Clin Invest* 58(3):731–41, 1976.

37. Boers, G. H., et al. Heterozygosity for homocystinuria in premature peripheral and cerebral occlusive arterial disease. *N Engl J Med* 313(12):709–15, 1985.

38. McCully, K. S.—interviewed in *Prevention* September, 1979, pp. 138–45.

39. Brattstrom, L., et al. Impaired homocysteine metabolism in early-onset cerebral and peripheral occlusive arterial disease. Effects of pyridoxine and folic acid treatment. *Atherosclerosis* 81(1):51–60, 1990.

40. Brattstrom, L. E., et al. Folic acid—an innocuous means to reduce plasma homocysteine. *Scand J Clin Lab Invest* 48:215–21, 1988.

41. Hoag, J. M., et al. Special communication: An approach to the management of hyperlipoproteinemia. *JAMA* 255(4):512–21, 1986.

42. Anonymous. *The Medical Letter.* Vol. 27, August 30, 1985.

43. Canner, P. L. *J Am Coll Cardiol* 5:442, 1985.

44. Rinehart, J. F., Greenberg, L. D. Vitamin B_6 deficiency in the Rhesus monkey. *Am J Clin Nutr* 4:318–25, 1956.

45. Gaddi, A., et al. Controlled evaluation of pantethine, a natural hypolipidemic compound, in patients with different forms of hypolipoproteinemia. *Atherosclerosis* 50(1):73–83, 1984.

46. Cattin, L., et al. Treatment of hypercholesterolemia with pantethine and fenofibrate: An open randomized study on 43 subjects. *Curr Ther Res* 38(3):386–95, 1985.

47. Horsey, J., et al. Ischaemic heart disease and aged patients: effects of ascorbic acid on lipoproteins. *J Human Nutr* 35:53–8, 1981.

48. Esk, C., et al. Correlation of plasma ascorbic acid with cardiovascular risk factors. *Clin Res* 38:A747, 1990.

49. Dobson, H. M., et al. The effect of ascorbic acid on the seasonal variations in serum cholesterol levels. *Scot Med J* 29(3):176–82, 1984.

50. Bordia, A., et al. Effect of vitamin C on platelet adhesiveness and platelet aggregation in coronary artery disease patients. *Clin Cardiol* 8(10):552–4, 1985.

51. Dalderup, L. M. Vitamin D, cholesterol, and calcium. *Lancet* 1:645–6, 1968.

52. Kummerow, F. A. Nutrition imbalance and angiotoxins as dietary risk factors in coronary heart disease. *Am J Clin Nutr* 32:58–83, 1979.

53. Hennig, B., Boissonneault, G. A. The roles of vitamin E and oxidized lipids in atherosclerosis. *Int Clin Nutr Rev* 8(3):134–9, 1988.

54. Gey, K. F., et al. Inverse correlation between plasma vitamin E and mortality from ischemic heart disease in cross-cultural epidemiology. *Am J Clin Nutr* 53:326S–34S, 1991.

55. Cloarec, M. J., et al. Alpha-tocopherol: Effect on plasma lipoproteins in hypercholesterolemic patients. *Isr J Med Sci* 23(8):869–72, 1987.

56. Jandak, J., et al. Reduction of platelet adhesiveness by vitamin E supplementation in humans. *Thrombosis Res* 49:393–404, 1988.

57. Creter, D., et al. Effect of vitamin E on platelet aggregation in diabetic retinopathy. *Acta Hematol* 62:74, 1979.

58. Albanese, A. A. *Nutr Rep Int* August, 1973.

59. Carlson, L. A., et al. Effect of oral calcium upon serum cholesterol and triglycerides in patients with hyperlipidemia. *Atherosclerosis* 14:391–400, 1971.

60. Yacowitz, H., et al. Calcium and lipid metabolism: effects of increased dietary calcium on atherosclerosis in rabbits. *Trans N Y Acad Sci* vol. 33(3):344–50, 1971.

61. Simonoff, et al. Low plasma chromium in patients with coronary artery and heart diseases. *Biol Trace Element Res* 6:431, 1984.

62. Railes, R., Albrink M. J. Effect of chromium chloride supplementation on glucose tolerance and serum lipids including high density lipoprotein of adult men. *Am J Clin Nutr* 34:2670–8, 1981.

63. Rasmussen, H. S., et al. Magnesium deficiency in patients with ischemic heart disease with and without acute myocardial infarction uncovered by intravenous loading test. *Arch Intern Med* 148:329–32, 1988.

64. Lauler, D. P., Ed. A symposium: magnesium deficiency—pathogenesis, prevalence, and strategies for repletion. *Am J Cardiol* 16(14):G1G–46G, 1989.

65. Dychner, T., Wester, P. O. Magnesium and potassium in serum and muscle in relation to disturbances of cardiac rhythm, in *Magnesium in Health and Disease*. Spectrum Publishing Company, 1980, pp. 551–7.

66. Seelig, M. S., Heggtveit, H. A. Magnesium interrelationships in ischemic heart disease: A review. *Am J Clin Nutr* 27(1):59–79, 1974.

67. Davis, W. H., et al. Monotherapy with magnesium increases abnormally low high density lipoprotein cholesterol: A clinical essay. *Curr Ther Res* 36:341, 1984.

68. Borgman, R. F. Dietary factors in essential hypertension. *Prog Food Nutr Sci* 9:109–47, 1985.

69. Kok, F. J., et al. Decreased selenium levels in acute myocardial infarction. *JAMA* 261(8):1161–4, 1989.

70. Stead, N. W., et al. Selenium (Se) balance in the dependent elderly. *Am J Clin Nutr* 39:677, 1984.

71. Schiavon, R., et al. Selenium enhances prostacyclin production by cultured epithelial cells: Possible explanation for increased bleeding times in volunteers taking selenium as a dietary supplement. *Thrombosis Res* 34:389, 1984.

72. Cherchi, A., et al. Effects of L-carnitine on exercise tolerance in chronic, stable angina: A multicenter, double-blind, randomized, placebo controlled crossover study. *Int J Clin Pharmacol Ther Toxicol* 23(10):569–72, 1985.

73. Kosolcharoen, P., et al. Improved exercise tolerance after administration of carnitine. *Curr Ther Res* November, 1981:753–64.

74. Abdel-Aziz, M. T., et al. Effect of carnitine on blood lipid pattern in diabetic patients. *Nutr Rep Internat* 29:1071, 1984.

75. Rossi, C. S., Silliprandi, N. Effect of carnitine on serum HDL cholesterol: Report of two cases. *Johns Hopkins Med J* 150:51–4, 1982.

76. Wright, J. V. *Dr. Wright's Guide to Healing with Nutrition*. Emmaus, PA, Rodale Press, 1984, Chapter 12, pp. 159–67.

77. Kamikawa, T., et al. Effects of coenzyme Q_{10} on exercise tolerance in chronic stable angina pectoris. *Am J Cardiol* 56:247, 1985.

78. Nakazawa, K., Murata, K. The therapeutic effect of chondroitin polysulphate in elderly atherosclerotic patients. *J Int Med Res* 693):217–25, 1978.

79. Morrison, L. M., Enrick, L. Coronary heart disease: reduction of death rate by chrondroitin sulfate A. *Angiology* 24:269–8766, 1973.

80. Simpson, H., et al. Low dietary intake of linoleic acid predisposes to myocardial infarction. *Br Med J* 285:684, 1982.

81. Rapley, C. H., et al. Fatty acid pattern and ischaemic heart disease. *Lancet* 1:1202, 1987.

82. Wood, D. A., et al. Adipose tissue and platelet fatty acids and coronary heart disease in Scottish men. *Lancet* 2:117–121, 1984.

83. Horrobin, D. F. The importance of gamma-linolenic acid and prostaglandin E1 in human nutrition and medicine. *J Holistic Med* 3:118–39, 1981.

84. Norell, S. E., et al. Fish consumption and mortality from coronary heart disease. *Br Med J* 293:426, 1986.

85. Terano, T., et al. Effects of eicosapentaenoic acid on platelet function, blood viscosity and red cell deformability in humans. *Atherosclerosis* 46:321–31, 1983.

86. Saynor, R., et al. The long-term effect of dietary supplementation with fish lipid concentrate on serum lipids, bleeding time, platelets and angina. *Atherosclerosis* 50:3–10, 1984.

87. Mehta, J. L., et al. Dietary supplementation with omega-3 polyunsaturated fatty acids in patients with stable coronary artery disease. *Am J Med* 84:45–52, 1988.

88. Fox, P. F., Dicorieto, P. E. Fish oils inhibit endothelial cell production of platelet-derived growth factor-like protein. *Science* 241:453–6, 1988.

89. Green, P., et al. Effect of fish-oil ingestion on cardiovascular risk factors in hyperlipidemic subjects in Israel: a randomized, double-blind crossover study. *Am J Clin Nutr* 52:1118–24, 1990.

90. Margolis, S., Dobbs, A. S. Nutritional management of plasma lipid disorders. *J Am Coll Nutr* 8 Suppl S:33S–45S, 1989.

91. Nieper, H. A. Effect of bromelain on coronary heart disease and angina pectoris. *Acta Med Empirica* 5:274–75, 1978.

92. Felton, G. E. Fibrinolytic and antithrombotic action of bromelain may eliminate thrombosis in heart patients. *Med Hypotheses* 6(11):1123–33, 1980.

Herpes Simplex

1. Cumming, C. Herpes: A nutritional approach. *Anabolism* November–December, 1982.

2. Lewin, S. *Vitamin C: Its Molecular Biology and Medical Potential.* New York, Van Nostrand Reinhold Co., 1973.

3. Kim, J. E., Shklar, G. The effect of vitamin E on the healing of gingival wounds in man. *J Periodontol* 54:305, 1983.

4. Starasoler, S., Haber, G. S. Use of vitamin E in primary herpes gingivostomatitis in an adult. *N Y State Dent J* 44(9):382–83, 1978.

5. Gordon, Y. J., et al. Irreversible inhibition of herpes simplex virus replication in BSC-1 cells by zinc ions. *Antimicrob Agents Chemother* 8(3):377–80, 1975.

6. Fitzherbert, J. Genital herpes and zinc. Letter. *Med J Aust* 1:399, 1979.

7. Eby, G. Use of topical zinc to prevent recurrent herpes simplex infection: Review of literature and suggested protocols. *Med Hypotheses* 17:157–65, 1985.

8. Brody, I. Topical treatment of recurrent herpes simplex and post-herpetic erythema multiforme with low concentrations of zinc sulphate solution. *Br J Dermatol* 104(2):191–94, 1981.

9. Finnerty, E. F. Topical zinc in the treatment of herpes simplex. *Cutis* 37(2):130–31, 1986.

10. Ziaie, Z., Kefalides, N. A. Lithium chloride restores host protein synthesis in herpes simplex virus–infection endothelial cells. *Biochem Biophys Res Commun* 160(3):1073–8, 1989.

11. Lieb, J. Remission of recurrent herpes infection during infection with lithium. Letter. *N Engl J Med* 301(17):942, 1979.

12. Amsterdam, J. D., et al. A possible antiviral action of lithium carbonate in herpes simplex virus infections. *Biol Psychiatry* 27(4):447–53, 1990.

13. Skinner, G. R. Lithium ointment for genital herpes. Letter. *Lancet* 2:288, 1983.

14. Terezhalmy, G. T., et al. The use of water-soluble bioflavonoid-ascorbic acid complex in the treatment of recurrent herpes labialis. *Oral Surg* 45:56–62, 1978.

15. Griffith, R. S., et al. Success of L-lysine therapy in frequently recurrent herpes simplex infection. *Dermatologica* 175:183–90, 1987.

16. McCune, M. A., et al. Treatment of recurrent herpes simplex infections with L-lysine monohydrochloride. *Cutis* 34(4):366–73, 1984.

17. Bricklin, M. Executive Editor. *Rodale's Encyclopedia of Natural Home Remedies*. Emmaus, PA, Rodale Press, 1982, p. 6.

18. Schmeisser, D. D., et al. Effect of excess dietary lysine on plasma lipids of the chick. *J Nutr* 113(9):1777–83, 1983.

19. Rapoport, L., Levine, W. I. Treatment of oral ulceration with Lactobacillus acidophillus tablets. Report of forty cases. *Oral Surg* 20(5):591–93, 1965.

20. Zimmerman, D. R. Self-treatment of cold sores with ice. Letter. *Lancet* 2:1260, 1978.

21. Response from a reader to an article by Dr. David R. Zimmerman in *Ladies Home Journal*—reported in *Better Nutrition*, July 1979.

22. VanderPlate, C., Kerrick, G. Stress reduction treatment of severe recurrent genital herpes. *Biofeedback Self Regul* 10(2):181–88, 1985.

High Blood Pressure

1. Anonymous. Nutrition and blood pressure: The effect of diet on hypertension. The Salt Institute, 1982.

2. Iacono, J. M., et al. Dietary polyunsaturated fat and hypertension. *Ann Med* 21(3):251–4, 1989.

3. Garcia-Palmieri, M. R., et al. Milk consumption, calcium intake, and decreased hypertension in Puerto Rico. Puerto Rico Heart Program study. *Hypertension* 6(3):322–28, 1984.

4. Anderson, J. W., Tietyen-Clark, J. Dietary fiber: hyperlipidemia, hypertension, and coronary heart disease. *Am J Gastroenterol* 81(10):907–19, 1986.

5. Ahrens, R. A. National Academy of Sciences, 1975-Summarized in H. G. Preuss, R. D. Fournier Minireview: Effects of sucrose ingestion on blood pressure. *Life Sci* 30:879–86, 1982.

6. Beevers, D. G., Maheswaran, R. Does alcohol cause hypertension or pseudo-hypertension? *Proc Nutr Soc* 47(2):111–14, 1988.

7. Myers, M. G. Effects of caffeine upon blood pressure. *Arch Intern Med* 148(5):1189–93, 1988.

8. Ophir, O., et al. Low blood pressure in vegetarians: The possible role of potassium. *Am J Clin Nutr* 37:755–62, 1983.

9. Margetts, R. M., et al. Vegetarian diet in mild hypertension: A randomized controlled trial. *Br Med J* 293:1468–71, 1986.

10. Grant, E. C. Food allergies and migraine. *Lancet* 2:966–69, 1979.

11. Price, A. S. The role of food allergy in hypertension: An experimental study. *Rev Gastroenterol* 10(5):233–45, 1943.

12. McCarron, D. A., Reusser, M. E. The integrated effects of electrolytes on blood pressure. *The Nutr Rep* 9(8), August, 1991.

13. Egan, B. Nutritional and lifestyle approaches to the prevention and management of hypertension. *Comprehen Therapy* 11(8):15–20, 1985.

14. Khaw, K. T., Barrett-Connor, E. The association between blood pressure, age, and dietary sodium and potassium: A population study. *Circulation* 77(1):53–61, 1988.

15. Smith, W. C. S., et al. Urinary electrolyte excretion, alcohol consumption, and blood pressure in the Scottish heart study. *Br Med J* 297:329–30, 1988.

16. McCarron, D. A. Is calcium more important than sodium in the pathogenesis of essential hypertension? *Hypertension* 7(4):607–27, 1985.

17. Harlan, W. K., et al. Blood pressure and nutrition in adults. The National Health and Nutrition Examination Survey. *Am J Epidemiol* 120:17–24, 1984.

18. Resnick, L. M. Alterations of dietary calcium intake as a therapeutic modality in essential hypertension. *Can J Physiol Pharmacol* 64(6):803–7, 1986.

19. Altura, B. M., Altura B. T. Magnesium ions and contraction of vascular smooth muscles: Relationship to some vascular diseases. *Fed Proc* 40(12):2672–9, 1981.

20. Joffres, M. R., et al. Relationship of magnesium intake and other dietary factors to blood pressure: the Honolulu heart study. *Am J Clin Nutr* 45(2):469–75, 1987.

21. Anonymous. Hypomagnesemia and hypertension. *Anabolism* 2(6) June, 1983.

22. Seelig, M. *Magnesium Deficiency in the Pathogenesis of Disease.* New York, Plenum Press, 1980.

23. Moore, T. J. The role of dietary electrolytes in hypertension. *J Am Coll Nutr* 8 Suppl S:68S–80S, 1989.

24. Yamori, Y., et al. Studies on stroke prevention in animal models, and their supportable epidemiological evidence, in H. Barnett, et al., Eds. *Cerebrovascular Diseases: New Trends in Surgical and Medical Aspects.* Amsterdam, Elsevier/North Holland, 1981, pp. 47–62.

25. Fujita, T., et al. Effects of increased adrenomedullary activity and taurine in young patients with borderline hypertension. *Circulation* 75:525, 1987.

26. Lehnert, H., et al. Effects of L-tryptophan on blood pressure in essential hypertensives. Abstract. *Clin Exp Theory Pract* A9(1):208, 1987.

27. Salonen, J. T., et al. Blood pressure, dietary fats, and antioxidants. *Am J Clin Nutr* 48:1226–32, 1988.

28. Bonaa, K. H., et al. Effect of eicosapentaenoic and docosahexaenoic acids on blood pressure in hypertension. *N Engl J Med* 322:795–801, 1990.

29. Iacono, J. M., et al. Effect of dietary fat on blood pressure in a rural Finnish population. *Am J Clin Nutr* 20(9):860, 1983.

30. Williams, P. T., et al. Associations of dietary fat, regional adiposity, and blood pressure in men. *JAMA* 257(23):3251–6, 1987.

31. Foushee, D. B., et al. Garlic as a natural agent for the treatment of hypertension: A preliminary report. *Cytobios* 34:145–52, 1982.

32. Barrie, S. A., et al. Effects of garlic oil on platelet aggregation, serum lipids and blood pressure in humans. *J Orthomol Med* 2(1):15–21, 1987.

33. Glauser, S. C. Blood cadmium levels in normotensive and untreated hypertensive humans. *Lancet* 1:717–18, 1976.

34. Schroeder, H. A., Buckman, J. Cadmium hypertension: Its reversal in rats by a zinc chelate. *Arch Environ Health* 14:693, 1967.

35. Peirkle, J. L., et al. The relationship between blood lead levels and blood pressure and its cardiovascular risk implications. *Am J Epidemiol* 121:246–58, 1985.

36. Wright, J. V. A case of cadmium-related high blood pressure, in Wright J.V., Ed. *Dr. Wright's Guide to Healing with Nutrition.* Emmaus, PA, Rodale Press, 1984, Chapter 16, pp. 198–205.

Hyperactivity

1. Kershner, J., Hawke, W. Megavitamins and learning disorders: A controlled double-blind experiment. *J Nutr* 109:819–26, 1979.

2. Stein, T. P., Sammaritano, A. M. Nitrogen metabolism in normal and hyperkinetic boys. *Am J Clin Nutr* 39(4):520–24, 1984.

3. Walker, S. III. Drugging the American child: We're too cavalier about hyperactivity. *J Learn Disabil* 8:354, 1975.

4. Benton, D. Dietary sugar, hyperactivity and cognitive functioning: a methodological review. *J Appl Nutr* 41(1):13–22, 1989.

5. Conners, C. K. George Washington U. School of Medicine—reported in *New Medical Science.* December, 1987.

6. Wells, K. C. Laboratory of Behavioral Medicine, Children's Hospital, Washington, D.C., quoted in *Prevention,* July, 1985.

7. Walker, op. cit.

8. Firestone, P., et al. The effects of caffeine on hyperactive children. *J Learn Disabil* 11(3):133–41, 1978.

9. Feingold, B. F. Hyperkinesis and learning disabilities linked to the ingestion of artificial food colors and flavors. *J Learn Disabil* 9(9):551–59, 1976.

10. Swain, A., et al. Salicylates, oligoantigenic diets, and behavior. Letter. *Lancet* July 6, 1985, pp. 41–42.

11. Egger, J., et al. Controlled trial of oligoantigenic treatment in the hyperkinetic syndrome. *Lancet* 1:540–45, 1985.

12. Feingold, op. cit.

13. Brenner, A. The effects of megadoses of selected B complex vitamins on children with hyperkinesis: Controlled studies with long-term follow-up. *J Learn Disabil* 15(5):258–64, 1982.

14. Hoffer, A. Vitamin B_3 dependent child. *Schizophrenia* 3:107–13, 1971.

15. Brenner, op. cit.

16. Ibid.

17. Coleman, M., et al. A preliminary study of the effect of pyridoxine administration in a subgroup of hyperkinetic children: A double-blind crossover comparison with methylphenidate. *J Biol Psych* 14(5):741–51, 1979.

18. Haslam, R. H., Dalby, J. T. Blood serotonin levels in the attention-deficit disorder. Letter. *N Engl J Med* 309(21):1328–9, 1983.

19. Walker, op. cit.

20. Pfeiffer, C. C., Mailloux, R. Excess copper as a factor in human diseases. *J Orthomol Med* 2(3):171–82, 1987.

21. Durlach, J. Clinical aspects of chronic magnesium deficiency, in M. S. Seelig, Ed. *Magnesium in Health and Disease.* New York, Spectrum Publications, 1980.

22. Ward, N. I., et al. The influence of the chemical additive tartrazine on the zinc status of hyperactive children—a double-blind placebo-controlled study. *J Nutr Med* 1:51–57, 1990.

23. Gibson, R. A. The effect of dietary supplementation with evening primrose oil on hyperkinetic children. *Proc Nutr Soc Aust* 10:196, 1985.

24. Colquhoun, I., Bunday, S. A lack of essential fatty acids as a possible cause of hyperactivity in children. *Med Hypotheses* 7:673–79, 1981.

25. Galland, L. Increased requirements for essential fatty acids in atopic individuals: A review with clinical descriptions. *J Am Coll Nutr* 5:213–28, 1986.

26. Howard, J. M. H. Clinical import of small increases in serum aluminum. *Clin Chem* 30(10):1722–23, 1984.

27. David, O., et al. Lead and hyperactivity. *Lancet* 2:900–03, 1972.

28. Gittleman, R., Eskenazi, B. Lead and hyperactivity revisited. An investigation of nondisadvantaged children. *Arch Gen Psychiatry* 40:827–33, 1983.

Infections

1. Chandra, R. K. Trace element regulation of immunity and infection. *J Am Coll Nutr* 4(1):5–16, 1985.

2. Beisel, W. R. Single nutrients and immunity. *Am J Clin Nutr* 35:417–68 (Suppl), 1982.

3. Sanchez, A. Role of sugars in human neutrophilic phagocytosis. *Am J Clin Nutr* 26:180, 1973.

4. Sommer, A., et al. Increased risk of respiratory disease and diarrhea in children with pre-existing mild vitamin A deficiency. *Am J Clin Nutr* 40:1090–5, 1984.

5. Beisel, op. cit.

6. Pinnock, C. B., et al. Vitamin A status in children who are prone to respiratory tract infection. *Aust Paediatr J* 22(2):95–99, 1986.

7. Stacpoole, P. W. The role of vitamin C in infectious disease and allergic reactions. *Med Hypotheses* 1:42–6, 1975.

8. Rawal, B. D., et al. Inhibition of Pseudomonas aeruginosa by ascorbic acid acting singly and in combination with antimicrobials: in-vitro and in-vivo studies. *Med J Aust* 1(6):169–74, 1974.

9. Schwerdt, P. R., Schwerdt, C. E. Effect of ascorbic acid on rhinovirus replication in WI-38 cells. *Proc Soc Biol Med* 148:1237, 1975.

10. Seah, S. K. Vitamin C and experimental toxoplasmosis. Letter to the Editor. *Trans R Soc Trop Med Hyg* 68(1):76–7, 1974.

11. Smith, L. H. *The Clinical Experiences of Frederick R. Klenner, M.D.: Clinical Guide to the Use of Vitamin C.* Life Sciences Press, 1988.

12. Cathcart, R. F. 3rd. Vitamin C: the nontoxic, nonrate-limited, antioxidant free radical scavenger. *Med Hypotheses* 18(1):61–77, 1985.

13. Baehner, R. L., Boxer, L. A. Role of membrane vitamin E and cytoplasmic glutathione in the regulation of phagocytic functions of neutrophils and monocytes. *Am J Pediatr Hematol Oncol* 191:71–6, 1979.

14. Nockels, C. F. Protective effects of supplemental vitamin E against infection. *Fed Proc* 38:2134–8, 1979.

15. Chavance, M., et al. Nutritional support improves antibody response to influenza virus in the elderly. Letter to the Editor. *Br Med J* November 9, 1985, pp. 1348–49.

16. Chandra, op. cit.

17. Beisel, op. cit.

18. Ibid.

19. Hershko, C., et al. Iron and infection. *Br Med J* 296:660–4, 1988.
20. Baer, M. T., et al. Nitrogen utilization, enzyme activity, glucose intolerance and leukocyte chemotaxis in human experimental zinc depletion. *Am J Clin Nutr* 41(6):1220–35, 1985.
21. Salvin, S. B., Robin, B. S. Resistance and susceptibility to infection in inbred murine strains. IV. Effects of dietary zinc. *Cellular Immunol* 87(2):546–52, 1984.
22. Chandra, R. K. Excessive intake of zinc impairs immune responses. *JAMA* 252(11):1443–6, 1984.
23. Srinivas, U., et al. Trace element alterations in infectious diseases. *Scand J Clin Lab Invest* 48(6):495–500, 1988.
24. Ryan, R. E. A double-blind clinical evaluation of bromelains in the treatment of acute sinusitis. *Headache* 7(1):13–17, 1967.
25. Lucerti, M., Vignali, M. Influence of bromelain on penetration of antibiotics in uterus, salpinx and ovary. *Drug Exp Clin Res* 4(1):45–8, 1978.
26. Pandromos, P. N., Brusch, C. A., Ceresia, G. C. Cranberry juice in the treatment of urinary tract infections. *Southwest Med* 47(1):17–20, 1968.
27. Gilman, A. G., Goodman, L. S., Gilman, A. *The Pharmacological Basis of Therapeutics,* Edition 6. New York, Macmillan Publishing Co., Inc., 1980, pp. 1120.
28. Sobota, A. Inhibition of bacterial adherence by cranberry juice in the treatment of urinary tract infections. *Southwest Med* 47:17, 1968.
29. Luettig, B., et al. Macrophage activation by the polysaccharide arabinogalactan isolated from plant cell cultures of Echinacea purpurea. *J Nat Cancer Inst* 81(9):669–75, 1989.
30. Weber, N., et al. Antiviral activity of Allium sativum (garlic). Abstract. *Ann Mtg Am Soc Microbiol* 88:22, 1988.
31. Adetumbi, M. A., Lau, B. H. Allium sativum (garlic): A natural antibiotic. *Med Hypotheses* 12(3):227–37, 1983.
32. Elnima, E. I., et al. The antimicrobial activity of garlic and onion extracts. *Pharmazie* 38(11):747–8, 1983.

Infertility

1. Green, B. B., et al. Risk of ovulatory infertility in relation to body weight. *Fertil Steril* 50(9):621–26, 1988.
2. Anderson, R. A. Jr., et al. Spontaneous recovery from ethanol-induced male infertility. *Alcohol* 2(3):479–84, 1985.
3. Mendleson, J. H. Alcohol effects on reproductive function in women. *Psychiatry Letter* 4(7):35–8, 1986.
4. Wilcox, A., et al. Caffeinated beverages and decreased fertility. *Lancet* 2:1473–76, 1988.
5. Casas, M., et al. Dopaminergic mechanism for caffeine induced decrease in fertility? Letter. *Lancet* 1:731, 1989.
6. Dawson, D. W., Sawers, A. H. Infertility and folate deficiency. Case reports. *Br J Obstet Gynaecol* 89:678–80, 1982.
7. Ibid.
8. Abraham, G. E., Hargrove, J. T.—reported in *Med World News* March 19, 1979.
9. Kidd, G. S., et al. The effects of pyridoxine on pituitary hormone secretion in amenorrhea-galactorrhea syndromes. *J Clin Endocrinol Metab* 54(4):872–75, 1982.

10. Gulden, K. D. Pernicious anemia, vitiligo, and infertility. *J Am Board Fam Pract* 3(3):217–20, 1990.

11. Dawson, E. B., et al. Effect of ascorbic acid on male fertility. *Ann N Y Acad Sci* 498:312–23, 1987.

12. Dawson, E. B., et al—reported in Gonzalez, E. R. Sperm swim singly after vitamin C therapy. Medical News. *JAMA* A249(20):2747, 2751, 1983.

13. Hargreave, T. B., et al. Randomised trial of mesterolone versus vitamin C for male infertility. *Br J Urol* 56(6):740–44, 1984.

14. Abel, B. J., et al. Randomised trial of clomiphene citrate treatment and vitamin C for male infertility. *Br J Urol* 54(6):780–84, 1982.

15. Abbasi, A. A., et al. Experimental zinc deficiency in man: Effect on testicular function. *J Lab Clin Med* 96(3):544–50, 1980.

16. Skandhan, K. P., et al. Semen electrolytes in normal and infertile subjects. II. Zinc. *Experientia* 34(11):1476–7, 1978.

17. Prasad, A. S. Zinc in growth and development and spectrum of human zinc deficiency. *J Am Coll Nutr* 7(5):377–84, 1988.

18. Tikkiwal, M., et al. Effect of zinc administration on seminal zinc and fertility of oligospermic males. *Indian J Physiol Pharmacol* 31(1):30–34, 1987.

19. Netter, A., et al. Effect of zinc administration on plasma testosterone, dehydrotestosterone and sperm count. *Arch Androl* 7(1):69–73, 1981.

20. Papp, G., et al. The role of basic amino acids of the seminal plasma in fertility. *Int Urol Nephrol* 15(2):195–203, 1983.

21. Schachter, A., et al. Treatment of oligospermia with the amino acid arginine. *J Urol* 110(3):311–13, 1973.

22. Pryor, J. P., et al. Controlled clinical trial of arginine for infertile men with oligospermia. *Br J Urol* 50:47–50, 1978.

23. Wright, J. V. A case of low sperm count. *Prevention* August 1983, pp. 66–69.

Inflammatory Bowel Disease

1. Grimes, D. S. Refined carbohydrate, smooth-muscle spasm and disease of the colon. *Lancet* 1:395–97, 1976.

2. Kruis, W., et al. Influence of diets high and low in refined sugar on stool qualities, gastrointestinal transit time and fecal bile acid excretion. *Gastroenterology* 92:1483, 1987.

3. Leo, S., et al. Ulcerative colitis in remission: is it possible to predict the risk of relapse? *Digestion* 44(4):217–21, 1989.

4. Riemann, J. F., Kolb, S. Zuckerarme und faserreiche Kost bei Morbus Crohn. *Fortschr Med* 102(4):67–70, 1984.

5. Järnerot, G., et al. Consumption of refined sugar by patients with Crohn's disease, ulcerative colitis, or irritable bowel syndrome. *Scand J Gastroenterol* 18(8):999–1002, 1983.

6. Segal, I., et al. The rarity of ulcerative colitis in South African blacks. *Am J Gastroenterol* 74(4):332–36, 1980.

7. Leo, et al, op. cit.

8. Brandes, J. W., Lorenz-Meyer, H. [Sugar free diet: a new perspective in the treatment of Crohn's disease?] *Z Gastroenterol* 19(1):1–12, 1981.

9. Heaton, K. W., et al. Treatment of Crohn's disease with an unrefined-carbohydrate, fibre-rich diet. *Br Med J* 2:764–66, 1979.

10. Davies, S., Stewart, A. *Nutritional Medicine*. London, Pan Books, 1987, pp. 221–2.

11. Hodgson, H. J. F. Inflammatory bowel disease and food intolerance. *J R Coll Physicians London* 20(1):45–48, 1986.

12. Bennet, J. D. Use of alpha-tocopherylquinone in ulcerative colitis. *Gut* 27(6):695–97, 1986.

13. Hood, R. P. Nonspecific ulcerative colitis: successful treatment with D-alpha tocopherhol. *Digest of Chiropractic Economics* Sept.–Oct. 1984.

14. De Liz, A. L.—reported in Shute, W. E. *Dr. Wilfrid E. Shute's Complete Updated Vitamin E Book*. New Canaan, CT, Keats Publishing, Inc., 1975, pp. 238–9.

15. Rosenberg, I. H., et al. Nutritional aspects of inflammatory bowel disease. *Ann Rev Nutr* 5:463–84, 1985.

16. Salomon, P., et al. Treatment of ulcerative colitis with fish oil n-3-omega fatty acid: an open trial. *J Clin Gastroenterol* 12(2):157–61, 1990.

17. Lorenz, R., et al. Supplementation with n-3 fatty acids from fish oil in chronic inflammatory bowel disease: a randomized, placebo-controlled, double-blind cross-over trial. *J Intern Med* Suppl 225(731):225–32, 1989.

Inner Ear Dysfunction

1. Yanick, P., Gosselin, E. J. Audiologic and metabolic findings in 90 patients with fluctuant hearing loss. *J Am Audiol Soc* 2:15–18, 1975.

2. Sikora, M. A., et al. Diet-induced hyperlipidemia and auditory dysfunction. *Acta Otolaryngol (Stockh)* 102(5–6):372–81, 1986.

3. Spencer, J. T., Jr. Hyperlipoproteinemia and inner ear disease. *J Int Acad Metabology* 4:38–42, 1975.

4. Browning, G. G., et al. Blood viscosity as a factor in sensorineural hearing impairment. *Lancet* 1:121–3, 1986.

5. Rosen, S., et al. Dietary prevention of hearing loss. *Acta Otolaryngol (Stockh)* 70(4):242–7, 1970.

6. Strome, M., et al. Hyperlipidemia in association with childhood sensorineural hearing loss. *Laryngoscope* 98(2):165–9, 1988.

7. Yanick, P. Solving problematic tinnitus. A clinical scientific approach. *Townsend Letter for Doctors*. February—March, 1985, p. 31.

8. Proctor, B., Proctor, C. Metabolic management in Ménière's disease. *Ann Otol Rhinol Laryngol* 90(6 Pt 1):615–18, 1981.

9. Goldman, H. Metabolic causes of fluctuant hearing loss. *Otolaryngol Clin North Am* 8:369–73, 1975.

10. Currier, W. D. Metabolic errors and sudden deafness. *Otolaryngol Clin North Am* 8:501–6, 1975.

11. Spencer, J. T., Jr. Hyperlipoproteinemia, hyperinsulinism and Ménière's disease. *South Med J* 74:1194–7, 1981.

12. Hoover, S. N. Food allergy and Ménière's disease. Annual Meeting Abstracts *AAOA News* 5(4):10, 1987.

13. Shambaugh, G. Allergy and the inner ear. *Ear Clin Int* 1:166–7, 1981.

14. Pang, L. Q. The importance of allergy in otolaryngology, in L. D. Dickey, Ed. *Clinical Ecology*. Springfield, Il, Charles C. Thomas, 1976.

15. Chole, Q. Vitamin A in the cochlea. *Arch Otorhinolaryngol* 124:379–82, 1978.

16. Lohle, E. The influence of chronic vitamin A deficiency on human and animal ears. *Arch Otorhinolaryngol* 234:167–73, 1982.

17. Lobel, M. J. *Arch Otolaryngol* May, 1951.

18. Tappel, Al. *Nutrition Today* July–August 1973.

19. Romeo, G. The therapeutic effect of vitamins A and E in neurosensory hearing loss. *Acta Vitaminol Enzymol* 7 Suppl:85–92, 1985.

20. Ikeda, K., et al. The effect of vitamin D deficiency on the cochlear potentials and the perilymphatic ionized calcium concentration of rats. *Acta Otolaryngol Suppl (Stockh)* 435:64–72, 1987.

21. Brookes, G. B. Vitamin D deficiency and otosclerosis. *Otolaryngol Head Neck Surg* 93(3):313–21, 1985.

22. Ibid.

23. Brookes, G. B. Vitamin D deficiency—a new cause of cochlear deafness. *J Laryngol Otol* 97(5):405–20, 1983.

24. Sun, A. H. A preliminary report on combined traditional Chinese and Western medicine in sernsorineural hearing loss. An analysis of 108 cases. *J Tradit Chin Med* 2:215–22, 1982.

25. Sun, A. H., et al. Iron deficiency and hearing loss. *ORL* 49:118–22, 1987.

26. Gersdorff, M., et al. A clinical correlation between hypozincemia and tinnitus. *Arch Otorhinolaryngol* 244(3):190–3, 1987.

27. Gersdorff, M., et al. [The zinc sulfate overload test in patients suffering from tinnitus associated with low serum zinc. Preliminary report.] *Acta Otorhinolaryngol Belg* 41(3):498–505, 1987.

28. Paaske, P. B., et al. [Zinc therapy of tinnitus. A placebo-controlled study.] *Ugeskr Laeger* 152(35):2473–5, 1990.

29. Moser, M., et al. A double-blind clinical trial of hydroxyethylrutosides in Ménière's disease. *J Laryngol Otol* 98(3):265–72, 1984.

30. Madej, S. [Treatment of sudden deafness of vascular etiology with venoruton.] *Otolaryngol Pol* 43(3):214–17, 1989.

31. Grontved, A., et al. Ginger root against seasickness. A controlled trial on the open sea. *Acta Otolaryngol* 105(1–2):45–9, 1988.

32. Grontved, A., Hentzer, E. Vertigo-reducing effect of ginger root. A controlled clinical study. *ORL J Otorhinolaryngol Relat Spec* 48(5):282–6, 1986.

33. Hardisty, E. K. Ginger vanquishes vertigo. Letter. *Prevention* October, 1989, p. 134.

34. Meyer, B. [A multicenter randomized double-blind drug vs. placebo study of Ginkgo biloba extract in the treatment of tinnitus.] *Presse Med* 15(31):1562–4, 1986.

35. Haguenauer, J. P., et al. [Treatment of equilibrium disorders with Ginkgo biloba extract. A multicenter double-blind drug vs. placebo study.] *Presse Med* 15(31):1569–72, 1986.

36. Dubreuil, C. [Therapeutic trial in acute cochlear deafness. A comparative study of Ginkgo biloba extract and nicergoline.] *Presse Med* 15(31):1559–61, 1986.

37. Claussen, C. F. [Diagnostic and practical value of craniocorpography in vertiginous syndromes.] *Presse Med* 15(31):1565–8, 1986.

Insomnia

1. Stone, B. M. Sleep and low doses of alcohol. *Electroencephalogr Clin Neurophysiol* 48(6):706–09, 1980.

2. Shirlow, M. J., Mathers, C. D. A study of caffeine consumption and symptoms: Indigestion, palpitations, tremor, headache and insomnia. *Int J Epidemiol* 14(2):239–48, 1985.

3. Karacan, I., et al. Dose-related sleep disturbances induced by coffee and caffeine. *Clin Pharmacol Ther* 20:682–89, 1976.

4. Kah, A., et al. Insomnia and cow's milk allergy in infants. *Pediatrics* 76(6):880–84, 1985.

5. Möhler, H., et al. Nicotinamide is a brain constituent with benzodiazepine-like actions. *Nature* 278:563–65, 1979.

6. Schneider-Helmet, D., Spinweber, C. L. Evaluation of L-tryptophan for treatment of insomnia: a review. *Psychopharmacology (Berlin)* 89(1):1–7, 1986.

7. Ibid.

8. Hartmann, E. L.—presented at a symposium sponsored by the Am. Med. Assoc. and quoted in *Clin Psychiatry News,* March, 1985.

9. Bricklin, Mark, Executive Editor, *Rodale's Encyclopedia of Natural Home Remedies.* Emmaus, PA, Rodale Press, 1982, p. 413.

10. Leathwood, P. D., et al. Aqueous extract of valerian root (Valeriana officinalis L.) improves sleep quality in man. *Pharmacol Biochem Behav* 17(1):65–71, 1982.

11. Lindahl, O., Lindwall, L. Double blind study of a valerian preparation. *Pharmacol Biochem Behav* 3294):1065–66, 1989.

12. Hobbs, C. Valerian. *HerbalGram* No. 21, Fall, 1989, pp. 19–34.

Irritable Bowel Syndrome

1. Grimes, D. S. Refined carbohydrate, smooth-muscle spasm and disease of the colon. *Lancet* 1:395–97, 1976.

2. Cook, I. J., et al. Effect of dietary fiber on symptoms and rectosigmoid motility in patients with irritable bowel syndrome. A controlled, crossover study. *Gastroenterology* 98(1):66–72, 1990.

3. Lucei, M. R., et al. Is bran efficacious in irritable bowel syndrome? A double-blind, placebo controlled, cross-over study. *Gut* 28:221, 1990.

4. Manning, A. P., et al. Wheat fibre and irritable bowel syndrome: A controlled study. *Lancet* 2:417, 1977.

5. Wright, J. V. *Dr. Wright's Book of Nutritional Therapy.* Emmaus, PA, Rodale Press, 1979, Chapter 9, pp. 80–8.

6. Rumessen, J. J., Gudmand-Hÿer, E. Functional bowel disease: Malabsorption and abdominal distress after ingestion of fructose, sorbitol, and fructose-sorbitol mixtures. *Gastroenterology* 95(3):694–700, 1988.

7. Kruis, W., et al. Influence of diets high and low in refined sugar on stool qualities, gastrointestinal transit time and fecal bile acid excretion. *Gastroenterology* 92:-1483, 1987.

8. Kellow, J. F., et al. Dysmotility of the small intestine in irritable bowel syndrome. *Gut* 29(9):1236–43, 1988.

9. Alun-Jones, V. A., et al. Food intolerance: A major factor in the pathogenesis of irritable bowel syndrome. *Lancet* 2:1115–17, 1982.

10. Finn, R., et al. Expanding horizons of allergy and the total allergy syndrome. *Clin Ecology* 3(3):129–31, 1985.

11. Petitpierre, M., et al. Irritable bowel syndrome and hypersensitivity to food. *Ann Allergy* 54:538–40, 1985.

12. Manahan, B. *Eat for Health*. Tiburon, CA, HJ Kramer, Inc., 1988, p. 145.

13. Rees, W. R. W., et al. Treating irritable bowel syndrome with peppermint oil. *Br Med J* 2:835–36, 1979.

14. Svendlund, J., et al. Controlled study of psychotherapy in irritable-bowel syndrome. *Lancet* 2:589–92, 1983.

15. Radnitz, C. L., Blanchard, E. B. Bowel sound biofeedback as a treatment for irritable bowel syndrome. *Biofeed Self Regl* 13(2):169–79, 1988.

16. Neff, D. F., Blanchard, E. B. A multi-component treatment for irritable bowel syndrome. *Behav Ther* 18:70–73, 1987.

17. Schwartz, S. P., et al. Behavioral treatment of irritable bowel syndrome: A 1-year follow-up study. *Biofeed Self Regl* 11:189–98, 1986.

18. Harvey, R. F., et al. Individual and group hypnotherapy in treatment of refractory irritable bowel syndrome. *Lancet* 1:424–25, 1989.

Kidney Stones

1. Blacklock, N. J. Influence of diet on the formation of bladder and kidney stones. *Nutr Health* 2:89–99, 1983.

2. Rao, P. N. Dietary habit and urolithiasis, in D. L. J. Freed, Ed. *Health Hazards of Milk*. London, Balliere Tindall, 1984.

3. Noda, S., et al. Oxalate crystallization in the kidney in the presence of hyperuricemia. *Scanning Microsc* 3(3):829–35, 1989.

4. Griffith, H. M., et al. A control study of dietary factors in renal stone formation. *Br J Urol* 53:416–20, 1981.

5. Smith, I. H., et al. Nutrition and urolithiasis. *N Engl J Med* 298:87–89, 1978.

6. Yoshida, O. Epidemiology of urolithiasis in Japan. *Jap U Urol* 70:975–83, 1979.

7. Blacklock, N. J. Sucrose and idiopathic renal stone. *Nutr Health* 5(1/2):9–17, 1987.

8. Fellström, B., et al. Dietary history and dietary records in renal stone patients and control. *Urol Res* 12:58, 1984.

9. Heaney, R. P., Recker, R. R. Effects of nitrogen, phosphorus, and caffeine on calcium balance in women. *J Lab Clin Med* 99:46–55, 1982.

10. Butz, M., et al. Dietary influence on serum and urinary oxalate in healthy subjects and oxalate stone formers. *Urol Int* 35:309–15, 1980.

11. Fellström, et al, op. cit.

12. Modlin. M. Urinary phosphorylated inositols and renal stone. *Lancet* 2:1113–14, 1980.

13. Noronha, I. L., et al. [Rice bran in the treatment of idiopathic hypercalciuria in patients with urinary calculosis.] *Rev Paul Med* 107(1):19–24, 1989.

14. Vahlensieck, W. Review: The importance of diet in urinary stones. *Urol Res* 14(6):283–88, 1986.

15. Sierakowski, R., et al. Stone incidence as related to water hardness in different geographical regions in the United States. *Urol Res* 7:157–60, 1979.

16. Gershoff, S. N., Prien, E. L. Excretion of urinary metabolites in calcium oxalate urolithiasis: Effect of tryptophan and vitamin B_6 administration. *Am J Clin Nutr* 8:812, 1960.

17. Grimm, U., et al. [Studies on tryptophan metabolism in calcium oxalate urolithiasis.] *Z Urol Nephrol* 81(5):299–303, 1988.

18. Mitwalli, A., et al. Control of hyperoxaluria with large doses of pyridoxine in patients with kidney stones. *Int J Nephrol* 20(4):353–59, 1988.

19. Gibbs, D. A., Watts, R. W. E. The action of pyridoxine in primary hyperoxaluria. *Clin Sci* 38:277–86, 1970.

20. Piesse, J. W. Nutritional factors in calcium containing kidney stones with particular emphasis on vitamin C. *Int Clin Nutr Rev* 5(3):110–29, 1985.

21. Pacifici, R., et al. Effect of Ca and vitamin D supplementation on urinary calcium excretion in the adult female population. Abstract. *J Am Coll Nutr* 6(5):430, 1987.

22. Wasserstein, A. The calcium stone former with osteoporosis. *JAMA* 257(16):2215, 1987.

23. Coe, F. L., et al. Effects of low-calcium diet on urine calcium excretion, parathyroid function and serum 1,25 $(OH)_2D_3$ levels in patients with idiopathic hypercalciuria and normal patients. *Am J Med* 72:25–32, 1982.

24. Brokis, J. G., et al. The effects of vegetable and animal protein diets on calcium, urate and oxalate excretion. *Br J Urol* 54(6):590–3, 1982.

25. Wasserstein, op. cit.

26. Hodkinson, A. *Proc Roy Soc Med* 51:970, 1958.

27. Goldwasser, B., et al. Calcium stone disease: An overview. *J Urol* 135:1, 1986.

28. Preminger, G., et al. Hypomagnesiuric hypocitraturia. An apparent new entity for calcium nephrolithiasis. *J Lithotripsy Stone Dis*, 1990.

29. Labeeuw, et al. Magnesium in the physiopathology and treatment of renal calcium stones. *Press Med* 16:25–7, 1987.

30. Johansson, G., et al. Effects of magnesium hydroxide in renal stone disease. *J Am Coll Nutr* 1(2):179–85, 1982.

31. Kaneko, K., et al. Urinary calcium and calcium balance in young women affected by high protein diet of soy protein isolate and adding sulfur-containing amino acids and/or potassium. *J Nutr Sci Vitaminol (Tokyo)* 36(2):105–16, 1990.

32. Conte, A., et al. On the relation between citrate and calcium in normal and stone-former subjects. *Int J Nephrol* 21(4):369–73, 1989.

33. Harvey, J. A., et al. Calcium citrate: Reduced propensity for the crystallization of calcium oxalate in urine resulting from induced hypercalciuria of calcium supplementation. *J Clin Endocrinol Metabol* 61(6):1223–25, 1985.

34. Pak, C. Y., Fuller, C. Idiopathic hypocitraturic calcium-oxalate nephrolithiasis successfully treated with potassium citrate. *Ann Intern Med* 104:33–37, 1986.

35. Pak, C. Y., Peterson, R. Successful treatment of hyperuricosuric calcium oxalate nephrolithiasis with potassium citrate. *Arch Intern Med* 146:863, 1986.

36. Light, I., et al. Urinary ionized calcium in urolithiasis. *Urology* 1(1):67–70, 1973.

37. Scott, R., et al. The importance of cadmium as a factor in calcified upper urinary stone disease—A prospective 7-year study. *Br J Urol* 54:584, 1982.

38. Axellson, B., Piscator, M. Renal change after prolonged exposure to cadmium. *Arch Environ Health* 12:360–72, 1969.

39. Eusebio, E., Elliot, J. S. Effect of trace metals on crystallisation of calicum oxalate. *Invest Urol* 4:431, 1967.

40. Elliot, J. S., Ribeiro, M. E. The urinary excretion of trace metals in patients with calcium oxalate urinary stone. *Invest Urol* 10:253–55, 1973.

41. Nath, R., et al. Molecular basis of cadmium toxicity. *Prog Food Nutr Sci* 8(1–2):109–63, 1984.

42. Wright, J. V. *Dr. Wright's Book of Nutritional Therapy.* Emmaus, PA, Rodale Press, 1979, Chapter 30, pp. 264–71.

Learning Disabilities

1. Benton, D. Dietary sugar, hyperactivity and cognitive functioning: a methodological review. *J Appl Nutr* 41(1):13–22, 1989.
2. Goldman, J. A., et al. Behavioral effects of sucrose on preschool children. *J Abnorm Child Psychol* 14(4):656–77, 1986.
3. Tamborlane, W. V., professor of pediatrics, Yale School of Medicine, and Jones, T. M., visiting scientist from Australia—reported in *The New York Times*, 1990.
4. Gilliland, K., Andress, D. Ad lib caffeine consumption, symptoms of caffeinism, and academic performance. *Am J Psychiatry* 138(4):512–14, 1981.
5. Challem, J. J., Lewin, R. The miracle of little Andy Alexander. *Let's Live* May, 1983, pp. 32–39.
6. Kubala, A. L., Katz, M. M. Nutritional factors in psychological test behavior. *J Genet Psychol* 96:343–52, 1960.
7. Vermiglio, F., et al. Defective neuromotor and cognitive ability in iodine-deficient schoolchildren of an endemic goiter region in Sicily. *J Clin Endocrinol Metab* 70(2):379–84, 1990.
8. Boyages, S. C., et al. Iodine deficiency impairs intellectual and neuromotor development in apparently-normal persons. A study of rural inhabitants of north-central China. *Med J Aust* 150(12):676–82, 1989.
9. Lozoff, B. Iron and learning potential in childhood. *Bull N Y Acad Med* 65(10):1050–66, 1989.
10. Durlach, J. Clinical aspects of chronic magnesium deficiency, in M. S. Selig, Ed. *Magnesium in Health and Disease.* New York, Spectrum Publications, 1980.
11. Grant, E. C. G., et al. Zinc deficiency in children with dyslexia: Concentrations of zinc and other minerals in sweat and hair. *Br Med J* 296:607–9, 1988.
12. Kronick, D. A case history: Sugar, fried oysters, and zinc. *Academ Therap* 11:119, 1975.
13. Schoenthaler, S. J. The impact of a low food additive and sucrose diet on academic performance in 803 New York City public schools. *Int J Biosocial Res* 8(2):185–95, 1986.
14. Baker, S. McD. A biochemical approach to the problem of dyslexia. *J Learn Disabil* 18(10):581–84, 1985.
15. Howard, J. M. H. Clinical import of small increases in serum aluminum. *Clin Chem* 30(10):1722–3, 1984.
16. Capel, I. D., et al. Comparison of concentrations of some trace, bulk, and toxic metals in the hair of normal and dyslexic children. *Clin Chem* 27(6):879–81, 1981.
17. Marlowe, M., et al. Hair mineral content as a predictor of learning disabilities. *J Learn Disabil* 17(7):418–21, 1984.
18. Thatcher, R. W., Lester, M. L. Nutrition, environmental toxins and computerized EEG: A mini-max approach to learning disabilities. *J Learn Disabil* 18(5):287–97, 1985.
19. Needleman, H. L., Gatsonis, C. A. Low-level lead exposure and the IQ of children. A meta-analysis of modern studies. *JAMA* 263(5):673–8, 1990.

20. Miller, G. D. Interactions between lead and essential elements: Behavioral consequences. *The Nutr Rep* 9(2), 1991.
21. Flora, S. J., Tandon, S. K. Preventative and therapeutic effects of thiamine, ascorbic acid and their combination in lead intoxication. *Acta Pharmacol Toxicol (Copenh)* 58(5):374–8, 1986.
22. Collipp, P. J., et al. Manganese in infant formulas and learning disability. *Ann Nutr Metab* 27:488–94, 1983.
23. Ibid.

Menopausal Symptoms

1. Shute, E. *J Obstet Gynecol Br Emp* 49:482, 1942.
2. McLaren, H. C. Vitamin E in the menopause. *Br Med J* 2:1378, 1949.
3. Finkler, R. S. The effect of vitamin E in the menopause. *J Clin Endocrinol Metab* 9:89–94, 1949.
4. Rubenstein, B. B. Vitamin E diminishes the vasomotor symptoms of menopause. Abstract. *Fed Proc* 7:106, 1948.
5. Blatt, M. H. G., et al. Vitamin E and climacteric syndrome: Failure of effective control as measured by menopausal index. *Arch Intern Med* 91:792–9, 1953.
6. Smith, C. J. Non-hormonal control of vaso-motor flushing in menopausal patients. *Chic Med* March 7, 1964.
7. Horoschak, A. *Del State Med J* January, 1959.
8. Anonymous. Editorial: Tryptophan and depression. *Br Med J* 1:242–3, 1976.
9. Ishihara, M. Effect of gamma oryzanol on serum peroxide level and climacteric disturbances. *Asia-Oceania J Obstet Gynaecol* 10(3):317, 1984.

Menstrual Cramps

1. Hudgins, A. P. Vitamins P, C and niacin for dysmenorrhea therapy. *West J Surg Gynecol* 62:610–11, 1954.
2. Butler, E. B., McKnight, E. Vitamin E in the treatment of primary dysmenorrhoea. *Lancet* 1:844–7, 1955.
3. Kryzhanovskï G. N., et al. [Endogenous opioid system in the realization of the analgesic effect of alpha-tocopherol.] *Biull Eksp Biol Med* 105(2):148–50, 1988.
4. Shafer, N. Iron in the treatment of dysmenorrhea: A preliminary report. *Curr Ther Res* 7(6):365–6, 1965.
5. Fontana-Klaiber, H., Hogg, B. [Therapeutic effects of magnesium in dysmenorrhea.] *Schweiz Rundsch Med Prax* 79(16):491–4, 1990.
6. Seifert, B., et al. [Magnesium—a new therapeutic alternative in primary dysmenorrhea.] *Zentralbl Gynakol* 111(11):755–60, 1989.
7. Colombo, D., Vescovini, R. Controlled trial of anthocyanosides from Vaccinium myrtillus in primary dysmenorrhea. *G Ital Obstet Ginecol* 7:1033–8, 1985.

Migraine Headaches

1. Mansfield, L. E. Food allergy and migraine: Whom to evaluate and how to treat. *Postgrad Med* 83(7):46–55, 1988.
2. Egger, J., et al. Is migraine food allergy?: A double-blind controlled trial of oligoantigenic diet treatment. *Lancet* 2:865–9, 1983.

3. Haningtron, E. Preliminary report on tyramine headache. *Br Med J* 2:550–1, 1967.

4. Sandler, M., et al. A phenylethylamine oxidising defect in migraine. *Nature* 250:335, 1974.

5. Graham, J. R. Headache related to a variety of medical disorders, in O. Appenzeller, Ed. *Pathogenesis and Treatment of Headache.* New York, Spectrum Publications, 1976.

6. Ratner, D., et al. Milk protein-free diet for nonseasonal asthma and migraine in lactase-deficient patients. *Isr J Med Sci* 19:806–9, 1983.

7. Shirlow, M. J., Mathers, C. D. A study of caffeine consumption and symptoms: Indigestion, palpitations, tremor, headache and insomnia. *Int J Epidemiol* 14(2):239–48, 1985.

8. Greden, J. F., et al. Caffeine-withdrawal headache: A clinical profile. *Psychosomatics* 21:411–18, 1980.

9. Harrison, D. P. Copper as a factor in the dietary precipitation of migraine. *Headache* 26(5):248–50, 1986.

10. Koehler, S. M., Glaros, A. The effect of aspartame on migraine headaches. *Headache* 28(1):10–14, 1988.

11. Gettis, A. Serendipity and food sensitivity: A case study. *Headache* 27:73–75, 1987.

12. Sicuteri, F. Endorphins, opiate receptors and migraine headaches. *Headache* 17:253–6, 1978.

13. Crook, M. Migraine: A biochemical headache? *Biochem Soc Trans* 9(4):351–7, 1981.

14. Unge, G., et al. Effects of dietary protein-tryptophan restriction upon 5-HT uptake by platelets and clinical symptoms in migraine-like headache. *Cephalalgia* 3(4):213–18, 1983.

15. Hasselmark, L., et al. Effect of a carbohydrate-rich diet, low in protein-tryptophan, in classic and common migraine. *Cephalalgia* 7:87–92, 1987.

16. Blau, J. N., Pike, D. A. Effect of diabetes on migraine. *Lancet* 2:241–3, 1970.

17. Anderson, J. W., Gustafson, N. J. Dietary fiber in disease prevention and treatment. *Compr Ther* 13(1):43–53, 1987.

18. Dexter, J. D., et al. The five hour glucose tolerance test and the effect of low sucrose diet in migraine. *Headache* 18:91–94, 1978.

19. Abraham, G. E., Lubran, M. M. Serum and red cell magnesium levels in patients with premenstrual tension. *Am J Clin Nutr* 34(11):2364–6, 1981.

20. Weaver, K. Magnesium and its role in vascular reactivity and coagulation. *Contemp Nutr* 12(3), 1987.

21. Glueck, C. J., et al. Amelioration of severe migraine with omega-3 fatty acids: A double-blind, placebo-controlled clinical trial. Abstract. *Am J Clin Nutr* 43:710, 1986.

22. McCarren, T., et al. *Am J Clin Nutr* 41:874a, 1985.

23. Murphy, J. J., et al. Randomised double-blind placebo-controlled trial of feverfew in migraine prevention. *Lancet* 2:188–92, 1988

24. Johnson, E. S., et al. Efficacy of feverfew as prophylactic treatment of migraine. *Br Med J* 291:653–60, 1982.

25. Heptinstall, S., et al. Extracts of feverfew inhibit granule secretion in blood platelets and polymorphonuclear leucocytes. *Lancet* 1:1071–4, 1985.

26. Johnson, et al, op. cit.

Mitral Valve Prolapse

1. Gërard, R., et al. [Mitral valve prolapse and spasmophilia in the adult.] *Arch Mal Coeur* 72(7):715–20, 1979.
2. Durlach, J., et al. Latent tetany and mitral valve prolapse due to chronic primary magnesium deficit, in Halpern and Durlach, Eds. *Magnesium Deficiency. First European Congress on Magnesium.* Karger, Basel, 1985.
3. Ibid.
4. Fernandes, J. S., et al. Therapeutic effect of a magnesium salt in patients suffering from mitral valve prolapse and latent tetany. *Magnesium* 4:283, 1985.
5. Trivellato, M., et al. Carnitine deficiency as the possible etiology of idiopathic mitral valve prolapse: Case study with speculative annotation. *Texas Heart Inst J* 11(4):370, 1984.
6. Oda, T. Effect of coenzyme Q$_{10}$ on stress-induced cardiac dysfunction in paediatric patients with mitral valve prolapse: A study by stress echocardiography. *Drugs Exp Clin Res* 11(8):557–76, 1985.

Muscle Cramps

1. Roberts, H. J. Spontaneous leg cramps and "restless legs" due to diabetogenic (functional) hypoinsulinism: A basis for rational therapy. *J Fla Med Assoc* 60(5):29–31, 1973.
2. Anderson, J. W., Gustafson, N. J. Dietary fiber in disease prevention and treatment. *Compr Ther* 13(1):43–53, 1987.
3. Ellis, J. M., Presley, J. *Vitamin B$_6$ The Doctor's Report.* New York, Harper & Row, 1973.
4. Ellis, J. M. *The Doctor Who Looked at Hands.* New York, Vantage Press, 1966, pp. 266–67.
5. Ayres, S. Jr., Mihan, R. Leg cramps (systremma) and "restless legs" syndrome. A progress report on response to vitamin E (tocopherol). *South Med J* 67(11):1308–12, 1974.
6. *Home Remedies for Everyday Health Problems.* Emmaus, PA, Rodale Press, 1987, p.5.
7. Hammar, M., et al. Calcium and magnesium status in pregnant women. A comparison between treatment with calcium and vitamin C in pregnant women with leg cramps. *Int J Vitam Nutr Res* 57(2):179–83, 1987.
8. Bricklin, M., Ed. *Rodale's Encyclopedia of Natural Home Remedies.* Emmaus, PA, Rodale Press, 1982, pp. 314–5.
9. Riss, R., et al. [Clinical aspects and treatment of calf muscle cramps during pregnancy.] *Geburtshilfe Frauenheilkd* 43(5):329–31, 1983.
10. Hammer, et al, op. cit.

Obesity

1. Morgan, S. L. Rational weight loss programs: A clinician's guide. *J Am Coll Nutr* 8(3):186–94, 1989.

2. Mirkin, G. B., Shore, R. N. The Beverly Hills diet: Dangers of the newest weight loss fad. *JAMA* 246(19):2235–7, 1981.

3. Rabast, U., et al. Comparative studies in obese subjects fed carbohydrate-restricted and high carbohydrate 1,000-calorie formula diets. *Nutr Metab* 22(5):269–77, 1978.

4. Friedman, R. B. Fad diets: Evaluation of five common types. *Postgrad Med* 89(1):249–58, 1986.

5. Ibid.

6. Yang, M. U., Van Itallie, T. B. A composition of weight loss during short-term weight reduction. *J Clin Invest* 58:722–30, 1976.

7. Astrup, Á., et al. Dietary fibre added to very low calorie diet reduces hunger and alleviates constipation. *Int J Obes* 14:105–12, 1990.

8. Wadden, T. A., et al. Responsible and irresponsible use of very-low-calorie diets in the treatment of obesity. *JAMA* 263(1):83–5, 1990.

9. Trubo, R. Fad diets: Unqualified hunger for miracles. *Med World News* August 11, 1986.

10. Fisler, J. S., Drenick, E. J. Starvation and semistarvation diets in the management of obesity. *Ann Rev Nutr* 7:465–84, 1987.

11. Apfelbaum, M., et al. [The composition of weight loss during the water diet. Effects of protein supplementation.] *Gastroenterologia* 108(3):121–34, 1967.

12. Blackburn, G. L. Fad reducing diets: Separating fads from facts. *Contemp Nutr* 8(7), 1983.

13. Smith, U. Dietary fibre, diabetes and obesity. *Int J Obes* 11 Suppl 1:27–31, 1987.

14. Lecomte, A. A double-blind study confirms the effects of weight of bean husk Arkocaps. *Revue de L'association Mondiale de Phytotherapie* 1:41–4, 1985.

15. Walsh, D. E., et al. Effect of glucomannan on obese patients: A clinical study. *Int J Obes* 8(4):289–93, 1984.

16. Spielman, A., et al. The effect of guar granules as an adjuvant to a self-help weight loss program. Abstract. *Am J Clin Nutr* 51:524, 1990.

17. Cairella, M., Godi, R. Clinical observations on the use of xanthan gum in obesity. *Clin Dietol* 13(1):37–40, 1986.

18. Douglass, J., et al. Effects of a raw food diet on hypertension and obesity. *South Med J* 78(7):841, 1985.

19. Fullerton, D. T., et al. Sugar, opioids and binge eating. *Brain Res Bull* 1496):673–80, 1985.

20. Rodin, J. Comparative effects of fructose, aspartame, glucose and water preloads on calorie and macronutrient intake. *Am J Clin Nutr* 51:428–35, 1990.

21. Dulloo, A. G., Miller, D. S. Obesity: A disorder of the sympathetic nervous system. *World Rev Nutr Diet* 50:1–56, 1987.

22. Schwarz, J-M., et al. Thermogenesis in men and women induced by fructose vs. glucose added to a meal. *Am J Clin Nutr* 49:667–74, 1989.

23. Dulloo, A. G., et al. Normal caffeine consumption: influence on thermogenesis and daily energy expenditure in lean and postobese human volunteers. *Am J Clin Nutr* 49:44–50, 1989.

24. Randolph, T. G. Masked food allergy as a factor in the development and persistence of obesity. *J Lab Clin Med* 32:1547, 1947.

25. Ibid.

26. O'Banion, D., Greenberg, M. Behavioral effects of food sensitivity, in D. R. O'Banion, Ed. *An Ecological and Nutritional Approach to Behavioral Medicine.* Springfield, IL, Charles C. Thomas, 1981.

27. Naylor, G. J., et al. A double blind placebo controlled trial of ascorbic acid in obesity. *Nutr Health* 1985, p. 425.

28. van Gaal, L., et al. Exploratory study of coenzyme Q_{10} in obesity, in K. Folkers, Y. Yamamura, Eds. *Biomedical and Clinical Aspects of Coenzyme Q.* Volume 4. Amsterdam, Elsevier Science Publishers, 1984, pp. 369–73.

29. Haslett, C., et al. A double-blind evaluation of evening primrose oil as an anti-obesity agent. *Int J Obes* 7(6):549–53, 1983.

30. Garcia, C. M., et al. Gamma linolenic acid causes weight loss and lower blood pressure in overweight patients with family history of obesity. *Swed J Biol Med* 4:8–11, 1986.

Osteoarthritis

1. Bjarnason, I., et al. Intestinal permeability and inflammation in rheumatoid arthritis: Effects of non-steroidal anti-inflammatory drugs. *Lancet* 2:1171–74, 1984.

2. Chao, I. T. Food incompatibility as a major cause of chronic arthritis of different forms. *Ann Allergy* 47(8):128, 1981.

3. Childers, N. F. A relationship of arthritis to the Solanaceae (nightshades). *J Int Acad Preventive Med* November, 1982:31–7.

4. Wright, J. V. Prevention clinics: A case of food-induced arthritis. *Prevention* October, 1979, pp. 55–59.

5. Kaufman, W. The use of vitamin therapy to reverse certain concomitants of aging. *J Am Geriatr Soc* 3:927, 1955.

6. Kaufman, W. Niacinamide: A most neglected vitamin. *J Int Acad Prev Med* Winter, 1983, pp. 5–25.

7. Schwartz, E. R. The modulation of osteoarthritic development by vitamins C and E. *Int J Vit Nutr Res* Suppl 26:141–46, 1984.

8. Krystal, G., et al. Stimulation of DNA synthesis by ascorbate in culture of articular chondrocytes. *Arthritis Rheum* 25:318–25, 1982.

9. Machtey, I., Ouaknine, L. Tocopherol in osteoarthritis: A controlled pilot study. *J Am Geriatr Soc* 26:328, 1978.

10. Schwartz, op. cit.

11. White, G. Vitamin E inhibition of platelet prostaglandin biosynthesis. *Fed Proc* 36:350, 1977.

12. deFabio, A. Treatment and prevention of osteoarthritis. *Townsend Letter for Doctors,* Feb.–March, 1990:143–8.

13. Newnham, R. E. Boron beats arthritis. *Proc ANZAAS,* Australian Academy of Science, Canberra, 1979.

14. Travers, R. L., Rennie, G. C., Newnham, R. E. Boron and arthritis: the results of a double-blind pilot study. *J Nutr Med* 1:127–32, 1990.

15. Sullivan, M. X., Hess, W. C. Cystine content of fingernails in arthritis. *J Bone Joint Surg* 16:185, 1935.

16. Osterberg, A. E., et al. Absorption of sulphur compounds during treatment by sulphur baths. *Arch Derm Syph* 20:156–66, 1929.

17. Woldenberg, S. C. The treatment of arthritis with colloidal sulphur. *J South Med Assoc* 28:875–81, 1935.

18. D'Ambrosio, E., et al. Glucosamine sulphate: A controlled clinical investigation in arthrosis. *Pharmatherapeutica* 2(8):504–8, 1981.

19. Vidal y Plana, R. R., et al. Articular cartilage pharmacology: I. In vitro studies on glucosamine and non-steroidal anti-inflammatory drugs. *Pharmacol Res Commun* 10(6):557–69, 1978.

20. Pujalte, J. M., et al. Double-blind and clinical evaluation of oral glucosamine sulphate in the basic treatment of osteoarthritis. *Curr Med Res Opin* 7(2):110–14, 1980.

21. di Padova, C. S-adenosylmethionine in the treatment of osteoarthritis. Review of the clinical studies. *Am J Med* 83(5A):60–65, 1987.

22. Flohë, L. Superoxide dismutase for therapeutic use: clinical experience, dead ends and hopes. *Mol Cell Biochem* 84(2):123–31, 1988.

23. Giri, S. N., Misra, H. P. Fate of superoxide dismutase in mice following oral route of administration. *Med Biol* 62(5):285–9, 1984.

24. Ordonez, L., Rothschild, P. R. Absorption study with SOD/CAT whole food antioxidant enzyme complex. Biotec Food Corporation, 1215 Center St., Honolulu, HI 96816-3226, 1989.

25. Rothschild, P. R., et al. Effect of oral antioxidant enzyme supplementation upon musculo-skeletal inflammation. Biotec Food Corporation, 1215 Center St., Honolulu, HI 96816-3226, 1989.

26. Randall, D., et al. Effect of oral Dismutase enzyme supplementation upon musculo-skeletal inflammation. Biotec Food Corporation, 1215 Center St., Honolulu, HI 96816–3226, 1989.

27. Kampf, R. *Schweizerische Apotheker-Zeitung* 114:337–42, 1976.

28. Pinget, M., Lecomte, A. [The effects of harpagophytum capsules (Arkocaps) in degenerative rheumatology.] *Medecine Actuelle* 12(4):65–67, 1985.

29. Gibson, R. G., et al. Perna canaliculus in the treatment of arthritis. *The Practitioner* 224:955–60, 1980.

30. Rauis, J.—reported in Walker M. Therapeutic effects of shark cartilage. *Townsend Letter for Doctors* June, 1989:288–91.

31. Orcasita, J. A—reported in Walker M. Therapeutic effects of shark cartilage. *Townsend Letter for Doctors* June, 1989:288–91.

Osteoporosis

1. Blank, R. P., et al. Calcium metabolism and osteoporotic ridge absorption: A protein connection. *J Prostet Dent* 58(5):590–5, 1987.

2. Weisner, N. M., in N. W. Solomons, I. H. Rosenberg, Eds. *Absorption and Malabsorption of Mineral Nutrients.* New York, Alan R. Liss, 1984, p. 15.

3. Barzel, U. S. Acid loading and osteoporosis. Letter to the Editor. *J Am Geriatr Soc* 30(9):613, 1982.

4. Marsh, A. G. Cortical bone density of adult lacto-ovo-vegetarian and omnivorous women. *J Am Diet Assoc* February, 1980, pp. 148–51.

5. Holl, M., Allen, L. Sucrose ingestion, insulin response and mineral metabolism. *J Nutr* 117:1229–33, 1987.

6. Pak, C. Y. C. Calcium metabolism. *J Am Coll Nutr* 8(S):46S–53S, 1989.

7. Diamond, T., et al. Ethanol reduces bone formation and may cause osteoporosis. *Am J Med* 86(3):282–8, 1989.

8. Heaney, R. P., Recker, R. R. Effects of nitrogen, phosphorus, and caffeine on calcium balance in women. *J Lab Clin Med* 99:46–55, 1982.

9. Hyams, D. E., Ross, E. J. Scurvy, megaloblastic anaemia and osteoporosis. *Br J Clin Pract* 17:332–40, 1963.

10. Eufemio, M. A. Vitamin D: Advances in the therapy of osteoporosis—Part VIII. *Geriatr Med Today* 9(11):37–49, 1990.

11. Nielsen, F. H., et al. Effect of dietary boron on mineral, estrogen, and testosterone metabolism in postmenopausal women. *FASEB J* 1:394–97, 1987.

12. Cauley, J. A., et al. Endogenous estrogen levels and calcium intakes in postmenopausal women. *JAMA* 260(21):3150–5, 1988.

13. Chan, G., et al. Effects of increased dietary calcium intake upon the calcium and bone mineral status of lactating adolescent and adult women. *Am J Clin Nutr* 46:319–23, 1987.

14. Tractenbarg, D. E. Treatment of osteoporosis: What is the role of calcium? *Postgrad Med* 87(4):263–70, 1990.

15. Eufemio, M. A. Fluoride therapy: Advances in the therapy of osteoporosis, part III. *Geriatr Med Today* 8(9):79–88, 1989.

16. Riggs, B. L., et al. Effect of fluoride treatment on the fracture rate in postmenopausal women with osteoporosis. *N Engl J Med* 322:802–9, 1990.

17. Spak, C-J., et al. Tissue response of the gastric mucosa after ingestion of fluoride. *Br Med J* 298:1686–7, 1989.

18. Angus, R. M., et al. Dietary intake and bone mineral density. *Bone Mineral* 4(3):265–78, 1988.

19. Cohen, L., Kitzes, R. Infrared spectroscopy and magnesium content of bone mineral in osteoporotic women. *Israel J Med Sci* 17:1123–25, 1981.

20. Krolner, B., et al. Physical exercise as prophylaxis against involutional vertebral bone loss: a controlled trial. *Clin Sci* 64(5):541–6, 1983.

Pain

1. Lebenthal, E., et al. Recurrent abdominal pain and lactose absorption in children. *Pediatrics* 67(6):828–32, 1981.

2. Rowe, A. H. Allergic fatigue and toxemia. *Ann Allergy* 17:9–18, 1959.

3. Boublik, J. H., et al. Coffee contains potent receptor binding activity. *Nature* 301:246–8, 1983.

4. Russell, L. C. Caffeine restriction as initial treatment for breast pain. *Nurse Pract* 14(2):36–7, 40, 1989.

5. Fu, Q. G., et al. B vitamins suppress spinal dorsal horn nociceptive neurons in the cat. *Neurosci Lett* 95(1–3):192–7, 1988.

6. Brüggemann, G., et al. [Results of a double-blind study of diclofenac and vitamin B_1, B_6, B_{12} versus diclofenac in patients with acute pain of the lumbar vertebrae. A multicenter study.] *Klin Wochenschr* 68(2):116–20, 1990.

7. Mazzoni, P., Valenti, F. Un nuovo anestetico generale per via endovenosa—la tiamina. *Acta Anesh (Padova)* 15:815–28, 1964.

8. Quirin, H. Pain and vitamin B_1 therapy. *Biblthca Nutr Dieta* (38):110–11, 1986.

9. Bernstein, A. L. Vitamin B_6 in neurology. *Ann N Y Acad Sci* 585:250–60, 1990.

10. Hanck, A., Weiser, H. Analgesic and anti-inflammatory properties of vitamins. *Int J Vitam Nutr Res* (suppl)27:189–206, 1985.

11. Hieber, H. Die dehandlung vertebragener schmerzen und sensibilitätsstörungen mit hochdosiertem hydroxocobalamin. *Med Monatsschr* 28:545–8, 1974.

12. Dettori, A. G., Ponari, O. Effecto antalgico della cobamide in corso di neuropatie periferiche di diversa etiopatogenesi. *Minerva Med* 64:1077–82, 1973.

13. Creagan, E. T., et al. Failure of high-dose vitamin C (ascorbic acid) to benefit patients with advanced cancer. *N Engl J Med* 301:687–90, 1979.

14. Kurz, D., Eyring, E. J. Effect of vitamin C on osteogenesis imperfecta. *Pediatrics* 54:56–61, 1974.

15. Lytle, R. L. Chronic dental pain: Possible benefits of food restriction and sodium ascorbate. *J Appl Nutr* 40(2):95–8, 1988.

16. Greenwood, J. R. Optimum vitamin C intake as a factor in the preservation of disc integrity. *Med Ann DC* 33:274, 1964.

17. Hanck, A., Weiser, H. Analgesic and anti-inflammatory properties of vitamins. *Int J Vitam Nutr Res* (suppl)27:189–206, 1985.

18. Bhathena, S., et al. Decreased plasma enkephalins in copper deficiency in man. *Am J Clin Nutr* 43:42–6, 1986.

19. van Rij, A. M., et al. Selenium deficiency in total parenteral nutrition. *Am J Clin Nutr* 32:2076–85, 1979.

20. Jameson, S., et al. *Läkaresällskapets Riksstämma,* 1985.

21. Jameson, S., et al. Pain relief and selenium balance in patients with connective tissue disease and osteoarthrosis: A double-blind selenium tocopherol supplementation study. *Nutr Res* Suppl 1:291–7, 1985.

22. Budd, K. Use of D-phenylalanine, an enkephalinase inhibitor, in the treatment of intractable pain. *Adv Pain Res Ther* 5:305–8, 1983.

23. Walsh, N. E., et al. Analgesic effectiveness of D-phenylalanine in chronic pain patients. *Arch Phys Med Rehabil* 6797):436–9, 1986.

24. Kitade, T., et al. Studies on the enhanced effect of acupuncture analgesia and acupuncture anesthesia by D-phenylalanine (2nd report)—schedule of administration and clinical effects in low back pain and tooth extraction. *Acupunct Electrother Res* 15(2):121–35, 1990.

25. Takeshirge, M., et al. Parallel individual variations in effectiveness of acupuncture, morphine analgesia, and dorsal PAG-SPA and their abolition by D-phenylalanine. *Adv Pain Res Ther* 5:563–8, 1983.

26. Hachisu, M., et al. Relationship between enhancement of morphine analgesia and inhibition of enkephalinase by 2S, 3R 3-amino-2-hydroxy-4-phenylbuanoic acid derivatives. *Life Sci* 30:1739–46, 1982.

27. Seltzer, S., et al. The effects of dietary tryptophan on chronic maxillofacial pain and experimental pain tolerance. *J Psychiatry Res* 17:181–6, 1982–3.

28. Shpeen, S. E., et al. The effect of tryptophan on postoperative endodontic pain. *Oral Surg Oral Med Oral Pathol* 58(4):446–9, 1984.

29. Lieberman, H. R., et al. Mood, performance and pain sensitivity: Changes induced by food constituents. *J Psychiatry Res* 17:135–45, 1983.

30. Lynn, B. Capsaicin: actions on nociceptive C-fibres and therapeutic potential. *Pain* 41(1):61–9, 1990.

31. Bernstein, J. E., et al. Topical capsaicin treatment of chronic posttherapeutic neuralgia. *J Am Acad Dermatol* 21(2 Pt 1):265–70, 1989.

32. Rayner, H. C., et al. Relief of local stump pain by capsaicin cream. Letter. *Lancet* 2:1276–7, 1989.

33. Watson, C. P. N., et al. The post-mastectomy pain syndrome and the effect of topical capsaicin. *Pain* 38:177–86, 1989.

34. Morgenlander, J. C., et al. Capsaicin for the treatment of pain in the Guillain-Barrë Syndrome. Letter. *Ann Neurol* 28(2):199, 1990.

Parkinson's Disease

1. Tsui, J., et al. The effect of dietary protein on the efficacy of L-dopa: A double-blind study. *Neurology* 39:549–52, 1989.

2. Clayton, P., et al. Subacute combined degeneration of the cord, dementia and parkinsonism due to an inborn error of folate metabolism. *J Neurol Neurosurg Psychiatry* 49:920–7, 1986.

3. Matthews, J., et al. Effect of therapy with vitamin B_{12} and folic acid on elderly patients with low concentrations of serum vitamin B_{12} or erythrocyte folate but normal blood counts. *Acta Haematologica* 79:84–7, 1988.

4. Frank, O., et al. Superiority of periodic intramuscular vitamins over daily oral vitamins in maintaining normal vitamin titers in a geriatric population. *Am J Clin Nutr* 30:630, 1977.

5. Bender, D. A., et al. Niacin depletion in Parkinsonian patients treated with L-dopa, benserazide and carbidopa. *Clin Sci* 56(1):89–93, 1979.

6. Black, M. J., Brandt, R. B. Nicotinic acid or N-methyl nicotinamide prolongs elevated brain dopa and dopamine in L-dopa treatment. *Biochem Med Metab Biol* 36(2):244–51, 1986.

7. Birkmayer, W., et al. Nicotinamidadenindinucleotide (NADH): The new approach in the therapy of Parkinson's disease. *Am Clin Lab Sci* 19:38–43, 1989.

8. Baker, A. B. Treatment of paralysis agitans with vitamin B_6. *JAMA* 116:2484, 1941.

9. Spies., T. D., Bean, W. B. Parkinson's disease (paralysis agitans). *Science* 91:10, 1940.

10. Reilly, D. K., et al. On-off effects in Parkinson's disease: a controlled investigation of ascorbic acid therapy. *Adv Neurol* 37:51–60, 1983.

11. Sacks, W., Simpson, G. M. Ascorbic acid in levodopa therapy. Letter. *Lancet* 1:527, 1975.

12. Golbe, L. I., et al. Case-control study of early life dietary factors in Parkinson's disease. *Arch Neurol* 45:1350–3, 1988.

13. Stern, G. M. Vitamin E and Parkinson's disease. Letter. *Lancet* 1:508, 1987.

14. Fahn, S. An open trial of high-dosage antioxidants in early Parkinson's disease. *Am J Clin Nutr* 53:380S–1S, 1991.

15. Birkmayer, W., Birkmayer, J. G. D. Iron, a new aid in the treatment of Parkinson patients. *J Neural Trans* 67:287–92, 1986.

16. Jellinger, K., et al. Brain iron and ferritin in Parkinson's and Alzheimer's diseases. *J Neural Transm Park Dis Demt Sect* 2(4):327–40, 1990.

17. Sofic, E., et al. Selective increase of iron in substantia nigra zona compacta of parkinsonian brains. *J Neurochem* 56(3):978–82, 1991.

18. Zayed, J., et al. [Environmental factors in the etiology of Parkinson's disease.] *Can J Neurol Sci* 17(3):286–91, 1990.

19. Mena, I., et al. Chronic manganese poisoning. Clinical picture and manganese turnover. *Neurology* 17:128–36, 1967.

20. Florence, T. M., Stauber, J. L. Neurotoxicity of manganese. Letter. *Lancet* 1:363, 1988.

21. Kunin, R. A. *Meganutrition.* New York, McGraw-Hill, 1980.

22. Meininger, V., et al. [L-methionine treatment of Parkinson's disease: preliminary results.] *Rev Neurol (Paris)* 138(4):297–303, 1982.

23. Smythies, J. R., Halsey, J. H. Treatment of Parkinson's disease with L-methionine. *South Med J* 77:1577, 1984.

24. Snider, S. R. Octacosanol in parkinsonism. Letter. *Ann Neurol* 16(6):723, 1984.

25. England, H. Octacosanol helped his Parkinson's disease. *Prevention* March, 1983.

26. Critchley, E. M. R. Evening primrose oil (Efamol) in parkinsonism and other tremors: A preliminary study, in D. F. Horrobin, Ed. *Clinical Uses of Essential Fatty Acids.* Montreal, Eden Press, 1982:205–8.

27. Fernandez Pardal, J., et al. *Ann Psig Biol* 3:234–6, 1974.

28. Heller, B., et al. Therapeutic action of D-phenylalanine in Parkinson's disease. *Arzneim-Forsch* 26:577–9, 1976.

29. Lehmann, J. Tryptophan malabsorption in levodopa-treated parkinsonian patients. *Acta Med Scand* 194:181–9, 1973.

30. Sandyk, R., Fisher, H. L-tryptophan supplementation in Parkinson's disease. *Int J Neurosci* 45(3–4):215–9, 1989.

31. Coppen, A., et al. Levodopa and L-tryptophan therapy in parkinsonism. *Lancet* 1:654–7, 1972.

32. Growdon, J. H., et al. Effects of oral L-tyrosine and homovanillic acid levels in patients with Parkinson's disease. *Life Sci* 30(10):827–32, 1982.

33. Lemoine, P., et al. [L-tyrosine: a long-term treatment of Parkinson's disease.] *C R Acad Sci [III]* 309(2):43–7, 1989.

34. Zayed, et al. op. cit.

35. Hirsch, E. C., et al. Iron and aluminum increase in the substantia nigra of patients with Parkinson's disease: an X-ray microanalysis. *J Neurochem* 56(2):446–51, 1991.

36. Ngim, C. H., Devathasan, G. Epidemiologic study on the association between body burden mercury level and idiopathic Parkinson's disease. *Neuroepidemiology* 8(3):128–41, 1989.

Peptic Ulcers

1. Ippoliti, A. F., et al. The effect of various forms of milk on gastric-acid secretion. *Ann Intern Med* 84:286–9, 1976.

2. Kumar, N., et al. Effect of milk on patients with duodenal ulcers. *Br Med J* 293:666, 1986.

3. Malhotra, S. L. A comparison of unrefined wheat and rice diets in the management of duodenal ulcer. *Postgrad Med J* 54:6–9, 1978.

4. Rydning, A., et al. Prophylactic effect of dietary fiber in duodenal ulcer disease. *Lancet* 2:736–9, 1982.

5. Lenz, H. J., et al. Wine and five percent ethanol are potent stimulators of gastric acid secretion in humans. *Gastroenterology* 85(5):1082–7, 1983.

6. McArthur, K., et al. Relative stimulatory effects of commonly ingested beverages on gastric acid secretion in humans. *Gastroenterology* 83:199–203, 1982.

7. Marotta, R. B., Floch, M. H. Diet and nutrition in ulcer disease. *Med Clin North Am* 75(4):967–9, 1991.

8. Katschinski, B. D., et al. Duodenal ulcer and refined carbohydrate intake: a case-control study assessing dietary fibre and refined sugar intake. *Gut* 31(9):993–6, 1990.

9. Yudkin, J. Eating and ulcers. Letter. *Br Med J* February 16, 1980, pp. 483–4.

10. Duroux, P., et al. Early dinner reduces nocturnal gastric acidity. *Gut* 30(8):1063–7, 1989.

11. Budagovskaia, V. N., Voïtko, N. E. [Allergic reactions in patients with peptic ulcer; incidence of food and drug allergy.] *Vopr Pitan* (3):30–3, 1984.

12. Kaess, H., Kellermann, M., Castro, A. Food intolerance in duodenal ulcer patients, non ulcer dyspepsia patients and healthy subjects. A prospective study. *Klin Wochenschr* 66(5):208–11, 1988.

13. Pollard, H. M., Stuart, G. J. Experimental reproduction of gastric allergy in human beings with controlled observations on the mucosa. *J Allergy* 13:467–73, 1942.

14. Siegel, J. Gastrointestinal ulcer—Arthus reaction! *Ann Allergy* 32:127–30, 1974.

15. Andre, C., et al. Evidence for anaphylactic reactions in peptic ulcer and varioliform gastritis. *Ann Allergy* 51:325–7, 1983.

16. Reimann, H. J., Ewin, J. Gastric mucosal reactions in patients with food allergy. *Am J Gastroenterol* 83(11):1212–19, 1988.

17. Siegel, J. Immunologic approach to the treatment and prevention of gastrointestinal ulcers. *Ann Allergy* 38:27–41, 1977.

18. Davies, S., Stewart, A. *Nutritional Medicine.* London, Pan Books, 1987, p. 210.

19. Patty, E., et al. Controlled trial of vitamin A in gastric ulcer. *Lancet* 2:876, 1982.

20. Mahmood, T., et al. Prevention of duodenal ulcer formation in the rat by dietary vitamin A supplementation. *JPEN J Parenter Enteral Nutr* 10(1):74–7, 1986.

21. Dubey, S. S., et al. Ascorbic acid, dehydroascorbic acid, glutathione and histamine in peptic ulcer. *Indian J Med Res* 76:859–62, 1982.

22. O'Connor, J. H., et al. Vitamin C in the human stomach: relation to gastric pH, gastroduodenal disease, and possible sources. *Gut* 30(4):436–42, 1989.

23. Portnoy, B., Wilkinson, J. P. Vitamin C deficiency in peptic ulceration and hematemesis. *Br Med J* 554–60, 1938.

24. Russell, R. L., et al. Ascorbic acid levels in leucocytes of patients with gastrointestinal hemorrhage. *Lancet* 2:603–6, 1968.

25. Smith, D. T., McConkey, M. Peptic ulcers (gastric, pyloric and duodenal) occurrence in guinea-pigs fed on a diet deficient in vitamin C. *Arch Intern Med* 51:413–26, 1933.

26. Debray, C., et al. [Treatment of gastro-duodenal ulcers with large doses of ascorbic acid.] *Semaine Therpeutic (Paris)* 44:393–8, 1968.

27. Miwa, M., et al. The therapeutics of peptic ulcers: Clinical evaluation of C-Fe therapy. *Tokai J Exp Clin Med* 5(1):41–4, 1980.

28. Litinskaia, E. V., et al. [The vitamin E concentration and lipid peroxidation status of patients with peptic ulcer undergoing laser therapy.] *Vrach Delo* (8):70–2, 1989.

29. Yoshikawa, T., et al. Vitamin E in gastric mucosal injury induced by ischemia-reperfusion. *Am J Clin Nutr* 53:210S–4S, 1991.

30. Ibid.

31. Litinskaia, et al. op. cit.

32. Arutiniunian, V. M., et al. [Use of alpha-tocopherol acetate (vitamin E) and

sodium nucleinate in the treatment of patients with stomach and duodenal ulcer.] *Klin Med (Mosk)* 6194):52–4, 1983.

33. Toteva, E. T., et al. [Use of alpha-tocopherol in the complex treatment of patients with peptic ulcer.] *Vrach Delo* (2):79–81, 1988.

34. Poynard, T., et al. Randomized double-blind clinical trial of aluminum phosphate versus rantidine in the acute treatment of duodenal ulcer. *Digestion* 47(2):105–10, 1990.

35. Graves, A. B., et al. The association between aluminum-containing products and Alzheimer's disease. *J Clin Epidemiol* 43(1):35–44, 1990.

36. Lotz, M., Zisman, E., Bartter, F. C. Evidence for a phosphorus-depletion syndrome in man. *N Engl J Med* 278(8):409–15, 1968.

37. McNulty, C. A. M., et al. Susceptibility of clinical isolates of Campylobacter pyloridis to 11 antimicrobial agents. *Antimicrob Agents Chemther* 28:837–8, 1985.

38. Gorbach, S. L. Bismuth therapy in gastrointestinal diseases. *Gastroenterology* 99(3):863–75, 1990.

39. McGuigan, J. E. Peptic ulcer, in K. J. Isselbacher, et al., Eds. *Harrison's Principles of Internal Medicine,* Ninth Edition. New York, McGraw-Hill Book Company, 1980.

40. Ibid.

41. Lotz, Zisman, Bartter, op. cit.

42. Cho, C. H., Ogle, C. W. A correlative study of the antiulcer effects of zinc sulphate in stressed rats. *Eur J Pharmacol* 70:241, 1978.

43. Oner, G., et al. The role of zinc ion in the development of gastric ulcers in rats. *Eur J Pharmacol* 70:241, 1981.

44. Frommer, D. J. The healing of gastric ulcers by zinc sulphate. *Med J Aust* 793–6, 1975.

45. Kassir, Z. A. Endoscopic controlled trial of four drug regimens in the treatment of chronic duodenal ulceration. *Ir Med J* 78:153–6, 1985.

46. Turpie, A. G., et al. Clinical trial of deglycyrrhizinate liquorice in gastric ulcer. *Gut* 10:299–303, 1969.

47. Rees, W. D. W., et al. Effect of deglycyrrhizinated liquorice on gastric mucosal damage by aspirin. *Scand J Gastroenterol* 14:605–7, 1979.

48. van Marle, J., et al. Deglycyrrhizinised liquorice (DGL) and the renewal of rat stomach epithelium. *Eur J Pharmacol* 72:219–25, 1981.

49. Cheney, G. *Calif Med,* January, 1956.

50. Bricklin, M. *Rodale's Encyclopedia of Natural Home Remedies.* Emmaus, PA, Rodale Press, 1982, p. 466.

Periodontal Disease

1. Sidi, A. D., Ashley, F. P. Influence of frequent sugar intakes on experimental gingivitis. *J Periodontol* 55(7):419–23, 1984.

2. Pack, A. R. C. Folate mouthwash: effect on established gingivitis in periodontal patients. *J Clin Periodontol* 11:619–28, 1984.

3. Vogel, R. I., et al. The effect of folic acid on gingival health. *J Periodontol* 47(11):667–8, 1976.

4. Thomson, M. E., Pack, A. R. C. Effects of extended systemic and topical folate

supplementation on gingivitis of pregnancy. *J Clin Periodontol* 9(3):275–80, 1982.

5. Jacob, R. A., et al. Experimental vitamin C depletion and supplementation in young men. Nutrient interactions and dental health effects. *Ann N Y Acad Sci* 498:333–46, 1987.

6. Woolfe, S. N., et al. Relationship of ascorbic levels of blood and gingival tissue with response to periodontal therapy. *J Clin Periodontol* 11(3):159–65, 1984.

7. Krook, L., et al. Human periodontal disease: Morphology and response to calcium therapy. *Cornell Vet* 62(1):32–53, 1972.

8. Wical, K. E., Brussee, P. Effects of a calcium and vitamin D supplement on alveolar ridge resorption in immediate denture patients. *J Prosthetic Dent* 41(1):4–11, 1979.

9. Krook, et al., op. cit.

10. Uhrbom, E., Jacobson, L. Calcium in periodontitis: clinical effect of calcium medication. *J Clin Periodontol* 11(4):230–41, 1984.

11. Hansen, I. L., et al. Bioenergetics and clinical medicine. IX. Gingival and leucocytic deficiencies of coenzyme Q_{10} in patients with periodontal disease. *Res Comm. Chem Pathol Pharmacol* 14:729, 1976.

12. Folkers, K., Yamamura, Y. *Biomedical and Clinical Aspects of Coenzyme Q,* Volume One. Amsterdam, Elsevier/North Holland Biomedical Press, 1977, pp. 294–311.

13. Wilkinson, E. G., et al. Treatment of periodontal and other soft tissue diseases of the oral cavity with coenzyme Q, in K. Folkers, Y. Yamamura, Eds. *Biomedical and Clinical Aspects of Coenzyme Q.* Volume One. Amsterdam, Elsevier/North Holland Biomedical Press, 1977.

14. Bliznakov, E. G., Hunt, G. L. *The Miracle Nutrient: Coenzyme Q_{10}.* New York, Bantam Books, 1986, pp. 3–4.

15. Harper, D. S., et al. Clinical efficacy of a dentifrice and oral rinse containing sanguinaria extract and zinc chloride during 6 months of use. *J Periodon* 6196):352–6, 1990.

16. Southard, G. L., et al. The relationship of sanguinaria extract concentration and zinc ion to plaque and gingivitis. *J Clin Periodontol* 14(6):315–9, 1987.

17. Ibid.

18. Siblerud, R. L. The relationship between mercury from dental amalgam and oral cavity health. *Ann Dent* 49(2):6–10, 1990.

19. Eggleston, D. W. Effect of dental amalgam and nickel alloys on T-lymphocytes: Preliminary report. *J Prosthet Dent* 51(5):617–23, 1984.

20. Brechner, J., Armstrong, W. D. Relation of gastric acidity to alveolar bone resorption. *Ann Intern Med* 66:917–23, 1967.

21. Ivanovich, P., et al. The absorption of calcium carbonate. *Ann Intern Med* 66:917–23, 1967.

Premenstrual Tension Syndrome (PMS)

1. Abraham, G. E. Management of the premenstrual tension syndrome: rationale for a nutritional approach, in J. Bland, Ed. *1986: A Year in Nutritional Medicine.* New Canaan, CT, Keats Publishing, Inc., 1986.

2. Goei, G. S., et al. Dietary patterns of patients with premenstrual tension. *J Appl Nutr* 34(1):4–11, 1982.

3. Abraham, G. E. Magnesium deficiency in premenstrual tension. *Magnesium Bull* 1:68–73, 1982.

4. Wurtman, J. J., et al. Effect of nutrient intake on premenstrual depression. *Am J Obstet Gynecol* 161(5):1228–34, 1989.

5. Abraham, *Year in Nutritional Medicine,* op. cit.

6. Oettle, G. J., et al. Glucose and insulin responses to manufactured and whole-food snacks. *Am J Clin Nutr* 45:86–91, 1987.

7. Seelig, M. Human requirement of magnesium: Factors that increase needs, in J. Durlach, Ed. *First International Symposium on Magnesium Deficiency in Human Pathol.* Paris, Springer-Verlag, 1973, p. 11.

8. Goldin, B. R., et al. Estrogen excretion patterns and plasma levels in vegetarian and omnivorous women. *N Engl J Med* 307:1542–7, 1982.

9. Kuchel, D., et al. Catecholamine excretion in 'idiopathic' edema: Decreased dopamine excretion, a pathologic factor. *J Clin Endocrinol Metab* 44:639, 1977.

10. Abraham, *Year in Nutritional Medicine,* op. cit.

11. Ferranini, E., et al. Sodium elevates the plasma glucose response to glucose ingestion in man. *J Clin Endocrinol Metab* 54:455, 1982.

12. Freinkel, N., Getzer, B. E. Oral glucose tolerance curve and hypoglycemias in the fed state. *N Engl J Med* 280:820–8, 1969.

13. Rossignol, A. M. Caffeine-containing beverages, total fluid consumption, and premenstrual syndrome. *Am J Public Health* 80(9):1106–10, 1990.

14. Boyd, N. F., et al. Effect of a low-fat high-carbohydrate diet on symptoms of cyclical mastopathy. *Lancet* 2:128–32, 1988.

15. Jones, D. V. Influence of dietary fat on self-reported menstrual symptoms. *Physiol Behav* 40(4):483–7, 1987.

16. Doll, H., et al. Pyridoxine (vitamin B_6) and the premenstrual syndrome: A randomized crossover trial. *J R Coll Gen Pract* 39:364–8, 1989.

17. Abraham, G. E., et al. Effect of vitamin B_6 on plasma and red blood cell magnesium levels in premenopausal women. *Ann Clin Lab Sci* 11(4):333–6, 1981.

18. London, R. S., et al. Efficacy of alpha-tocopherol in the treatment of premenstrual syndrome. *J Reprod Med* 32(6):400–4, 1987.

19. London, R. S., et al. The effect of alpha-tocopherol on premenstrual symptomatology: A double-blind study. *J Am Coll Nutr* 2(2):115–22, 1983.

20. Goei, et al, op. cit.

21. Abraham, *Magnesium Bull,* op. cit.

22. Abraham, G. E. Nutritional factors in the etiology of the premenstrual syndrome. *J Reprod Med* 28:446–64, 1983.

23. Thys-Jacobs, S., et al. Calcium supplementation in premenstrual syndrome: a randomized crossover trial. *J Gen Intern Med* 4(3):183–9, 1989.

24. Spencer, H., et al. *Magnesium in Health and Disease.* Jamaica, NY, SP Medical and Scientific Books, 1980, pp. 911–19.

25. Sherwood, R. A., et al. Magnesium and the premenstrual syndrome. *Ann Clin Biochem* 23(6):667–70, 1986.

26. Nicholas, A. [Treatment of premenstrual syndrome and dysmenorrhea by the magnesium ion], in J. Durlach, Ed. *First International Symposium on Magnesium Deficiency in Human Pathology.* Paris, Springer-Verlag, 1973, pp. 261–3.

27. Stebbing, J. B., et al. Reactive hypoglycaemia and magnesium. *Magnesium Bull* 4(2):131–4, 1982.

28. Cantin, M. [Hyperaldosteronism secondary to the course of a magnesium deficit.], in J. Durlach, Ed. *First International Symposium on Magnesium Deficit in Human Pathology.* Paris, F. Vitel, 1973, pp. 451–60.

29. Redmond, D. E., et al. Menstrual cycle and ovarian hormone effects on plasma and platelet monamine oxidase (MAO) and plasma dopamine-hydroxylase activities in the Rhesus monkey. *Psychosom Med* 37:417, 1975.

30. Barbeau, A., et al. [Deficiency of magnesium and cerebral dopamine], in J. Durlach, Ed. *First International Symposium on Magnesium Deficit in Human Pathology.* Paris, F. Vitel, 1973, pp. 149–52.

31. Brown, R. C., Bidlack, W. R. Regulation of glucuronyl transferase by intracellular magnesium, in *Proceedings of the International Symposium on Magnesium and Its Relationship to Cardiovascular, Renal and Metabolic Disorders.* Los Angeles, 1985, p. 24.

32. Curry, D. L., et al. Magnesium modulation of glucose-induced insulin secretion by the perfused rat pancreas. *Endocrinology* 101:203, 1977.

33. Davies, S., Stewart, A. *Nutritional Medicine.* London, Pan Books, 1987, p. 316.

34. Brush, M. G., et al. Abnormal essential fatty acid levels in plasma of women with premenstrual syndrome. *Am J Obstet Gynecol* 150(4):363–6, 1984.

35. Oekerman, P. A., et al. Evening primrose oil as a treatment of the premenstrual syndrome. *Recent Adv Clin Nutr* 2:404–5, 1986.

36. Bates, C. *Essential Fatty Acids and Immunity in Mental Health.* Tacoma, WA, Life Sciences Press, 1987, p. 71.

37. Lagrue, G., et al. Idiopathic cyclic edema. The role of capillary hyperpermeability and its correction by Ginkgo biloba extract. *Presse Med* 15(31):1550–3, 1986.

38. Young, P. C. M., et al. Effect of metal ions on the binding of 17-beta-estradiol to human endometrial cystol. *Fertil Steril* 28:312–18, 1972.

39. Abraham, G. E., Elsner, C. W., Lucas, L. A. Hormonal and behavioral changes during the menstrual cycle. *Senologia* 3:33–38, 1978.

40. Van Praag, H. M. Neuroendocrine disorders in depressions and their significance for the monoamine hypothesis of depression. *Acta Psychiatr Scand* 57:389–404, 1978.

41. Hanson, M. A., et al. Hair tissue concentration of minerals, trace elements, and toxic metals in normal women and patients with premenstrual tension syndromes, in M. Abdulla et al., Eds. *Health Effects and Interactions of Essential and Toxic Elements.* New York, Pergamon Press, 1983, pp. 608–11.

42. Fine, B. P., et al. Influence of magnesium on the intestinal absorption of lead. *Environ Res* 12:224, 1976.

43. Krall, A. R., et al. Effects of magnesium infusions on the metabolism of calcium and lead, in M. Cantin, M. S. Seelig, Eds. *Magnesium in Health and Disease.* New York, Spectrum Publications, 1980, pp. 941–8.

Prostate Enlargement

1. Györkey, F., Sato, C. S. In vitro 65-Zinc-binding capacities of normal, hyperplastic and carcinomatous human prostate gland. *Exp Mol Pathol* 8:216–24, 1968.

2. Bush, I. M. Zinc and the prostate. Presented at the annual meeting of the American Medical Association. Chicago, 1974.

3. Fahim, M. S., et al. Zinc treatment for the reduction of hyperplasia of the prostate. *Fed Proc* 35:361, 1976.

4. Van Fleet, J. K. *A Doctor's Private Healing Secrets*. Parker Publishing Company, 1977.

5. Dumrau, F. Benign prostatic hyperplasia: Amino acid therapy for symptomatic relief. *Am J Geriatr* 10:426–30, 1962.

6. Feinblatt, H. M., et al. Palliative treatment of benign prostatic hypertrophy: Value of glycine, alanine, glutamic acid combination. *J Maine Med Assoc* 46:99–102, 1958.

7. Klein, L. A., Stoff, J. S. Prostaglandins and the prostate: An hypothesis on the etiology of benign prostatic hyperplasia. *Prostate* 4(3):247–51, 1983.

8. Hart, J. P., Cooper, W. L. Vitamin F in the treatment of prostatic hyperplasia. Report Number 1, Lee Foundation for Nutritional Research, Milwaukee, WI, 1941.

9. Buck, A. C., et al. Treatment of outflow tract obstruction due to benign prostatic hyperplasia with the pollen extract, Cernilton. A double-blind, placebo-controlled study. *Br J Urol* 66(4):398–404, 1990.

10. Maekawa, M., et al. [Clinical evaluation of Cernilton on benign prostatic hypertrophy—a multiple center double-blind study with Paraprost.] *Hinyokika Kiyo* 36(4):495–516, 1990.

11. Barlet, A., et al. [Efficacy of Pygeum africanum extract in the medical therapy of urination disorders due to benign prostatic hyperplasia: evaluation of objective and subjective parameters. A placebo-controlled double-blind multicenter study.] *Wien Klin Wochenschr* 102(22):667–73, 1990.

12. Champault, G., et al. A double-blind trial of an extract of the plant Serenoa repens in benign prostatic hyperplasia. *Br J Clin Pharmacol* 18:461–2, 1984.

13. Duvia, R., et al. Advances in the phytotherapy of prostatic hypertrophy. *Med Praxis* 4:143–8, 1983.

14. Gaby, A. B. Literature review and commentary. *Townsend Letter for Doctors,* May, 1990.

15. Habib, F. K., et al. Metal-androgen interrelationships in carcinoma and hyperplasia of the human prostate. *J Endocrinol* 71(1):133–41, 1976.

16. Lahtonen, R. Zinc and cadmium concentrations in whole tissue and in separated epithelium and stroma from human benign prostatic hypertrophic glands. *Prostate* 6(2):177–83, 1985.

17. Hoffman, L., et al. Carcinogenic effects of cadmium on the prostate of the rat. *J Cancer Res Clin Oncol* 109(3):193–9, 1985.

18. Webber, M. M. Selenium prevents the growth stimulatory effects of cadmium on human prostatic epithelium. *Biochem Biophys Res Commun* 127(3):871–7, 1985.

Psoriasis

1. Schamberg, J. F. The dietary treatment of psoriasis. *JAMA* 98:1633, 1932.

2. Newborg, B. Disappearance of psoriatic lesions on the rice diet. *N Carolina Med J* 47:253–5, 1986.

3. Lithell, H., et al. A fasting and vegetarian diet treatment trial on chronic inflammatory disorders. *Acta Derm Venereol (Stockh)* 63(5):397–403, 1983.

4. Buckley, L. D. Diet and hygiene in diseases of the skin. *JAMA* 59:535, 1912.

5. Monk, B. E., Neill, S. M. Alcohol consumption and psoriasis. *Dermatologica* 173(2):57–60, 1986.

6. Douglass, J. M. Psoriasis and diet. Letter. *Calif Med* 133(5):450, 1980.

7. Majewski, S., et al. Decreased levels of vitamin A in serum of patients with psoriasis. *Arch Dermatol Res* 280:499–501, 1989.

8. Kaplan, R. P., et al. Etretinate therapy for psoriasis: clinical responses, remission times, epidermal DNA and polyamine responses. *J Am Acad Dermatol* 8(1):95–102, 1983.

9. Cohen, E. L. Vitamin B_{12} in psoriasis. Letter. *Br Med J* 1:125, 1963.

10. Sneddon, J. B. Vitamin B_{12} in psoriasis. Letter. *Br Med J* 1:328, 1963.

11. Carslaw, R. W., Neill, J. Vitamin B_{12} in psoriasis. Letter. *Br Med J* 1:611, 1963.

12. Staberg, B., et al. Abnormal vitamin D metabolism in patients with psoriasis. *Acta Derm Venereol (Stockh)* 67:65–8, 1987.

13. Morimoto, S., Yoshikawa, K. Psoriasis and vitamin D_3. A review of our experience. *Arch Dermatol* 125(2):231–4, 1989.

14. Dochao, A., et al. [Therapeutic effects of vitamin D and vitamin A in psoriasis: A 20-year experiment.] *Actas Dermosfiliogr* 66(3–4):121–30, 1975.

15. Wright, J. V. Psoriasis and 'activated' vitamin D. *Let's Live* April, 1989.

16. Fairris, G. M., et al. The effect of supplementation with selenium and vitamin E in psoriasis. *Ann Clin Biochem* 26 (Pt 1):83–8, 1989.

17. Broglund, E., Enhamre, A. Treatment of psoriasis with topical selenium sulphide. Letter. *Br J Dermatol* 117(5):665–6, 1987.

18. Lassus, A., et al. Effects of dietary supplementation with polyunsaturated ethyl-ester lipids (angiosan) in patients with psoriasis and psoriatic arthritis. *J Int Med Res* 18:68–73, 1990.

19. Ziboh, V. A., et al. Effects of an 8-week dietary supplementation of eicosapentaenoic acid in serum, PMNs and epidermal fatty acids of psoriatic subjects. *Clin Res* 33:699A, 1985.

20. Bittiner, S. B., et al. A double-blind, randomised, placebo-controlled trial of fish oil in psoriasis. *Lancet* 1:378–80, 1988.

21. Dewsbury, C. E., et al. Topical eicosapentaenoic acid in the treatment of psoriasis. *Br J Dermatol* 120:581, 1989.

22. Ellis, C. N., et al. Experimental therapies for psoriasis. *Sem Dermatol* 4(4):313–19, 1985.

23. Hebborn, P., et al. Action of topically applied arachidonic acid on the skin of patients with psoriasis. *Arch Dermatol* 124:387–91, 1988.

24. Nugteren-Huying, W. M., et al. [Fumaric acid therapy in psoriasis: a double-blind, placebo-controlled study.] *Ned Tijdschr Geneeskd* 134(49):2387–91, 1990.

25. Nieboer, C., et al. Systemic therapy with fumaric acid derivatives: new possibilities in the treatment of psoriasis. *J Am Acad Dermatol* 20(4):601–8, 1989.

26. Sax, A., Ed. *Psoriasis Researcher Newsletter* February, 1987.

27. Bernstein, J. E., et al. Effects of topically applied capsaicin on moderate and severe psoriasis vulgaris. *J Am Acad Dermatol* 15(3):504–7, 1986.

28. Shore, R. N. Clearing of psoriatic lesions after the application of tape. Letter. *N Engl J Med* 312(4):246, 1985.

29. Wollina, U., et al. [Occlusive therapy of psoriasis—comparison of clinical effectiveness of short-term and prolonged use.] *Z Hautkr* 65(8):737–9, 1990.

Rheumatoid Arthritis

1. Lucas, C., Power, L. Dietary fat aggravates rheumatoid arthritis. *Clin Res* 29(4):754A, 1981.

2. Darlington, L. G., et al. Placebo-controlled, blind study of dietary manipulation therapy in rheumatoid arthritis. *Lancet* February 1, 1986, pp. 236–38.

3. Williams, R. Rheumatoid arthritis and food: A case study. Letter to the Editor. *Br Med J* 283:563, 1981.

4. Bjarnason, I., et al. Intestinal permeability and inflammation in rheumatoid arthritis: Effects of non-steroidal anti-inflammatory drugs. *Lancet* 2:1171–73, 1984.

5. Barton-Wright, E. C., Elliott, W. A. The pantothenic acid metabolism of rheumatoid arthritis. *Lancet* 2:862–3, 1963.

6. Calcium pantothenate in arthritic conditions. A report from the General Practitioner Research Group. *Practitioner* 224:208–11, 1980.

7. Oldroyd, K. G., Dawes, P. T. Clinically significant vitamin C deficiency in rheumatoid arthritis. *Br J Rheumatol* 24:362–63, 1985.

8. Gabor, M. Pharmacologic effects of flavonoids on blood vessels. *Angiologica* 9:355–74, 1972.

9. Conforti, A., et al. Serum copper and ceruloplasmin levels in rheumatoid arthritis and degenerative joint disease and their pharmacological implications. *Pharmacol Res Commun* 15(9):859–76, 1983.

10. Niedermeier, W. Concentration and chemical state of copper in synovial fluid and blood serum of patients with rheumatoid arthritis. *Ann Rheum Dis* 24:544, 1965.

11. Sorenson, J., in *The Anti-inflammatory Activities of Copper Complexes. Metal Ions and Biological Systems.* Marcel Dekker, 1982:77–125.

12. Walker, W. R., Keats, D. M. An investigation of the therapeutic value of the "copper bracelet." *Agents Actions* 6:454, 1976.

13. Sorenson, J. Copper aspirinate: A more potent anti-inflammatory and anti-ulcer agent. *J Int Acad Prev Med* 1980:7–21.

14. Okuyama, S., et al. Copper complexes of non-steroid antiinflammatory agents: Analgesic activity and possible receptor activation. *Agents Actions* 21(1–2):130–44, 1987.

15. Simkin, P. A. Treatment of rheumatoid arthritis with oral zinc sulfate. *Agents Actions* 8:587–96, 1981 (Suppl).

16. Cohen, A., Goldman, J. Bromelains therapy in rheumatoid arthritis. *Pennsyl Med J* 67:27–30, 1964.

17. Tulleken, J. E., et al. N-3 polyunsaturated acids, interleukin-1 and tumor necrosis factor. Letter to the Editor. *N Engl J Med* 321(1):55, 1989.

18. Gibson, R. G., et al. Perna canaliculus in the treatment of arthritis. *The Practitioner* 224:955–60, 1980.

Index

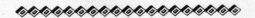

ABOUT THE AUTHOR

Born in New York City, Melvyn Werbach was educated at Columbia College, Tufts University School of Medicine, the National Institute of Mental Health, and the Cedars-Sinai Medical Center. In 1972, one year after completing his residency in psychiatry, Dr. Werbach launched one of the country's first clinical biofeedback programs, aimed at finding alternative methods of treating patients unresponsive to traditional care. In 1985 the Biofeedback Society of California awarded Dr. Werbach its Certificate of Honor for contributing to the development of biofeedback.

The following year Dr. Werbach published the first of his five books. His interest in nutritional medicine led him to write his most highly-acclaimed book to date, *Nutritional Influences on Illness,* hailed as a milestone in nutritional medicine by the president of the British Society for Nutritional Medicine.

Dr. Werbach, a member of the American College of Nutrition, writes a monthly column on nutritional medicine for the *International Journal of Alternative and Complementary Medicine* and is a member of the editorial board of the *Journal of Nutritional Medicine.* A diplomate of the American Board of Psychiatry and Neurology, he holds a faculty appointment in psychiatry at the UCLA School of Medicine. He lives in Los Angeles with his wife Gail and has two sons, Adam and Kevin.